THE
ILLUSTRATED
ENCYCLOPEDIA OF
ESSENTIAL
OILS

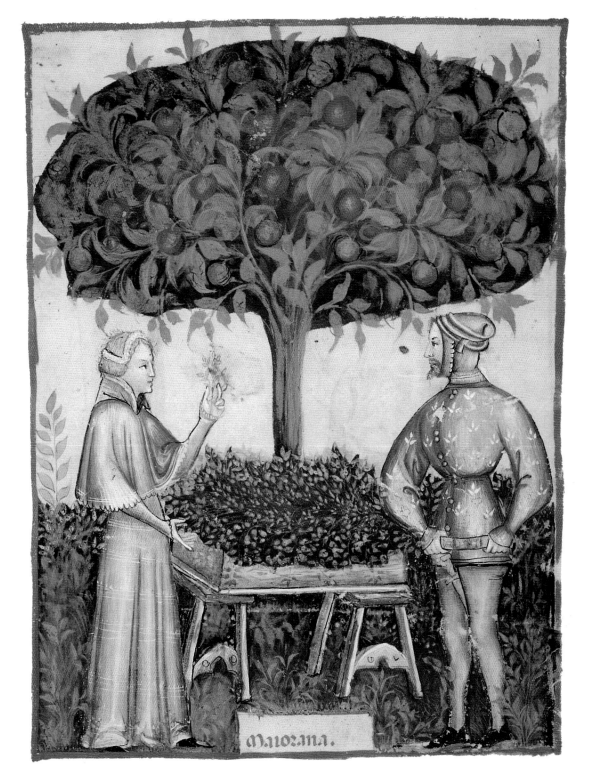

MAIORANA.

*Plants like marjoram have been
valued for centuries for their medical
and aromatherapy applications.*

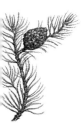
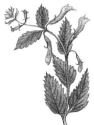

THE ILLUSTRATED ENCYCLOPEDIA OF ESSENTIAL OILS

*The Complete Guide
to the Use of Oils
in Aromatherapy
and Herbalism*

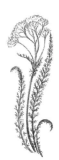

JULIA LAWLESS

ELEMENT

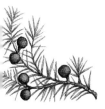
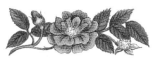
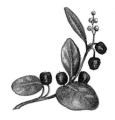

BY THE SAME AUTHOR:

Aromatherapy and the Mind
Home Aromatherapy
Lavender Oil
Rose Oil
Tea Tree Oil

Element
An Imprint of HarperCollins*Publishers*
77–85 Fulham Palace Road
Hammersmith, London W6 8JB

First published in Great Britain in 1995 by
Element Books Limited

3 5 7 9 10 8 6 4 2

ISBN 1 85230 7218

Printed and bound in Singapore by Imago

NOTE FROM THE PUBLISHER
Any information given in this book is not intended to be
taken as a replacement for medical advice. Any person with
a condition requiring medical attention should consult a
qualified practitioner or therapist.

Designed and created for Element Books with
The Bridgewater Book Company Ltd

Art Director: Terry Jeavons
Layout/page make-up: Michael Whitehead and Lee Forster
Editor: Joanne Jessup
Picture research: Vanessa Fletcher

Acknowledgments

My own interest in essential oils and herbal remedies derives from the maternal side of my family who came from Finland, where home 'simples' retained popularity long after they had vanished from most parts of Britain. My Finnish grandmother knew a great deal about herbs and wild plants, which she passed on to my mother. As she recalls: 'Mama's most important herb was parsley, which along with dill, marjoram, hops and others, were dried in bunches in the autumn, dangling at the ends of short lengths of cotton thread, all strung on a long length of thin rope stretching right across the kitchen stove.' As scents are very evocative for remembering old things, I remember it so well – the strong and heady smell emanating from these herbs when they were hung up, and the stove was warm.

Later, as a biochemist, my mother became involved with the research of essential oils and plants, and helped inspire in me a fascination for herbs and the use of natural remedies. Without her early enthusiasm and guidance, I'm sure this book would never have been written.

I should like to sincerely thank the following people who have made the book possible by contributing their time and energy in various ways: Barbara Austin MNIMH of the Herbal Treatment Centre, Cheltenham, for her creative criticism and suggestions regarding the relationship between aromatherapy and medical herbalism; John Black and Roger Dyer for their valuable expertise and careful corrections concerning the production and chemistry of essential oils; Jill Harvey and John Hughes BAALA of the Gloucestershire County Library for helping sort through all the early herbals in the 'Hartland' collection; and Merilyn King RMN of Coney Hill Hospital, Gloucester, for her painstaking work on the medical terminology and usage.

I would also like to thank all my friends who have been so encouraging, especially my father for all his help; Judith Allan for her editorial notes; Cara Denman for her guidance; Jill Purce for her initial assistance; and last but not least my husband Alec, for his constant support, and our daughter Natasha, for putting up with me.

My appreciation also goes to the services of the British Library, the Chelsea Physic Garden, the Royal Horticultural Society and my local Minchinhampton Library in Gloucestershire. It is my hope that this book will contribute a little to the current knowledge about aromatic plants and essential oils, and help bridge the gap between their different areas of application.

CONTENTS

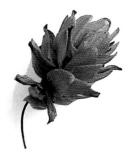

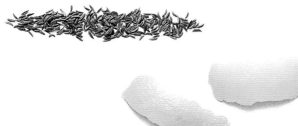

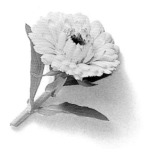

marigold flower

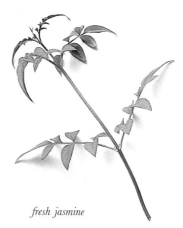

fresh jasmine

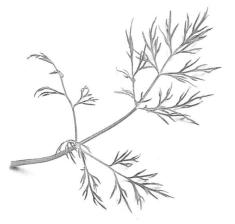

fresh dill

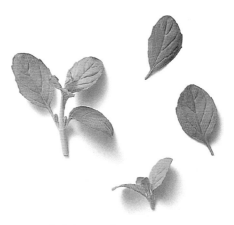

fresh pennyroyal

PREFACE

The last two decades have seen a growing interest in complementary healing methods and the use of naturally derived products such as essential oils. Since 1992, when *The Encyclopedia of Essential Oils* was first published, this interest has continued to flourish throughout the world.

Aromatherapy, once considered a fringe practice, has become so generally accepted and respected that it is increasingly on offer to hospital patients as part of their treatment. More and more, manufacturers of health products, cosmetics and perfumes are recognizing the value of essential oils in enhancing the quality and appeal of their products. At the same time, the home use of essential oils has risen dramatically as people discover for themselves the therapeutic benefits and unique aesthetic enjoyment of the oils.

Current scientific research into the chemistry and medicinal use of certain essential oils has helped confirm and clarify their precise healing potential. The demand for tea tree oil, for example, has expanded enormously over the last few years as a result of detailed analytical trials – in Australia it has even been hailed as the 'antiseptic of the future'! Such studies have highlighted the benefits of essential oils and the need for further research. Cultivation methods, climate, location, precise botanical species, extraction techniques and handling have all been found to have a profound influence on the final make-up of an oil, thus affecting its fragrance, purity and therapeutic value.

This revised and lavishly illustrated edition of *The Encyclopedia* adds an entirely new dimension to the original book. The botanical plates are both visually pleasing and informative while the photographic images of the oils themselves are quite striking in their variations of colour. The fresh layout allows a whole page for each essential oil and the text has been updated to include information that was unavailable when it was first compiled in 1992. This is in keeping with the original aim of the book, which was to present a truly comprehensive survey of essential oils in an up-to-date and accurate manner. Our success in this endeavour was confirmed in 1993 when the International Therapy Examination Council unanimously voted *The Encyclopedia of Essential Oils* the recommended text book for use on aromatherapy training courses in the UK.

It is my hope that this new *Illustrated Encyclopedia of Esssential Oils* will give pleasure to both the general reader and the specialist by adding a little more to their current knowledge of essential oils and helping to further their interest in the vast potential of aromatic plants.

JULIA LAWLESS

How to Use This Book

The *Illustrated Encyclopedia of Essential Oils* is divided into three parts:
Part I is a *general introduction to aromatics*, showing their changing role throughout history, from their ritual role in ancient civilizations to modern-day applications in aromatherapy, herbalism and perfumery.

Part II is a *therapeutic index* that lists common complaints with information on how they can be treated using aromatherapy oils.

Part III is a *systematic survey of over 160 essential oils* shown in alphabetical order according to the Latin names of the plants from which they are derived.

This book can be used in several ways:

1. As a *concise reference guide* to a wide range of aromatic plants and oils, like a herbal guide.

2. As a *self-help manual*, showing how to use aromatherapy oils for healing and to promote well-being.

3. It can be read from cover to cover as a *comprehensive textbook* on essential oils.

AS A REFERENCE GUIDE to essential oils, the name of the plant or oil may be found in the Botanical Index at the back of the book (pp. 248–53), where it is listed under:

    a) common name: e.g., frankincense

    b) Latin or botanical term: *Boswellia carteri*

    c) essential oil trade name: olibanum

    d) folk names: gum thus.

Other varieties, such as Indian frankincense *(Boswellia serrata)*, may be found in the Botanical Classification section under their common family name 'Burseraceae', along with related species such as elemi, linaloe, myrrh and opopanax. Less common essential oils, such as blackcurrant, do not appear in the main body of the book but are included in the Botanical Classification section under their common family name, in this case 'Grossulariaceae'.

AS A SELF-HELP MANUAL on aromatherapy, it is best to consult the Therapeutic Index in Part II, where common complaints are

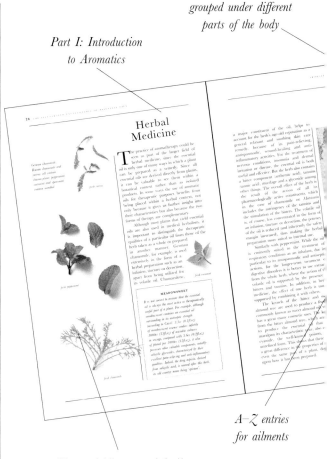

Part I: Introduction to Aromatics

Common complaints grouped under different parts of the body

A–Z entries for ailments

Plants yielding essential oils also used in medical herbalism

grouped according to different parts of the body: Skin Care; Circulation, Muscles and Joints; Respiratory System; Digestive System; Genito-urinary and Endocrine Systems; Immune System; Nervous System.

If, for example, you have developed a painful cramp in your neck, you should turn to the section on Circulation, Muscles and Joints where you will find the heading 'Muscular Cramp and Stiffness'. Of the essential oils listed, those shown in italics are generally considered to be the most useful and/or readily available; in this case, allspice, lavender, marjoram, rosemary and black pepper.

The choice of which oil to use depends on what is to hand, and on assessing the quality of each oil by consulting their entry in Part III of the book. **Special attention**

Most useful essential oils in italics

Part II: Therapeutic Index

Part III: The Oils

Vital safety data

Herbal tradition and uses as a folk remedy

Latin and common name of each plant

Specially commissioned photographs

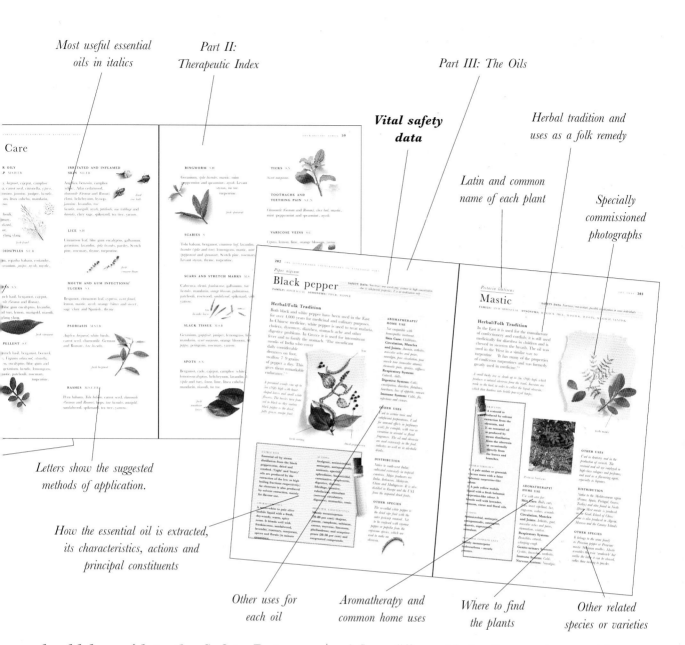

Letters show the suggested methods of application.

How the essential oil is extracted, its characteristics, actions and principal constituents

Other uses for each oil

Aromatherapy and common home uses

Where to find the plants

Other related species or varieties

should be paid to the Safety Data on each oil. On the basis of this assessment, we may choose to use lavender, marjoram and a little black pepper, which would make an excellent blend. Some of the principles behind blending oils can be found in Chapter 5, Creative Blending. The methods of application are indicated by the letters M, massage; B, bath; etc. Turn to Chapter 4, How to Use Essential Oils at Home, to find instructions on making up a massage oil, etc. Information on how essential oils work in specific cases can be found in Chapter 3, The Body – Actions and Applications.

AS A COMPREHENSIVE TEXTBOOK, this book shows the development of aromatics and their relationship with other herbal products. It defines different kinds of aromatic materials, methods of extraction and areas of production. And it includes information on their chemistry, pharmacology and safety levels. The 'Actions' ascribed to each plant refer to the properties of the whole herb or parts of it, or to the essential oil. Difficult technical terms are explained in the General Glossary at the end.

However, since the therapeutic guidelines are aimed primarily at the lay person without medical qualifications, the section on the aromatherapy application of essential oils at home is limited to the treatment of common complaints only. References to the medical and folk use of particular plants in herbal medicine and their actions are intended to provide background information only, and are not intended as a guide for self-treatment.

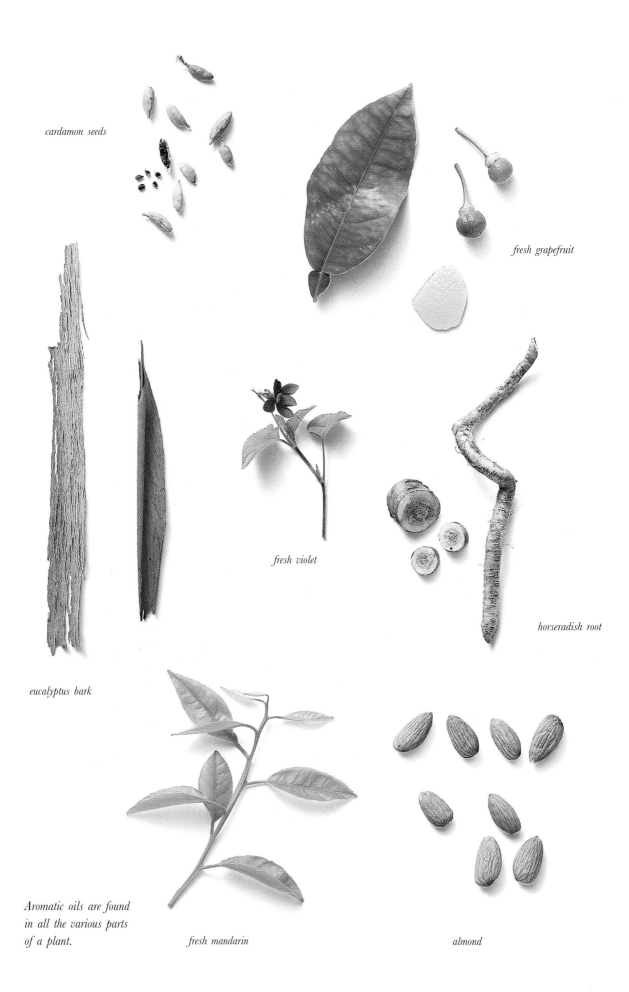

cardamon seeds

fresh grapefruit

eucalyptus bark

fresh violet

horseradish root

Aromatic oils are found
in all the various parts
of a plant.

fresh mandarin

almond

AN INTRODUCTION TO AROMATICS

1. HISTORICAL ROOTS

Natural Plant Origins

When we peel an orange, walk through a rose garden or rub a sprig of lavender between our fingers, we are all aware of the special scent of that plant. But what exactly is it that we can smell? Generally speaking, it is essential oils that give spices and herbs their specific scent and flavour, flowers and fruit their perfume. The essential oil in the orange peel is not difficult to identify; it is found in such profusion that it actually squirts out when we peel it. The minute droplets of oil contained in tiny pockets or glandular cells in the outer peel are very volatile; that is, they easily evaporate, infusing the air with their characteristic aroma.

But not all plants contain essential or volatile oils in such profusion. The aromatic content in the flowers of the rose is so very small that it takes one ton(ne) of petals to produce 300g (10½oz) of rose oil. It is not fully understood why some plants contain essential oils and others not. It is clear that the aromatic quality of the oils plays a role in the attraction or repulsion of certain insects or animals. It has also been suggested that they play an important part in the transpiration and life processes of the plant itself, and as a protection against disease. They have been described as the 'hormone' or 'life-blood' of a plant because of their highly concentrated and essential nature.

Aromatic oils can be found in all the various parts of a plant, including the seeds, bark, root, leaves, flowers, wood, balsam and resin. The bitter orange tree, for example, yields orange oil from the fruit peel; petitgrain from the leaves and twigs; and neroli oil from the orange blossoms. The clove tree produces different types of essential oil from its buds, stalks and leaves, whereas the Scotch pine yields distinct oils from its needles, wood and resin. The wide range of aromatic materials obtained from natural sources and the art of their extraction and use have developed slowly over the course of time, but their origins reach back to the very heart of the earliest civilizations.

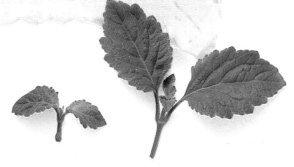

Ancient Civilizations

Aromatic plants and oils have been used for thousands of years, as incense, perfumes and cosmetics and for their medical and culinary applications. Their ritual use constituted an integral part of the tradition in most early cultures, where their religious and therapeutic roles became inextricably intertwined. This type of practice is still in evidence: for example, in the East, sprigs of juniper are burned in Tibetan temples as a form of purification; in the West, frankincense is used during the Roman Catholic mass.

In the ancient civilizations, perfumes were used as an expression of the animist and cosmic conceptions, responding above all to the exigencies of a cult ... associated at first with theophanies and incantations, the perfumes made by fumigation, libation and ablution, grew directly out of the ritual, and became an element in the art of therapy.[1]

The Vedic literature of India, dating from around 2000 BC, lists over 700 substances including cinnamon, spikenard, ginger, myrrh, coriander and sandalwood. But aromatics were considered to be more than just perfumes; in the Indo-Aryan tongue, 'atar' means smoke, wind, odour and essence, and the *Rig Veda* codifies their use for both liturgical and therapeutic purposes. The manner in which it is written reflects a spiritual and philosophical outlook, in which humanity is seen as a part of nature, and the handling of herbs as a sacred task: 'Simples, you who have existed for so long, even before the Gods were born, I want to understand your seven hundred secrets! . . . Come, you wise plants, heal this patient for me.'[2] Their understanding of plant lore developed into the traditional Indian or Ayurvedic system of medicine, which has enjoyed an unbroken transmission up to the present day.

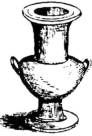

An alabaster vase from ancient Egypt used to store ointments.

The Chinese also have an ancient herbal tradition that accompanies the practice of acupuncture, the earliest records being in the *Yellow Emperor's Book of Internal Medicine* dating from more than 2000 years BC. Among the remedies are several aromatics such as opium and ginger, which, apart from their therapeutic applications, are known to have been utilized for religious purposes since the earliest times, as in the Li-ki and Tcheou-Li ceremonies. Borneo camphor is still used extensively in China today for ritual purposes.

But perhaps the most famous and richest associations concerning the first aromatic materials are those surrounding the ancient Egyptian civilization. Papyrus manuscripts dating back to the reign of Khufu, around 2800 BC, record the use of many medicinal herbs, while another papyrus written about 2000 BC speaks of 'fine oils and choice perfumes, and the incense of temples, whereby every god is gladdened'.[3] Aromatic gums and oils such as cedar and myrrh were employed in the embalming process, and the Egyptians were experts in cosmetology and renowned for their herbal preparations and ointments.

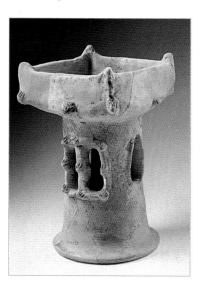

This pottery perfume burner was used in Syria in the thirteenth century BC.

An ancient Egyptian banquet scene, from the fifteenth century BC, shows women wearing perfume cones on their heads. As the heat melted the cones, their hair and bodies would be waxed and scented.

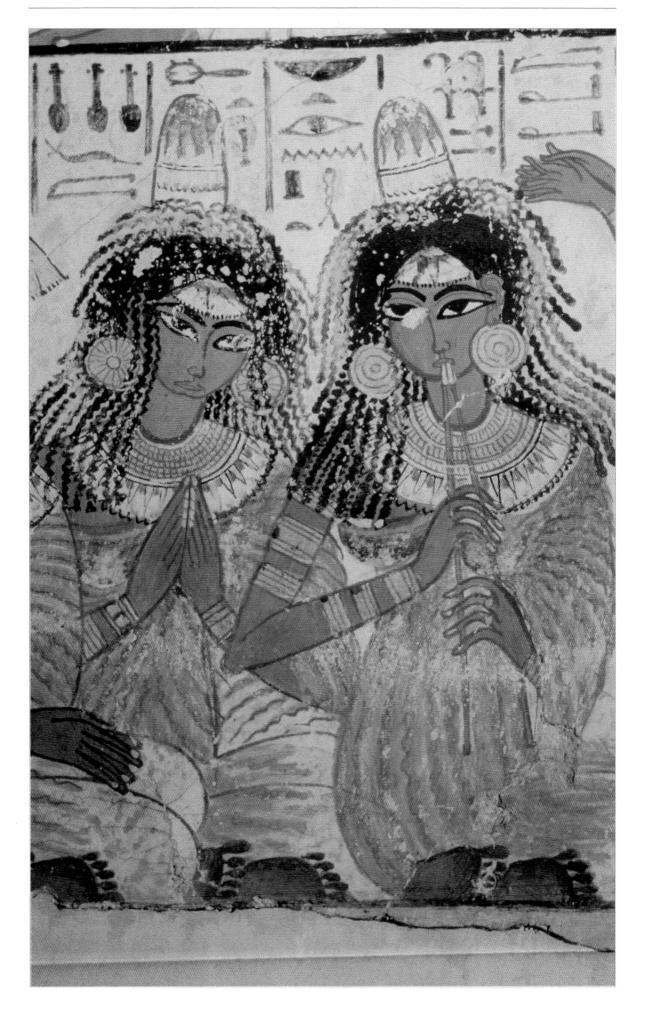

Treasures from the East

Natural aromatics and perfume materials constituted one of the earliest trade items of the ancient world, being rare and highly prized. When the Jewish people began their exodus from Egypt to Israel around 1240 BC, they took with them many precious gums and oils together with knowledge of their use. On their journey, according to the Book of Exodus, the Lord transmitted to Moses the formula for a special anointing oil, which included myrrh, cinnamon, calamus, cassia and olive oil among its ingredients. This holy oil was used to consecrate Aaron and his sons into priesthood, which continued from generation to generation. Frankincense and myrrh, as treasures from the East, were offered to Jesus at his birth.

In the East, aromatics and perfumes were highly valued commodities used in sacred rites and offered in homage to the gods. This painting by Albrecht Dürer shows the Magi bringing gifts of frankincense and myrrh to the baby Jesus.

The Phoenician merchants also exported their scented oils and gums to the Arabian peninsula and gradually throughout the Mediterranean region, particularly Greece and Rome. They introduced the West to the riches of the Orient: they brought camphor from China, cinnamon from India, gums from Arabia and rose from Syria, always ensuring that they kept their trading routes a closely guarded secret.

The Greeks especially learned a great deal from the Egyptians; Herodotus and Democrates, who visited Egypt during the fifth century BC, were later to transmit what they had learned about perfumery and natural therapeutics. Herodotus was the first to record the method of distillation of turpentine, in about 425 BC, as well as furnishing the first information about perfumes and numerous other details regarding odorous materials. Dioscorides made a detailed study of the sources and uses of plants and aromatics employed by the Greeks and Romans, which he compiled into a five-volume materia medica, known as the *Herbarius*.

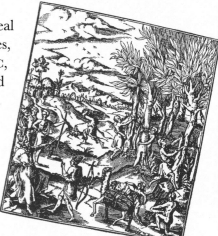

Harvesting cinnamon in India to be exported to Europe.

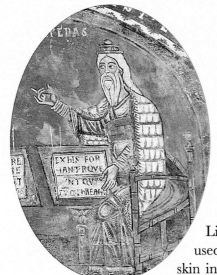

Hippocrates, probably the most famous of physicians, prescribed perfumed fumigations and fomentations as part of his medical treatments.

Hippocrates, who was born in Greece about 460 BC and universally revered as the 'father of medicine', also prescribed perfumed fumigations and fomentations; indeed 'from Greek medical practice there is derived the term "iatralypte", from the physician who cured by the use of aromatic unctions'.[4] One of the most famous of these Greek preparations, made from myrrh, cinnamon and cassis, was called 'megaleion' after its creator Megallus. Like the Egyptian 'kyphi', it could be used both as a perfume and as a remedy for skin inflammation and battle wounds.

The Romans were even more lavish in their use of perfumes and aromatic oils than the Greeks. They used three kinds of perfumes: 'ladysmata', solid unguents; 'stymmata', scented oils; and 'diapasmata', powdered perfumes. They were used to fragrance their hair, their bodies, their clothes and beds; large amounts of scented oil were used for massage after bathing. With the fall of the Roman Empire and the advent of Christianity, many of the Roman physicians fled to Constantinople taking the books of Galen, Hippocrates and Dioscorides with them. These great Graeco-Roman works were translated into Persian, Arabic and other languages, and at the end of the Byzantine Empire, their knowledge passed on to the Arab world. Europe, meanwhile, entered the so-called Dark Ages.

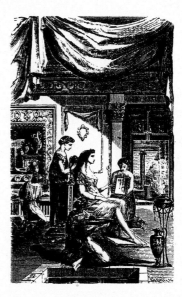

The Romans, like the Greeks and Egyptians, used fragrant oils in ceremonies and rituals, but they were particularly extravagant in their use of oils in baths, massage and as a scent for the hair and body.

Alchemy

Between the seventh and thirteenth centuries the Arabs produced many great men of science, among them Avicenna (AD 980–1037). This highly gifted physician and scholar wrote over a hundred books in his lifetime, one of which was devoted entirely to the flower most cherished by Islam, the rose. Among his discoveries, he has been credited with the invention of the refrigerated coil, a breakthrough in the art of distillation, which he used to produce pure essential oils and aromatic water. However, in 1975 Dr Paolo Rovesti led an archeological expedition to Pakistan to investigate the ancient Indus Valley civilization. There, in the museum of Taxila at the foot of the Himalayas, he found a perfectly preserved distillation apparatus made of terracotta. The presence of perfume containers also exhibited in the museum dating from the same period, about 3000 BC, confirmed its use for the preparation of aromatic oils.

Rose water became one of the most popular scents and came to the West at the time of the Crusades, along with other exotic essences, and the method of distillation. By the thirteenth century, the 'perfumes of Arabia'

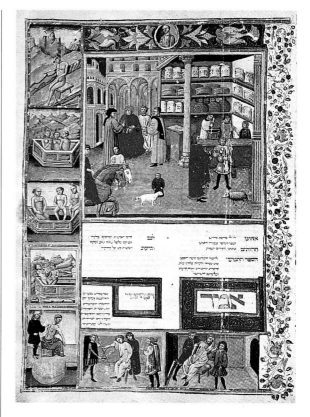

A fifteenth-century Hebrew edition of Avicenna's Canon of Medicine *showing a pharmacy and some typical medical treatments of the time.*

An alchemy master preparing his ingredients (right).

Archeological evidence from the Indus Valley suggests that people were preparing aromatic oils over 4,000 years ago (below).

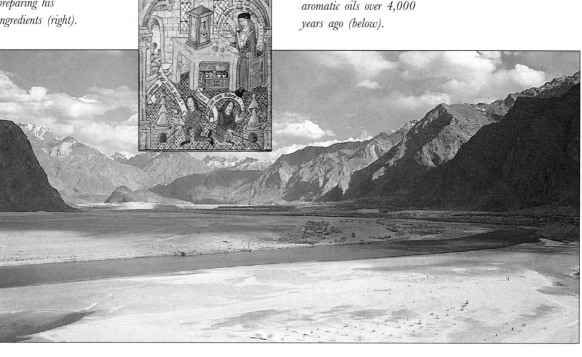

*'Alchemy was the bridge across which the rich symbolism of the ancient world – Arab, Greek, Gnostic – was transported into our own era… thus symbolism fell from the rarefied heights into the melting-pot, and began to be tested in continuous, dynamic interactions with the findings of chemistry.'*⁵

Volatile oils can be equated with the purified human psyche or 'quintessence' of the alchemists.

were famous throughout Europe. During the Middle Ages, floors were strewn with aromatic plants, and little herbal bouquets were carried as a protection against plague and other infectious diseases. Gradually the Europeans, lacking the gum-yielding trees of the Orient, began to experiment with their own native herbs such as lavender, sage and rosemary. By the sixteenth century lavender water and essential oils known as 'chymical oils' could be bought from the apothecary, and, following the invention of printing, the period 1470 to 1670 saw the publica-

This engraving from Brucschwig's sixteenth-century manuscript 'The Art of Distillation' shows the instruments and plants used by the alchemist. The stag and fountain are archetypal images associated with alchemy.

tion of many herbals such as the *Grete Herball* published in 1526, some of which included illustrations of the retorts and stills used for the extraction of volatile oils.

In the hands of the philosophers, the art of distillation was employed in the practice of alchemy, the hermetic pursuit dedicated to the transformation of base metals into gold. It was primarily a religious quest in which the stages of the distillation process were equated with stages of an inner psychic transmutation. Just as aromatic material could be distilled to produce a pure essence, so the human emotions could be refined to reveal their true nature.

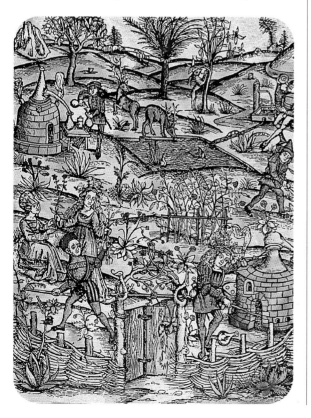

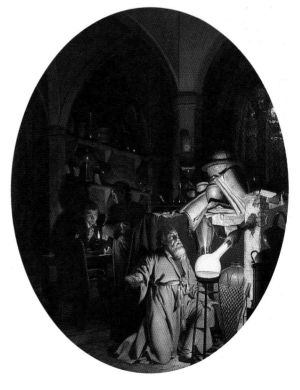

This eighteenth-century painting by Joseph Wright gives an accurate portrayal of the alchemist's equipment.

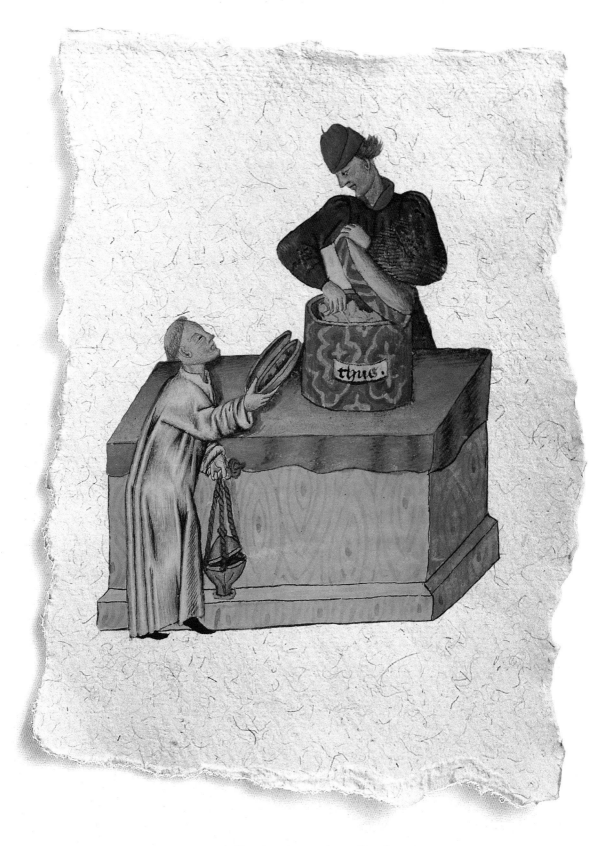

A fifteenth-century merchant selling thyme.

The Scientific Revolution

Throughout the Renaissance period, aromatic materials filled the pharmacopoeias, which for many centuries remained the main protection against epidemics. Over the next few centuries the medicinal properties and application of increasing numbers of new essential oils were analysed and recorded by the pharmacists. The list included both well-established aromatics such as cedar, cinnamon, frankincense, juniper, rose, rosemary, lavender and sage, but also essences such as artemisia, cajeput, chervil, orange flower, valerian and pine.

The perfumery and distillation industries attracted illustrious names of the day, and in the northern countries of Europe, especially at Grasse in France, flourishing commercial enterprises sprang up. By the end of the seventeenth century, the profession of perfumery broke away from the allied fields, and a distinction was made between perfumes and the aromatics that had become the domain of the apothecary.

Alchemy gave way to technical chemistry, and with it went the interest in the

The reception room of a master apothecary. For many centuries, the apothecaries of Europe analysed and recorded the medicinal properties of many new essential oils.

interrelatedness of matter and spirit, and the interdependence of medicine and psychology. There developed the idea of combating speculation with logic and deductive reason. With the scientific revolution of the early nineteenth century, chemists were able to identify for the first time the various constituents of the oils, and give them specific names such as 'geranoil', 'citronellol' and 'cineol'. In the *Yearbook of Pharmacy and Transactions of the British Pharmaceutical Conference* in 1907, we find, for example:

> *A pilea of undetermined botanical species has yielded a white essential oil with an odour of turpentine . . . A small amount of pinene was detected but its other constituents have not yet been identified. This oil is of interest as being the first instance of an essential oil derived from the family Uricacaea.*[6]

It is ironic that this enthusiastic research laid the ground for the development of the oils' synthetic counterparts, and the growth of the modern drug industry. Herbal medicine and aromatic remedies lost their credibility as methods of treatment went out of the hands of the individual and into those of professionals. By the middle of the twentieth century, the role of essential oils had been reduced almost entirely to their employment in perfumes, cosmetics and foodstuffs.

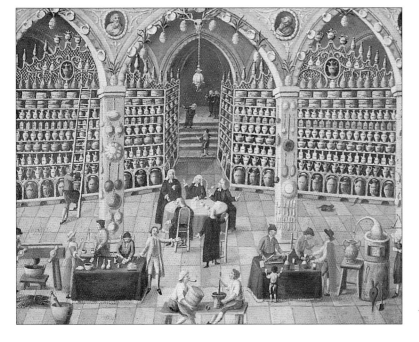

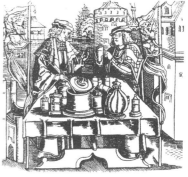

This sixteenth-century engraving shows perfumers at work with their chemical apparatus. By the end of the seventeenth century, perfumery had become a profession in its own right, and a distinction was made between perfumes and the aromatics used by the apothecary.

2. AROMATHERAPY AND MEDICAL HERBALISM
The Birth of Aromatherapy

The term 'aromatherapy' was first coined in 1928 by René-Maurice Gattefossé, a French chemist working in his family's perfumier business. He became fascinated with the therapeutic possibilities of the oils after discovering by accident that lavender was able to heal a severe burn on his hand quite rapidly and help prevent scarring. He also found that many of the essential oils were more effective in their totality than their synthetic substitutes or their isolated active ingredients. As early as 1904 Cuthbert Hall had shown that the antiseptic power of eucalyptus oil in its natural form was stronger than its isolated main active constituent, 'eucalyptol' or 'cineol'.

Another French doctor and scientist, Dr Jean Valnet, used essential oils as part of a programme by which he successfully treated specific medical and psychiatric disorders, the results of which were published in 1964 as *Aromatherapie*.

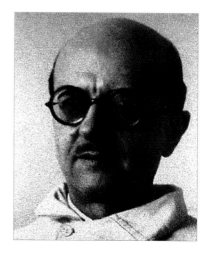

The French chemist René-Maurice Gattefossé devoted much of his life to the study of aromatherapy.

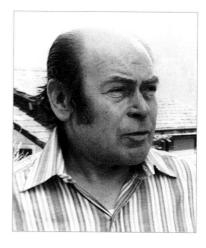

In his work Dr Jean Valnet has shown that there need not be a gulf between the traditional, natural approach to healing and the modern, analytical one.

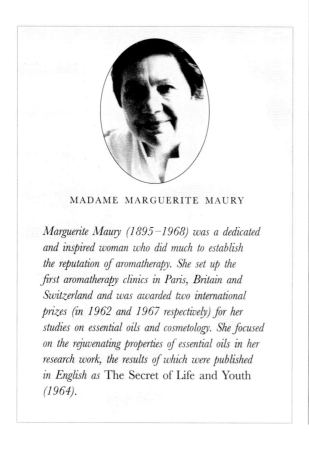

MADAME MARGUERITE MAURY

Marguerite Maury (1895–1968) was a dedicated and inspired woman who did much to establish the reputation of aromatherapy. She set up the first aromatherapy clinics in Paris, Britain and Switzerland and was awarded two international prizes (in 1962 and 1967 respectively) for her studies on essential oils and cosmetology. She focused on the rejuvenating properties of essential oils in her research work, the results of which were published in English as The Secret of Life and Youth *(1964).*

The work of Valnet was studied by Madame Marguerite Maury, who applied his research to her beauty therapy, in which she aimed to revitalize her clients by creating a 'strictly personal aromatic complex which she adapted to the subject's temperament and particular health problems. Hence, going far beyond any simple esthetic objective, perfumed essences when correctly selected, represent many medicinal agents.'[7]

In some respects, the word 'aromatherapy' can be misleading because it suggests that it is a form of healing that works exclusively through the sense of smell, and on the emotions. This is not the case, for apart from its scent, each essential oil has an individual combination of constituents that interacts with the body's chemistry in a direct manner, which then in turn affects certain organs or systems as a whole. For example, when the oils are used externally in the form of a massage treatment, they are easily absorbed via the skin and transported throughout the body. This can be demonstrated by rubbing a clove of garlic on the soles of the feet; the volatile oil content will be taken into the blood and the odour will appear on the breath a little while later. Different essential oils are absorbed through the skin at varying rates, for example:

TURPENTINE: *20 mins.*

EUCALYPTUS AND THYME: *20–40 mins.*

ANISE, BERGAMOT AND LEMON: *40–60 mins.*

CITRONELLA, PINE, LAVENDER AND

GERANIUM: *60–80 mins.*

CORIANDER, RUE AND PEPPERMINT:

100–120 mins.

It is therefore important to recognize that essential oils have three distinct modes of action with regard to how they interrelate with the human body: pharmacological, physiological and psychological. The pharmacological effect is concerned with the chemical changes that take place when an essential oil enters the bloodstream and reacts with the hormones and enzymes, etc.; the physiological mode with the way in which an essential oil affects the system of the body, whether they are sedated or stimulated, etc.; the psychological effect takes place when an essence is inhaled, and an individual responds to its odour. On the first two points, aromatherapy has much in common with the tradition of medical herbalism or phytotherapy – in other words, it is not simply the aroma that is important but also the chemical interaction between the oils and the body, and the physical changes that are brought about.

HOW AIR-BORNE AROMATIC OIL MOLECULES INTERACT WITH THE SYSTEMS OF THE BODY

Odour signals are passed *directly* to the limbic system of the *brain* evoking an *immediate* emotional or instinctual response.

Aromatic molecules enter the *lungs* and are absorbed via the alveoli into the blood.

The blood is carried to the *heart* and transported throughout the body via the circulatory system.

Different oils have affinities with specific parts of the body – e.g. spices particularly affect the *digestion*.

Waste and toxins are processed by the *liver and kidneys* and eliminated mainly via the lungs, but also in the urine and sweat.

Herbal Medicine

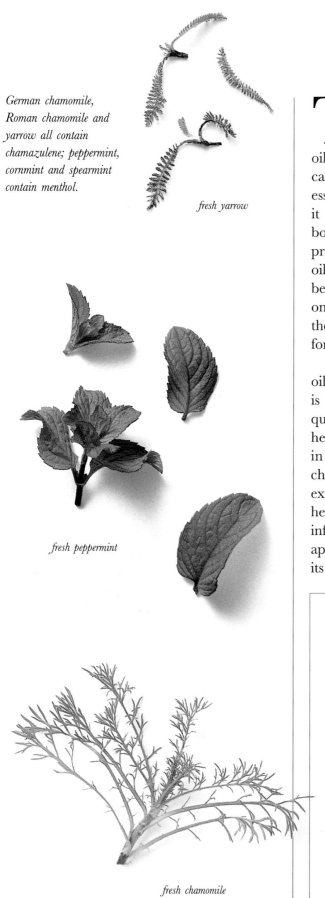

German chamomile, Roman chamomile and yarrow all contain chamazulene; peppermint, cornmint and spearmint contain menthol.

fresh yarrow

fresh peppermint

fresh chamomile

The practice of aromatherapy could be seen as part of the larger field of herbal medicine, since the essential oil is only one of many ways in which a plant can be prepared as a remedy. Since all essential oils are derived directly from plants, it can be valuable to see them within a botanical context rather than as isolated products. In some ways the use of aromatic oils for therapeutic purposes benefits from being placed within a herbal context, not only because it gives us further insight into their characteristics but also because the two forms of therapy are complementary.

Although most plants that yield essential oils are also used in medical herbalism, it is important to distinguish the therapeutic qualities of a particular oil from those of the herb taken as a whole or prepared in another manner. German chamomile, for example, is used extensively in the form of a herbal preparation such as an infusion, tincture or decoction, apart from being utilized for its volatile oil. Chamazulene,

fresh cornmint

MEADOWSWEET

It is not correct to assume that the essential oil is always the most active or therapeutically useful part of a plant. For example, although meadowsweet contains an essential oil outstanding in its antiseptic strength (according to Cavel,[8] 3.3cc (0.1fl.oz) of meadowsweet essence renders infertile 1000cc (35fl.oz) of microbic cultures in sewage, compared with 5.6cc (0.2fl.oz) of phenol per 1000cc (35fl.oz), it also possesses other valuable components, notably salicylic glycosides, characterized by their excellent pain-relieving and anti-inflammatory qualities. Indeed, the drug aspirin, derived from salicylic acid, is named after this herb, its old country name being 'spiraea'.

a major constituent of the oil, helps to account for the herb's age-old reputation as a general relaxant and soothing skin care remedy, because of its pain-relieving, antispasmodic, wound-healing and anti-inflammatory activities. For the treatment of nervous conditions, insomnia and dermal irritation or disease, the essential oil is both useful and effective. But the herb also contains a bitter component (anthemic acid), tannins (tannic acid), mucilage and a glycoside among other things. The overall effect of the herb is the result of the action of all its pharmacologically active constituents, which in the case of chamomile or *Matricaria* includes the astringency of the tannins and the stimulation of the bitters. The volatile oil is, of course, less concentrated in the form of an infusion, tincture or decoction, the potency of the oil is reduced (and inherently the safety margin increased), thus making the herbal preparation more suited to internal use.

Similarly with peppermint. While the oil is eminently suited to the treatment of respiratory conditions as an inhalant, due in particular to its antispasmodic and antiseptic actions, for the longer-term treatment of digestive disorders it is better to use extracts from the whole herb, where the action of the volatile oil is supported by the presence of bitters and tannins. In addition, in herbal medicine, the effect of one herb is usually supported by combining it with others.

The kernels of the (bitter and sweet) almond tree are used to produce a fixed oil commonly known as sweet almond oil, which has a great many cosmetic uses. The kernels from the bitter almond tree, which are used to produce the essential oil that gives marzipan its characteristic taste, also contain cyanide, the well-known poison, in its unrefined form. This shows that there can be a great difference in the properties of a plant, even the same part of a plant, depending upon how it has been prepared.

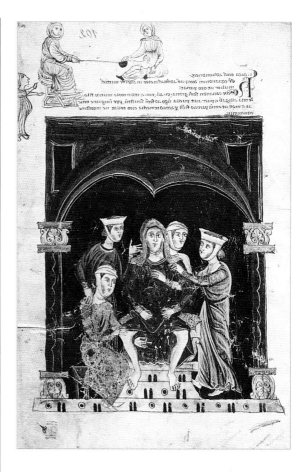

In this thirteenth-century manuscript miniature the women attending a birth are using coriander seed to hasten delivery. The drawings at the top show other uses of the herb.

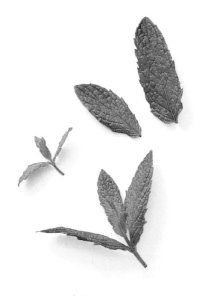

fresh spearmint

Therapeutic Guidelines

As a general rule that is in line with the present-day aromatherapy 'code of practice', it is best to use essential oils as external remedies only. This is due mainly to the high concentration of the oils and the potential irritation or damage that they can cause to the mucous membranes and delicate stomach lining in undiluted form. There even seems to be some kind of natural order in this scheme, in that volatile oils mix readily with oils and ointments suited to external application, which are absorbed readily through the skin and vaporize easily for inhalation. When inhaled, they can affect an individual's mood or feelings, and at the same time cause physiological changes in the body.

Herbs, on the other hand, yield up many of their qualities to water and alcohol and are appropriate for internal use. But, because they lack the concentrated aromatic element, they do not have the same subtle effects on the mind and emotions.

These are only superficial guidelines, for there are always exceptions to the rule. Plantain, for example, is an excellent wound-healing herb valuable for external use, although it does not contain any essential oil. Nor can we ignore the fact that a great many aromatic oils are used for flavouring our food and beverages and are consumed daily in minute amounts. Peppermint oil, for example, is used in a wide variety of alcoholic and non-alcoholic beverages, confectionery and

---

SAFETY GUIDELINES

In general, those essential oils which are commonly available are safe to use for aromatherapy or household purposes. However, due to their high concentration and potency, it is necessary to be aware of the following safety measures and take some precautions into account.
The safety data – *Always check the specific safety data before using a new oil (see individual entries in Part III).*
Internal use – DO NOT TAKE ESSENTIAL OILS INTERNALLY! *This rule is in accordance with the guidelines of safety recommended by the International Federation of Aromatherapy. Essential oils do not mix with water, and in an undiluted form they may damage the lining of the digestive tract. In addition, some essential oils are toxic if taken internally.*
Storage: *Store in dark bottles, away from light and heat, and well out of reach of children and pets.*

---

prepared savoury foods, although the highest average use does not exceed 0.104 per cent. The mint oils, which include spearmint and cornmint, are also used extensively by the pharmaceutical and cosmetic industries in products such as toothpaste, cough and cold remedies, and as fragrance components in soaps, creams, lotions, as well as colognes and perfumes. In addition, cornmint is frequently used as the starting material for the production of 'menthol' for use in the drug industry.

It can be seen that the use of essential oils covers a wide and varied spectrum. On the one hand, they share the holistic qualities of natural plant remedies, although it is true that some herbalists view essential oils in much the same light as they regard synthetic drugs, being a 'part' of the whole, rather than the entire herb. On the other hand, they play an active role in the pharmaceutical industry, either in their entirety or in the form of isolated constituents like 'phenol' or 'menthol'.

It is not the aim of this book to glorify natural remedies (some of which are in fact highly toxic) at the expense of scientific progress, nor to uphold the principles of our present-day drug-orientated culture, but simply to provide information about the oils themselves in their multifaceted nature.

BABIES AND CHILDREN

Always increase the dilution for babies and infants to at least half the recommended amount. For babies, avoid the possibly toxic and irritant oils altogether.
Babies 0–12 months: *use only 1 drop of lavender, rose or chamomile (German or Roman) essential oil, diluted in 1 tsp carrier oil for massage or bathing.*
Infants 1–5 years: *use only 2-3 drops of the 'safe' oils, i.e. those which are non-toxic and non-irritant, diluted in 1 tsp carrier oil for massage or bathing.*
Children 6–12 years: *use as for adults but in half the stated concentration.*
Children over 12 years: *use as directed for adults.*

SAFETY GUIDELINES

HAZARDOUS OILS

Some essential oils can be hazardous, especially in inexperienced hands, either due to high toxicity levels or because they can cause severe dermal irritation. The oils which should be avoided in this context are: **bitter almond, arnica, boldo, broom, buchu, calamus, camphor (brown and yellow), cassia, chervil, cinnamon (bark), costus, deertongue, elecampane, fennel (bitter), horseradish, jaborandi, melilotus, mugwort, mustard, oregano, pennyroyal, pine (dwarf), rue, sage (common), santolina, sassafras, savine, savory, tansy, thuja, thyme (red), tonka, wintergreen, wormseed and wormwood.** *These oils should not be used at all therapeutically!*

TOXICITY

Essential oils which should be used in moderation (only in dilution and for a maximum of two weeks at a time) because of toxicity levels are: **ajowan, anise star, aniseed, basil (exotic), bay laurel, bay (West Indian), calamintha, camphor (white), cascarilla bark, cassie, cedarwood (Virginian), cinnamon (leaf), clove (bud), coriander, eucalyptus, fennel (sweet), hops, hyssop, juniper, nutmeg, parsley, pepper (black), sage (Spanish), tagetes, tarragon, thyme (white), tuberose, turmeric, turpentine, valerian.**

NEAT APPLICATION

In general, essential oils should not be applied neat to the skin – always dilute them in a carrier oil or cream first. There are exceptions to this rule, such as the use of neat lavender for cuts, spots, burns etc. Certain non-irritant essential oils may be applied neat to the skin as a perfume, such as **ylang ylang** or **sandalwood** (check safety data in Part III). Always do a patch test first, and keep well away from the eyes.

PATCH TEST

Before applying any new oil neat to the skin, even as a perfume, always do a patch test. Put a few drops on the back of your wrist, cover with a plaster and leave for an hour or more. If irritation or redness occurs, bathe the area with cold water. For future use, reduce the concentration level by half or avoid altogether.

DERMAL/SKIN IRRITATION

Oils which may irritate the skin, especially if used in a high concentration are: **ajowan, allspice, aniseed, basil (sweet), black pepper, borneol, cajeput, caraway, cedarwood (Virginian), cinnamon (leaf), clove (bud), cornmint, eucalyptus, garlic, ginger, lemon, parsley, peppermint, pine needle (Scotch and longleaf), thyme (white) and turmeric.** These oils should be used in half the usual recommended dilutions. Always mix them first in a base oil, cream or gel before applying to the skin and do not use more than 3 drops in the bath.

SENSITIZATION

Some oils may cause skin irritation only in those people with very sensitive skins or can cause an allergic reaction in some individuals. Even some very common oils, such as tea tree or jasmine, have been known to cause 'sensitization' in a few cases. It is important for those with sensitive skins always to do a patch test before using a new oil to check for individual sensitization. Oils which may cause sensitization include: **basil (French), bay laurel, benzoin, cade, cananga, cedarwood (Virginian), chamomile (Roman and German), citronella, garlic, geranium, ginger, hops, jasmine, lemon, lemongrass, lemon balm (melissa), litsea cubeba, lovage, mastic, mint, orange, Peru balsam, pine (Scotch and longleaf), styrax, tea tree, thyme (white), Tolu balsam, turmeric, turpentine, valerian, vanilla, verbena, violet, yarrow and ylang ylang.**

PHOTOTOXICITY

Some oils are phototoxic i.e. they cause skin pigmentation if exposed to direct sunlight. Do not use the following oils either neat or in dilution on the skin, if the area will be exposed to the sun: **angelica root, bergamot (except bergapten-free type), cumin, ginger, lemon, lime, lovage, mandarin, orange and verbena.**

PREGNANCY

During pregnancy, use essential oils in half the usual stated amount, because of the sensitivity of the growing child. Oils which are potentially toxic or have emmenagogue properties (i.e stimulate the uterine muscles), are contra-indicated. The following oils should be avoided altogether: **ajowan, angelica, anise star, aniseed, basil, bay laurel, calamintha, cedarwood (all types), celery seed, cinnamon leaf, citronella, clary sage, clove, cumin, fennel (sweet), hyssop, juniper, labdanum, lovage, marjoram, myrrh, nutmeg, parsley, snakeroot, Spanish sage, tarragon and thyme (white).** These oils are best avoided during the first 4 months of pregnancy: **peppermint, rose and rosemary.**

HIGH BLOOD PRESSURE

Avoid the following oils in cases of high-hypertension: **hyssop, rosemary, sage (Spanish and common) and**

EPILEPSY

thyme.
Avoid the following oils in cases of epilepsy, due to their powerful action on the nervous system: **fennel (sweet),**

DIABETES

hyssop, rosemary and sage (all types).

HOMEOPATHY

Avoid **angelica** oil in cases of diabetes.
Homeopathic treatment is not compatible with the following: **black pepper, camphor, eucalyptus and peppermint.**

3. THE BODY – ACTIONS AND APPLICATIONS
How Essential Oils Work

The therapeutic potential of essential oils, like other plant-derived remedies, has yet to be fully realized. Although numerous medical herbs have been utilized since antiquity, many of which have been exploited to provide the biologically active compounds that form the basis for most of our modern drugs (such as quinine and cocaine), there is still a great deal to be learned about their precise pharmacology.

This is particularly true of aromatic oils, which by their very nature have such a concentrated yet multifaceted make-up. In addition, 'only a small proportion of the world flora has been examined for pharmacologically active compounds, but with the ever-increasing danger of plants becoming extinct, there is a real risk that many important plant sources may be lost'.[9]

Modern research has largely confirmed the traditionally held beliefs regarding the therapeutic uses of particular plants, although with time the terminology has changed. A herb such as basil, at one time described as a 'protection against evil', or 'good for the heart' whose scent 'taketh away sorrowfulness', may in modern usage be described as an excellent prophylactic, nerve tonic and antidepressant. Like herbal remedies, an essential oil can cover a wide field of activities; indeed the same herb or oil (such as lemon balm) can stimulate certain systems of the body while sedating or relaxing others. In order to gain a clearer understanding of the way essential oils work, and some of their particular areas of activity, it may be helpful to take an overall view of the systems of the human body.

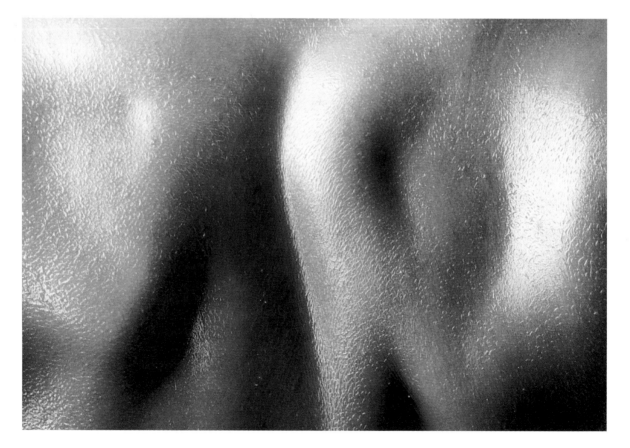

*An essential oil can have different effects on different parts of
the body, stimulating certain systems while relaxing others.*

The Skin

Skin problems are often the surface manifestation of deeper conditions, such as build-up of toxins in the blood, hormonal imbalance or nervous and emotional difficulties. In this area the versatility of essential oils is particularly valuable because they are able to combat such complaints on a variety of levels. Since essential oils are soluble in oil and alcohol and impart their scent to water, they provide the ideal ingredient for cosmetics and general skin care as well as for the treatment of specific diseases.

Within this context the following activities are of particular benefit:

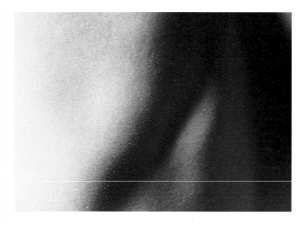

Essential oils can be used in numerous ways to treat skin complaints and conditions.

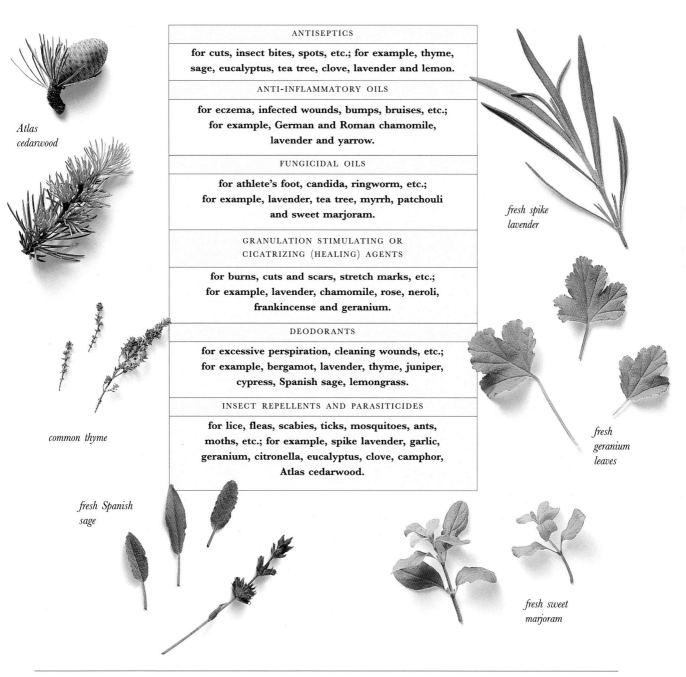

Atlas cedarwood

fresh spike lavender

common thyme

fresh geranium leaves

fresh Spanish sage

fresh sweet marjoram

ANTISEPTICS
for cuts, insect bites, spots, etc.; for example, thyme, sage, eucalyptus, tea tree, clove, lavender and lemon.
ANTI-INFLAMMATORY OILS
for eczema, infected wounds, bumps, bruises, etc.; for example, German and Roman chamomile, lavender and yarrow.
FUNGICIDAL OILS
for athlete's foot, candida, ringworm, etc.; for example, lavender, tea tree, myrrh, patchouli and sweet marjoram.
GRANULATION STIMULATING OR CICATRIZING (HEALING) AGENTS
for burns, cuts and scars, stretch marks, etc.; for example, lavender, chamomile, rose, neroli, frankincense and geranium.
DEODORANTS
for excessive perspiration, cleaning wounds, etc.; for example, bergamot, lavender, thyme, juniper, cypress, Spanish sage, lemongrass.
INSECT REPELLENTS AND PARASITICIDES
for lice, fleas, scabies, ticks, mosquitoes, ants, moths, etc.; for example, spike lavender, garlic, geranium, citronella, eucalyptus, clove, camphor, Atlas cedarwood.

The Circulation, Muscles and Joints

Essential oils are easily absorbed via the skin and mucosa into the bloodstream, affecting the nature of the circulation as a whole. Oils with a rubefacient or warming effect not only cause better local blood circulation but also influence the inner organs. They bring a warmth and glow to the surface of the skin and can provide considerable pain relief through their analgesic or numbing effect. Such oils can relieve local inflammation by setting free mediators in the body, which in turn cause the blood vessels to expand, so the blood is able to move more quickly and the swelling is reduced. Some oils, such as hyssop, tend to have a balancing or regulating effect on the circulatory system as a whole, reducing the blood pressure if it is too high or stimulating the system if it is sluggish.

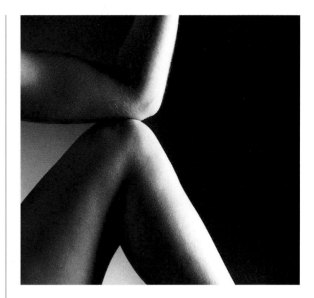

Once absorbed into the bloodstream, essential oils can be highly beneficial to the circulatory system.

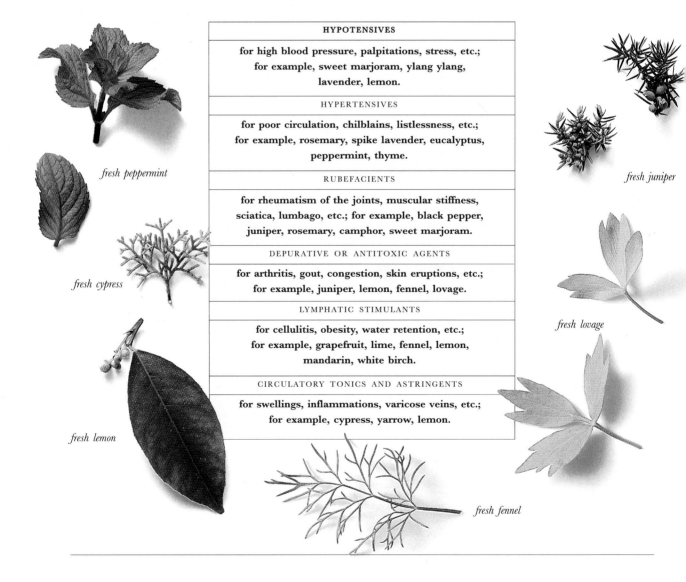

fresh peppermint

fresh cypress

fresh lemon

fresh juniper

fresh lovage

fresh fennel

HYPOTENSIVES
for high blood pressure, palpitations, stress, etc.; for example, sweet marjoram, ylang ylang, lavender, lemon.
HYPERTENSIVES
for poor circulation, chilblains, listlessness, etc.; for example, rosemary, spike lavender, eucalyptus, peppermint, thyme.
RUBEFACIENTS
for rheumatism of the joints, muscular stiffness, sciatica, lumbago, etc.; for example, black pepper, juniper, rosemary, camphor, sweet marjoram.
DEPURATIVE OR ANTITOXIC AGENTS
for arthritis, gout, congestion, skin eruptions, etc.; for example, juniper, lemon, fennel, lovage.
LYMPHATIC STIMULANTS
for cellulitis, obesity, water retention, etc.; for example, grapefruit, lime, fennel, lemon, mandarin, white birch.
CIRCULATORY TONICS AND ASTRINGENTS
for swellings, inflammations, varicose veins, etc.; for example, cypress, yarrow, lemon.

The Respiratory System

Nose, throat and lung infections are conditions that respond very well to treatment with essential oils. Inhalation is a very effective way of utilizing their properties, for 'although after arriving in the bronchi the main part will be exhaled directly by the lungs, they cause an increased bronchial secretion (a protective reaction) which is beneficial for many respiratory ailments'.[10] By inhalation they are absorbed into the blood circulation even faster than by oral application. In addition, most essential oils that are absorbed from the stomach are then excreted via the lungs, only a small part in the urine.

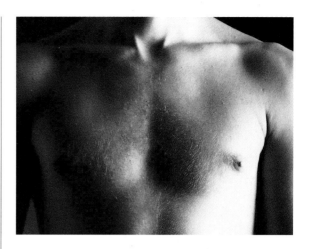

Inhalation of essential oils is an effective way to treat nose, throat and lung ailments.

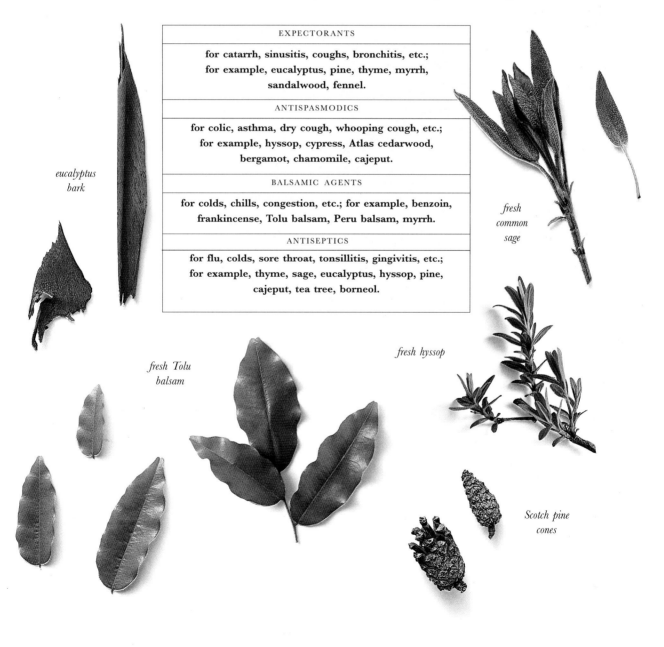

EXPECTORANTS
for catarrh, sinusitis, coughs, bronchitis, etc.; for example, eucalyptus, pine, thyme, myrrh, sandalwood, fennel.
ANTISPASMODICS
for colic, asthma, dry cough, whooping cough, etc.; for example, hyssop, cypress, Atlas cedarwood, bergamot, chamomile, cajeput.
BALSAMIC AGENTS
for colds, chills, congestion, etc.; for example, benzoin, frankincense, Tolu balsam, Peru balsam, myrrh.
ANTISEPTICS
for flu, colds, sore throat, tonsillitis, gingivitis, etc.; for example, thyme, sage, eucalyptus, hyssop, pine, cajeput, tea tree, borneol.

eucalyptus bark

fresh common sage

fresh Tolu balsam

fresh hyssop

Scotch pine cones

The Digestive System

Although it is not recommended that essential oils be taken orally, they can by external application effect certain changes in the digestive processes. However, whereas herbal medicine has many remedies at its disposal for a wide variety of stomach, gall bladder and liver complaints, such as dandelion, marshmallow, chamomile and meadowsweet, much of their effectiveness is based on a combination of aromatic components, together with bitters, tannins and mucilage, which are absent in the volatile oil alone. The external application of essential oils in problems of the digestive system, though effective, is consequently somewhat limited compared with the internal use of herbal remedies.

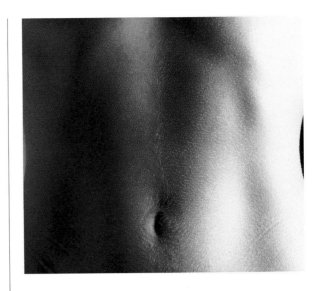

Essential oils may be applied externally for stomach and digestive complaints.

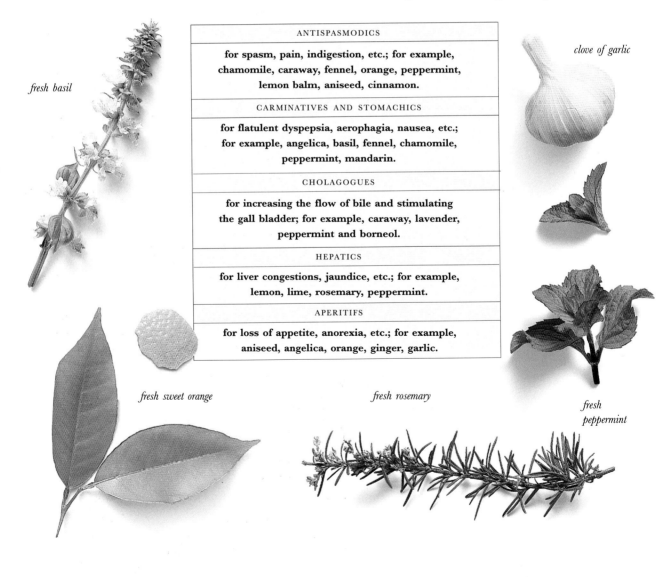

fresh basil

clove of garlic

ANTISPASMODICS
for spasm, pain, indigestion, etc.; for example, chamomile, caraway, fennel, orange, peppermint, lemon balm, aniseed, cinnamon.
CARMINATIVES AND STOMACHICS
for flatulent dyspepsia, aerophagia, nausea, etc.; for example, angelica, basil, fennel, chamomile, peppermint, mandarin.
CHOLAGOGUES
for increasing the flow of bile and stimulating the gall bladder; for example, caraway, lavender, peppermint and borneol.
HEPATICS
for liver congestions, jaundice, etc.; for example, lemon, lime, rosemary, peppermint.
APERITIFS
for loss of appetite, anorexia, etc.; for example, aniseed, angelica, orange, ginger, garlic.

fresh sweet orange

fresh rosemary

fresh peppermint

Genito-urinary/Endocrine Systems

Like the digestive system, the reproductive organs can be affected by absorption via the skin into the bloodstream, as well as through hormonal changes. Some essential oils such as rose and jasmine have an affinity for the reproductive system, having a strengthening effect as well as helping to combat specific complaints such as menstrual problems, genital infections and sexual difficulties. Other oils contain plant hormones that mimic the corresponding human hormones; oils such as hops, sage and fennel have been found to contain a form of estrogen that influences the menstrual cycle,

lactation and secondary sexual characteristics.

Other essential oils are known to influence the levels of hormone secretion of other glands, including the thyroid gland (which governs growth and metabolism), the adrenal medulla (which deals with stress reactions) and the adrenal cortex (which governs processes including the production of estrogen and androgen, the male sex hormone).

With regard to the kidneys, bladder and urinary system, it is difficult to bring about results simply by using essential oils. According to recent research, 'the diuretic effects of essential oils are virtually non-existent.'[11]

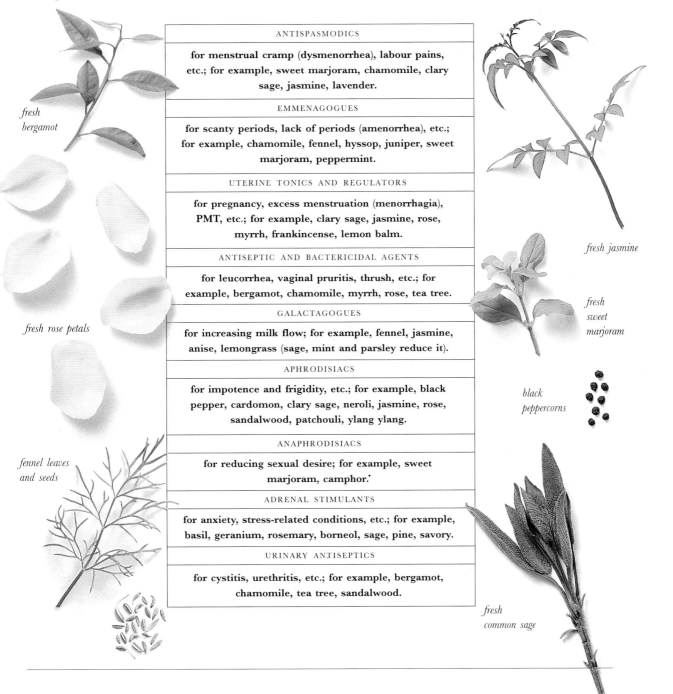

fresh bergamot

fresh rose petals

fennel leaves and seeds

ANTISPASMODICS

for menstrual cramp (dysmenorrhea), labour pains, etc.; for example, sweet marjoram, chamomile, clary sage, jasmine, lavender.

EMMENAGOGUES

for scanty periods, lack of periods (amenorrhea), etc.; for example, chamomile, fennel, hyssop, juniper, sweet marjoram, peppermint.

UTERINE TONICS AND REGULATORS

for pregnancy, excess menstruation (menorrhagia), PMT, etc.; for example, clary sage, jasmine, rose, myrrh, frankincense, lemon balm.

ANTISEPTIC AND BACTERICIDAL AGENTS

for leucorrhea, vaginal pruritis, thrush, etc.; for example, bergamot, chamomile, myrrh, rose, tea tree.

GALACTAGOGUES

for increasing milk flow; for example, fennel, jasmine, anise, lemongrass (sage, mint and parsley reduce it).

APHRODISIACS

for impotence and frigidity, etc.; for example, black pepper, cardomon, clary sage, neroli, jasmine, rose, sandalwood, patchouli, ylang ylang.

ANAPHRODISIACS

for reducing sexual desire; for example, sweet marjoram, camphor.

ADRENAL STIMULANTS

for anxiety, stress-related conditions, etc.; for example, basil, geranium, rosemary, borneol, sage, pine, savory.

URINARY ANTISEPTICS

for cystitis, urethritis, etc.; for example, bergamot, chamomile, tea tree, sandalwood.

fresh jasmine

fresh sweet marjoram

black peppercorns

fresh common sage

The Immune System

Virtually all essential oils have bactericidal properties, and by promoting the production of white blood cells, they can help prevent and treat infectious illness. It is these properties that gave aromatic herbs and oils such high repute with regard to infections such as malaria and typhoid in the tropics and epidemics of plague in the Middle Ages. 'People who use essential oils all the time . . . mostly have a high level of resistance to illness, catching fewer colds, etc., than average and recovering quickly if they do.'[12]

BACTERICIDAL AND ANTIVIRAL AGENTS (PROPHYLACTICS)
for protection against colds, flu, etc.; for example, tea tree, cajeput, niaouli, basil, lavender, eucalyptus, bergamot, camphor, clove, rosemary.
FEBRIFUGE AGENTS
for reducing fever and temperature, etc.; for example, angelica, basil, peppermint, thyme, sage, lemon, eucalyptus, tea tree.
SUDORIFICS AND DIAPHORETICS
for promoting sweating, eliminating toxins, etc.; for example, rosemary, thyme, hyssop, chamomile.

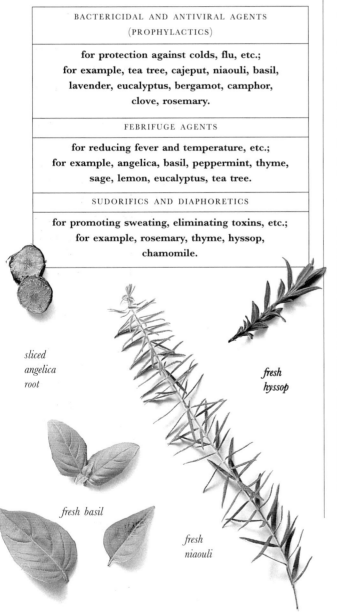

sliced angelica root

fresh hyssop

fresh basil

fresh niaouli

The Nervous System

Recent research shows that the properties of many oils correspond to the traditionally held views: chamomile, bergamot, sandalwood, lavender and sweet marjoram were found to have a sedative effect on the central nervous system; jasmine, peppermint, basil, clove and ylang ylang were found to have a stimulating effect. Neroli was found to be stimulating, and lemon to be sedating, contrary to popular belief. Some oils are known to be 'adaptogens', that is, they have a balancing or normalizing effect on the systems of the body: geranium and rosewood were either sedative or stimulating according to each situation and individual.

Words like 'relaxing' and 'uplifting' often have more to do with odour description and emotional response rather than physiological effect – although the two are related. Consequently, oils such as bergamot, lemon balm and lemon can be sedating to the nervous system but reviving to the 'spirit'. But oils such as jasmine, ylang ylang and neroli can be nerve stimulants yet soothing and relaxing on a more subtle emotional level.

SEDATIVES
for nervous tensions, stress, insomnia, etc.; for example, chamomile, bergamot, sandalwood, lavender, sweet marjoram, lemon balm, hops, valerian, lemon.
STIMULANTS
for convalescence, lack of strength, nervous fatigue, etc.; for example, basil, jasmine, peppermint, ylang ylang, neroli, angelica, rosemary.
NERVE TONICS (NERVINES)
for strengthening the nervous system as a whole; for example, chamomile, clary sage, juniper, lavender, marjoram, rosemary.

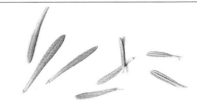

true lavender leaves

The Mind

This area is perhaps the most discussed and yet least understood area of activity regarding essential oils. There is no doubt that throughout history aromatic oils have been used for their power to influence the emotions and states of mind: this is the basis for their employment as incense for religious and ritualistic purposes. It is already known that two olfactory nerve tracts run right into the limbic system (the part of the brain concerned with memory and motion), which means that scents can evoke an immediate and powerful response that defies rational analysis.

Recent research at Warwick University, England, and Toho University, Japan, has aimed to put these traditionally held beliefs and applications into a scientific context. They came up with two types of reactions to odours which they called a 'hard-wired' response or a 'soft-wired' response: the first type is ingrained from before birth and is purely instinctual; the second is learned or acquired later on.

But to what extent is the effect of a particular oil dependent upon its chemical or physiological make-up, and to what extent does it rely upon a belief or an association? In dealing with the psychological or emotional responses to the scent of a particular oil, this kind of classification becomes much more difficult: surely here it is more appropriate to consider the temperament of each individual within a given context, rather than predict a set reaction.

At the Psychology of Perfumery Conference 1991, it was generally agreed that 'while pharmacological effects may be very similar from one person to another, psychological effects are bound to be different'.[13] The effect of an odour on a human being was dependent on a variety of factors, which include:

1. *how the odour was applied*
2. *how much was applied*
3. *the circumstances in which it was applied*
4. *the person to whom it was applied (age, sex, personality type)*

'We must, therefore, seek odoriferous substances which present affinities with the human being we intend to treat, those which will compensate for his deficiencies and those which will make his faculties blossom. It was by searching for this remedy that we encountered the individual prescription (IP), which on all points represents the identity of the individual.'[14]

5. *what mood they were in to start with*
6. *what previous associations they may have with the odour*
7. *anosmia, or inability to smell (certain scents).*

When we begin to consider individual needs, essential oils start to demonstrate the versatility of their nature. The rose is a good example: a flower associated with beauty, love, and spiritual depth in folklore and religious texts, but also with a long tradition of usage for physical conditions such as skin problems, regulating the female cycle, promoting the circulation, purifying the blood and as a heart tonic. When we smell the fragrance of the rose, it carries all these rich associations with it, affecting our mind and body simultaneously, as the effect is moulded by personal experience.

'The general trend of modern thought is strictly dualistic; psychic and somatic happenings are treated as mutually exclusive rather than inclusive.'[15] Trying to disentangle spirit from matter leads nowhere; as David Hoffmann says, 'Mind and Matter are mutually enfolded projections of a higher reality which is neither matter nor consciousness.'[16]

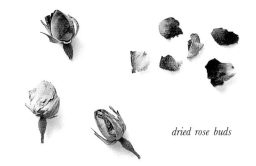

dried rose buds

4. HOW TO USE ESSENTIAL OILS AT HOME
Methods of Application

Essential oils can be used simply and effectively at home in a variety of ways, both for their scent and for their cosmetic and medicinal qualities. They can be used as perfumes and to revive pot pourris; they can be added to the bath and used to make individual beauty preparations. They can also be employed in the treatment of minor first aid cases and to help prevent and relieve many common complaints such as headaches, colds, period pains and aching muscles (see Therapeutic Index p. 55). They should always be stored in a cool place in dark bottles to protect them from photo-oxidation with as little contact with air as possible, and kept out of reach of children.

Some home uses for many essential oils can be found in the main body of the book, but the following pages suggest a few possible uses for individual essences and show some of the ways in which they can be applied.

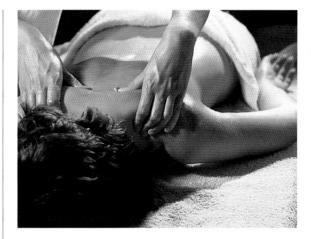

An aromatherapy massage being given across the shoulders, aimed at relieving tension.

A few drops of essential oil added to dried flower petals and seed-heads makes a fragrant pot-pourri.

WARNING

Essential oils should not be used at home to treat serious medical or psychological problems.

Massage

This is the method favoured by professional aromatherapists, who usually carry out a full body massage. Specific essential oils are chosen to suit the condition and temperament of the patient, and blend with a base oil, such as sweet almond oil or grapeseed oil.

The essential oil content in a blend should usually be between 1 per cent and 3 per cent depending on the type of disorder. Physical ailments like rheumatism or indigestion demand a stronger concentration than the more emotional or nervous conditions. Twenty drops of essential oils is roughly equivalent to one millilitre ($\frac{1}{4}$ tsp), so to make a blend it is possible to use the following proportions:

ESSENTIAL OIL	BASE OIL
20 to 60 drops	*100ml (3½ fl oz)*
7 to 25 drops	*25ml (1 fl oz)*
3 to 5 drops	*5ml (1 tsp)*

Massage is a relaxing and nourishing experience in itself, not least because of the unspoken communication based on touch, but it also ensures that the oils are effectively absorbed through the skin and into the bloodstream. For general well-being it is beneficial to practise self-massage on specific areas of the body, especially on the feet and hands. It is also useful to rub those particular parts of the body that are causing discomfort; for example, peppermint (in dilution) can be rubbed on the stomach in a clockwise direction to ease indigestion; marjoram can help to relax the neck and shoulders if they are stiff.

Skin Oils and Lotions

The essential oils are prepared much as they would be for a massage, except that the base oil should include the more nourishing oils such as jojoba, avocado or apricot kernel oil. The emphasis is on treating the skin itself and dealing with particular problems. A gentle circular movement of the fingers is often enough for the oils to be absorbed; it is important not to drag on the skin, especially in the delicate areas of the neck and around the eyes. Rose and neroli are good for dry or mature complexions; geranium, bergamot and lemon can help combat acne and greasy skin.

STEP-BY-STEP MASSAGE

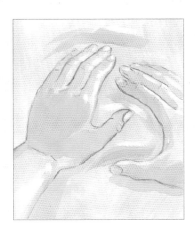
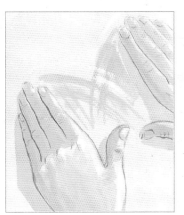

1. EFFLEURAGE
(STROKING MOVEMENTS)
*Soothing and comforting, this
is the most useful type of
movement for aromatherapy
massage. Always make sure
the hands (and oil) are slightly
warm before beginning. Then,
using slow, rhythmic strokes
and keeping the hands in
contact with the body, rub the
oil well into the skin. Excellent
for large areas such as the
back, but also good for delicate
regions, including the face.*

2. PETRISSAGE
(KNEADING MOVEMENTS)
*This technique is particularly
beneficial for areas of muscular
tightness or tension, such as the
shoulders or neck. It is usually
done with both hands, using
a firm but gentle kneading
movement, squeezing and rolling
the surface skin together with
the layers beneath. It helps
ease knotted muscles, stimulates
the circulation and also aids
the breakdown of fatty and
fibrous tissue.*

3. FRICTION
(CIRCULAR MOVEMENTS)
*Warming and stimulating,
friction is especially beneficial
for areas of cold, numbness
and poor circulation. Using the
flat palms of the hands, rub
the skin firmly in a vigorous,
circular movement so that
the surface of the skin moves
together with the pressure of the
hand. A light circular movement
(clockwise) may also be used
gently on the stomach area
to aid digestion.*

A few drops of essential oil can also be mixed into a bland cream or lotion, or added to a basic face mask, which might include oatmeal, honey or clay together with the pulp of various fruits. In some conditions, such as cold sores (herpes) and athlete's foot, it is better to use an alcohol-based lotion rather than an oil or cream. This can be made by adding 6 drops of essential oil to 5ml (1tsp) of iso-propyl alcohol or vodka. This mixture can be further diluted in a litre (1¾ pt) of boiled and cooled water for treating open cuts or sores, such as those caused by chickenpox or genital herpes.

Hot and Cold Compresses

This is a very effective way of using essential oils to relieve pain and reduce inflammation. A hot compress can be made by filling a bowl with very hot water, then adding 4 or 5 drops

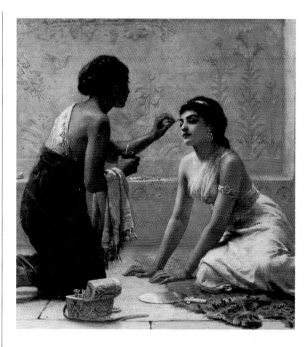

Since ancient times perfumes and cosmetics have been used to enhance appearance.

DIFFERENT SKIN TYPES

1. OILY SKIN
Oily skin is prone to congestion, often resulting in spots and blackheads. Hygiene is very important, but care should be taken not to disturb the natural pH balance of the skin. Astringent and antiseptic essential oils are indicated, such as tea tree, bergamot or geranium. Generally, the base oils should be kept light so that they can be absorbed easily – apricot kernel, peach kernel or jojoba are ideal.

2. DRY SKIN
A dry complexion becomes wrinkled more easily than oily skin, especially if it is exposed to too much sun or the effects of central heating. It therefore needs to be moisturized thoroughly and regularly. Dry skin also often tends to be sensitive, so mild essences such as sandalwood, chamomile and rose are indicated. Rich, nourishing base oils, like hazelnut, avocado and evening primrose oil, are valuable hydrating agents.

3. MATURE SKIN
Ageing is inevitable, but essential oils can do much to slow down the effects. The regular use of facial treatments containing cytophylactic oils (those that stimulate new cell growth and prevent wrinkles) is vital – such oils include lavender, neroli and frankincense. Base oils rich in Vitamin E, notably borage and wheatgerm, are especially beneficial for promoting cell regeneration; rosehip seed oil is also indicated.

true lavender

geranium

rose petals

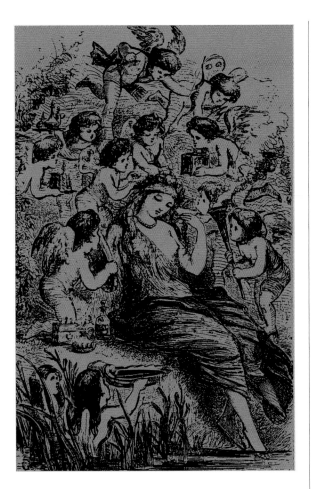

'Here first she bathes and round her body pours
Soft oils of fragrance, and ambrosial showers.'
HOMER, ILIAD, XIV

of essential oil. Dip a folded piece of cotton cloth, cotton wool or a face cloth into the bowl, squeeze out the excess water and place the cloth on the affected area until it has cooled to blood heat, then repeat. Hot compresses are particularly useful for backache, rheumatism and arthritis, abscesses, earache and toothache.

Cold compresses are made in a similar way, using ice cold rather than hot water. This type of compress is useful for headaches (apply to forehead or back of neck), sprains, strains and other hot, swollen conditions.

Hair Care

The hair can also be enhanced by the use of a few drops of essential oils in the final hair rinse or added straight to a mild shampoo.

An alcohol-based scalp rub can be made by adding 5ml (1tsp) of an essential oil to 100ml (3½ fl oz) of vodka – this method can be used to condition the hair or to get rid of unwanted parasites such as lice and fleas. An excellent conditioning treatment for different types of hair can be made by adding about 3 per cent (or 60 drops) of an essential oil to a nourishing base oil such as olive oil with jojoba or sweet almond oil, massaging it into the scalp, then wrapping the hair in warm towels for an hour to two. Oils such as rosemary, West Indian bay and chamomile all help to condition and encourage healthy hair growth; lavender can be used to repel lice and fleas; while bergamot and tea tree can help to control dandruff.

Flower Waters

It is possible to make toilet or flower water at home by adding about 20 to 30 drops of essential oil to a 100ml (3½ fl oz) bottle of spring or de-ionized water, leaving if for a few days in the dark and then filtering it using a coffee filter paper. Although essential oils do not dissolve in water, they do impart their scent to it as well as their properties.

This method can be very helpful in the prevention and treatment of skin conditions such as acne, dermatitis and eczema, and to tone and cleanse the complexion. Almost any oil can be used, but the more traditional ones include rose, orange blossom, lavender and petitgrain; or blended flower waters can be made to suit specific complexions.

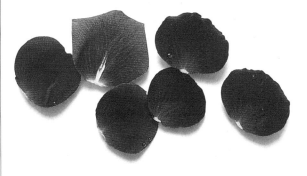

Rose oil, extracted from the petals, makes
a pleasant flower water or bath essence.

Baths

One of the easiest and most pleasurable ways of using essential oils is to add 5 to 10 drops of oil to the bath water when the tub is full. Aromatic bathing has traditionally been used as an enjoyable and sensual experience, especially by the Romans, but also to treat a wide range of complaints, including irritating skin conditions, muscular aches and pains, rheumatism and arthritis. An essence such as ylang ylang can be enjoyed as a euphoric aromatic experience in itself; chamomile or lavender can help to relieve stress-related complaints such as anxiety or insomnia; rosemary or pine can help soothe aching limbs. Take care to avoid those oils that may be irritating to the skin.

Vaporization

A delightful way to scent a room, free of the dust or smoke that can be caused by incense, is to use an oil burner or aromatic diffuser. Alternatively, a few drops of oil can be placed on a light bulb ring or added to a small bowl of water placed on a radiator. Specific oils can be chosen to create different atmospheres: frankincense and cedarwood have been used traditionally in a ritual context to create a peaceful and relaxed mood. Vaporized oils such as citronella or lemongrass also provide an excellent way of keeping insects at bay or clearing the air of unwanted smells such as cigarette smoke.

At one time, the leaves of juniper and rosemary were burned to help control

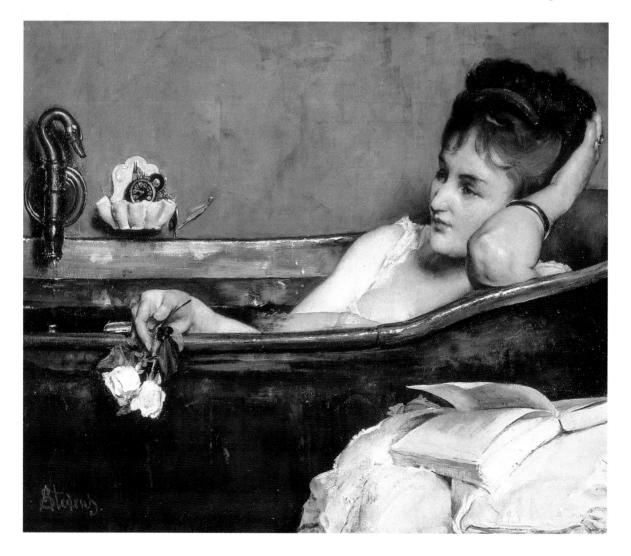

'The Bath' by Alfred George Stevens. Aromatic bathing has long been a popular way of enjoying essential oils.

epidemics and purify the air. Such coils can help keep the environment free of germs and inhibit the development of infections like the common cold or flu. An oil such as myrtle or eucalyptus can be used in the bedroom at night to relieve breathing difficulties or children's coughs. A few drops may also be put on the pillow or onto a handkerchief for use throughout the day.

Always ensure that the oil burner is in a safe place and out of reach of children or pets.

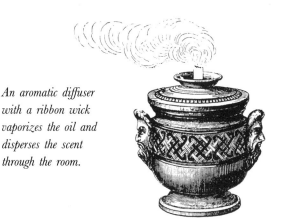

An aromatic diffuser with a ribbon wick vaporizes the oil and disperses the scent through the room.

Douche

This can be useful to help combat common genito-urinary infections such as thrush, cystitis or pruritis. In the case of candida or thrush, add between 5 and 10 drops of tea tree to a litre (1¾ pt) of warm water and shake well. This mixture can either be used in a sitz bath, bidet or put into an enema/douche pot, which can be bought from some pharmacies. Certain oils such as lavender and cypress can also aid the healing process after childbirth.

Neat Application

Generally speaking, essential oils are not applied to the skin in an undiluted form. However, there are some exceptions to the rule: lavender, for example, can be applied undiluted to burns, cuts and insect bites; tea tree to spots; and lemon to warts. Certain essential oils such as sandalwood, jasmine or rose make excellent perfumes, dabbed neat on the skin. Beware of those oils that are known to be phototoxic (discolour the skin

when exposed to direct sunlight) such as bergamot; irritants such as red thyme; or skin sensitizers such as cinnamon bark.

It can also be interesting to make an individual fragrance by blending a selection of oils – see Chapter 5. Certain oils may also be used to perfume linen and clothes or rejuvenate pot pourris.

Internal Use

Due to the high concentration of essential oils (and the high toxicity of a handful of essences), it is not recommended that they be taken at home in this manner. The International Federation of Aromatherapists also advises against this method of application. However, since essential oils are readily absorbed through the skin, they can affect the internal organs and systems of the body by external use.

In a condition such as arthritis, for example, which indicates a build up of toxins in the joints, the use of dietary measures and herbal remedies can be greatly enhanced by the external application of oils such as juniper and white birch.

STEAM INHALATION

This method is especially suited to sinus, throat and chest infections. Add about 5 drops of an oil such as peppermint or thyme to a bowl of hot water, cover the head and bowl with a towel and breathe deeply for a minute – then repeat. Sitting in a steaming hot bath is another way of inhaling a certain amount of essential oil, but obviously it is not as concentrated. This type of application can also act as a kind of facial sauna: oils like lemon or tea tree can help to unclog the pores and clear the complexion.

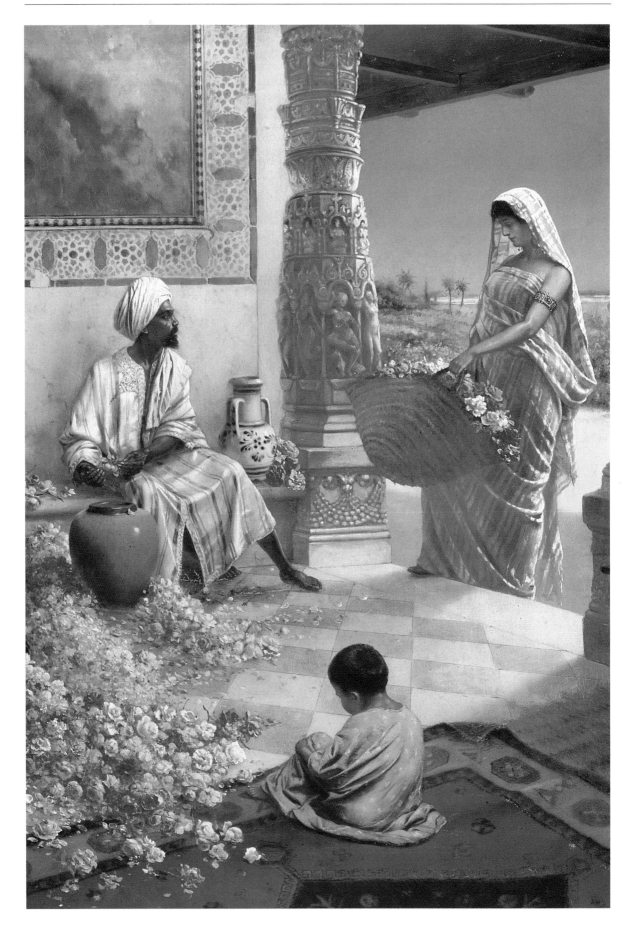

'The Perfume Makers' (detail)
by Rudolph Ernst, 1854–1920

5. CREATIVE BLENDING
Therapeutic and Esthetic Properties

Essential oils are blended principally for two reasons: for their medical effects or to create a perfume. When we are using pure essential oils, these are not two different categories but rather two ends of a scale. At one end of the scale we are dealing with the therapeutic action on a purely physical condition such as backache – at the other end, with an emotional or esthetic response to a particular odour. But, of course, the individual who is suffering from lumbago also has a psychic or emotional disposition of which they may or may not be aware, which will naturally respond in a more subtle way to a particular blend of oils. Similarly, when we create a personal perfume that expresses the unique personality of an individual through fragrance, it has a generally remedial effect on the person as a whole.

Therefore, when we are blending oils, even if it is principally for their medicinal properties, it is worth keeping the fragrance in mind. It is more pleasing to use a remedy that smells attractive to the individual concerned. Some scents can be quite incompatible – a predominantly floral blend, for example, would be unacceptable to most men. How to choose the oils and combine them is a matter of personal choice, but there are some useful guidelines to keep in mind.

Correct proportions are important in blending essential oils, as are individual perfume preferences.

Correct Proportions
For therapeutic purposes, essential oils are usually diluted before being applied to the skin. To make a massage or body oil the essential oil or oils should first be mixed with a light base oil such as grapeseed or sweet almond oil. (See also Chapter 4. How to Use Essential Oils at Home.) Other oils that could be used for the base include sunflower, hazelnut, safflower, peanut, soya or corn oil – mineral oils, however, are best avoided. The more nourishing and generally thicker oils, which include jojoba, avocado, peach or apricot kernel, borage, olive, sesame, and some infused oils such as calendula or St John's wort, can also be included (up to about 10 per cent) in the treatment of specific conditions. If a little wheatgerm oil (about 5 per cent) is added to the blend, this will help to preserve it.

The essential oil content in a blend should usually be between 1 and 3 per cent depending on the type of disorder; physical ailments demand a stronger concentration than the more emotional or nervous conditions. Some oils, such as the high-quality florals, have a more diffusive power than most other essences – this means that a very small percentage is all that is needed to have a powerful effect.

bitter almonds

Synergies

The proportions of each essential oil in a blend can also be vital to the effectiveness of the remedy as a whole (many aromatherapy books contain exact recipes for specific disorders). Some oils blended together have a mutually enhancing effect upon one another, so that the whole is greater than the sum of the parts: for example, the anti-inflammatory action of chamomile is supported by being mixed with lavender. When the blended oils are working harmoniously together, then the combination is called a 'synergy'. 'In order to create a good synergy, you must take into account not only the symptom to be treated but also the underlying cause of the disorder, the biological terrain, and the psychological or emotional factors involved.'[17]

This is very much the conclusion that Madame Maury reached when she prescribed an IP (or Individual Prescription) for her patients, in which the blended essences were matched not only to their physical requirements but also to their circumstances and temperament.

In general, oils of the same botanical family blend well together. Also those that share common constituents usually mix well, such as the camphoraceous oils containing a good percentage of cineol, which includes all the members of the Myrtacease group (eucalyptus, tea tree, cajeput, myrtle, etc.) but also many herbs including spike lavender, rosemary and Spanish sage. Most floral fragrances blend well together, as do the woods, balsams, citrus oils and spices, etc. Rosewood and linaloe combine well together, although they belong to different botanical families, since they both contain a high proportion of linalol and linalyl acetate.

Some oils such as rose, jasmine, oakmoss and lavender seem to enhance just about any blend, and can be found (mainly in an adulterated form) among the ingredients of most commercial perfumes – 'no perfume without rose'.

Some combinations, on the other hand, have an inhibiting power over one another. It is a matter of getting to know the 'character' of each essential oil and trusting the intuition.

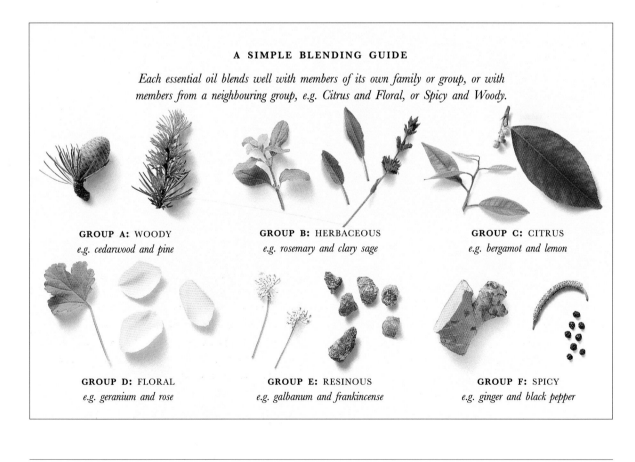

A SIMPLE BLENDING GUIDE

Each essential oil blends well with members of its own family or group, or with members from a neighbouring group, e.g. Citrus and Floral, or Spicy and Woody.

GROUP A: WOODY
e.g. cedarwood and pine

GROUP B: HERBACEOUS
e.g. rosemary and clary sage

GROUP C: CITRUS
e.g. bergamot and lemon

GROUP D: FLORAL
e.g. geranium and rose

GROUP E: RESINOUS
e.g. galbanum and frankincense

GROUP F: SPICY
e.g. ginger and black pepper

Fragrant Harmony

In the nineteenth century, a Frenchman called Piesse instigated a new approach to perfumery work by classifying odours according to the notes in a musical scale. He transposed the idea of musical harmony into the realm of fragrances where the corresponding notes to each scent formed perfectly balanced chords or harmonics when they were combined together.

The purist vision of Piesse has long since been discarded but continues to provide inspiration in perfumery work today since the oils are still divided into 'top', 'middle' and 'base' notes.

The *top note* has a fresh, light quality that is immediately apparent, due to the fast evaporation rate.

The *middle note* is the heart of the fragrance, which usually forms the bulk of the blend, whose scent emerges some time after the first impression.

The *base note* is a rich, heavy scent that emerges slowly and lingers. It also acts as a fixative to stop the lighter oils from dispersing too quickly.

Ylang ylang is said to be a well-balanced perfume oil in its own right. It could be described as having a very powerful sweet floral top note, a creamy-rich middle note, and a soft floral, slightly spicy base note.

For the sake of simplicity, each essential oil is also classified in this way according to its dominant character – although there are many different opinions on the matter!

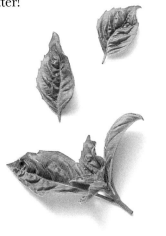

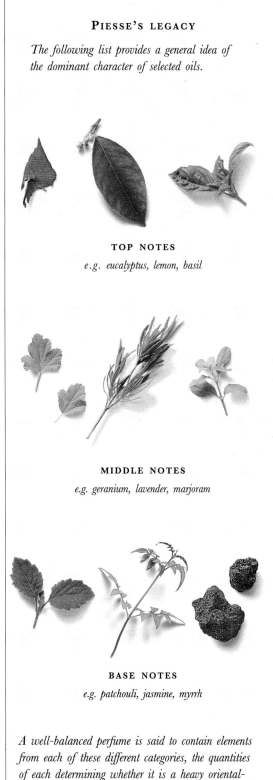

PIESSE'S LEGACY

The following list provides a general idea of the dominant character of selected oils.

TOP NOTES

e.g. eucalyptus, lemon, basil

MIDDLE NOTES

e.g. geranium, lavender, marjoram

BASE NOTES

e.g. patchouli, jasmine, myrrh

A well-balanced perfume is said to contain elements from each of these different categories, the quantities of each determining whether it is a heavy oriental-type scent or a light floral aroma. Although this theory is used primarily in fragrance work, the same principles can also be applied to aromatherapy and personalized remedies.

Personal Perfumes

Creating a perfume or an individual fragrance is like painting a picture or making a meal: it needs the correct balance of colours or flavours, neither too sparse nor too crowded; it also generally has a theme. A perfume should have a focus around which other fragrances unite. For example, if we want to create an oriental fragrance or a heart-warming, elevating type of blend, then woody or musky oils and balsams will play a central role. The exotic perfume 'Shalimar' by Guerlain contains a predominance of such oils, containing among its ingredients Peru balsam, benzoin, opopanax, vanilla, patchouli, rose, jasmine, orris and vetiver as well as rosewood, lemon, bergamot and mandarin.

The overall character of a perfume also benefits from unusual or diverse combinations which can help to give personality to an otherwise 'flat' fragrance. A floral fragrance with a hint of spice such as clove or cinnamon can add depth and interest, but the percentage of such additions is critical because they can easily upset the balance.

A skilled perfumier can identify some 30,000 different odours, but to begin with it is best to become familiar with a few common oils and develop from there. By initially

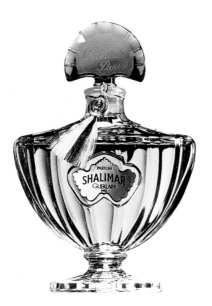

'Shalimar' by Guerlain contains a combination of woody or musky oils and balsams.

HOME PERFUMES

Home perfumes need not be complex: rose and benzoin (base notes), rosewood (middle note) and bergamot (top note) would together make a pleasing combination with an uplifting, warming quality. Rosewood is an oil that can be used to round off sharp edges, as well as providing a good bridge between citrus and floral or woody-balsamic notes.

keeping to a maximum of three or four oils per blend it is possible to keep in touch with their individual scents and qualities, and then slowly build up a personal vocabulary of odours.

Most commercial perfumes are diluted in alcohol; a typical eau de cologne contains no more than 3–5 per cent aromatic material, usually synthetic. Home-made perfumes are best made up simply of pure essences, which last longer and may be used neat on the skin or in the bath, etc.

Personal experimentation is the only way to really find out what works, for the unique quality of essential oils is that they possess an array of therapeutic possibilities complemented by a vast spectrum of fragrances that can be mixed in endless combinations! In the words of John Steele:

Creative blending is an aesthetic alchemical process... learning to 'listen through the nose'. To listen is to be receptive, to be empty. Every drop shifts the orchestrations of olfactory vibrations, the 'song of the blend'. A blend is not made at once, rather it evolves, it organically grows and interacts not only within the essential oils, but also with the blender.[18]

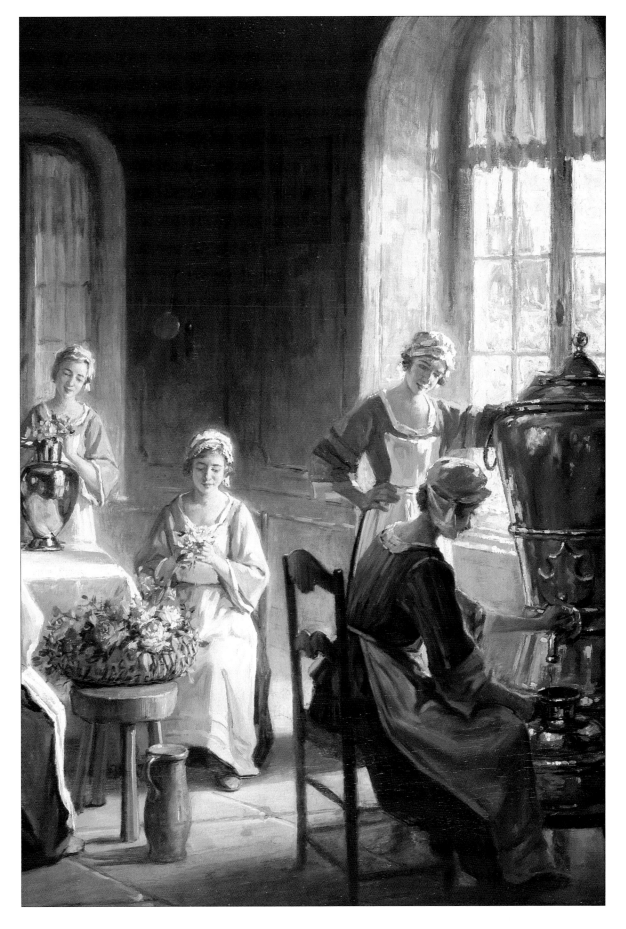

'The Perfume Makers' by Albert Sorkau presents
an idealized portrait of the perfume industry in
the early years of the twentieth century.

6. A GUIDE TO AROMATIC MATERIALS
Habitat

Over thirty families of plants, with some ninety species, represent the main oil-producing group. The majority of spices (allspice, cardomon, clove, nutmeg, ginger, etc.) originate in tropical countries; conversely, the majority of herbs grow in temperate climates (bay, cumin, dill, marjoram, fennel, lavender, rosemary, thyme, etc.). The same plant grown in a different region and under different conditions can produce essential oils of widely diverse characteristics, which are known as 'chemotypes'.

Common thyme *(Thymus vulgaris)*, for example, produces several chemotypes depending on the conditions of its growth and dominant constituent, notably the citral or linalol types, the thyuanol type, and the thymol or carvacrol type. It is therefore important not only to know the botanical name of the plant from which an oil has been produced but also its place of origin and main constituents.

One of the principal ways of defining the qualities of a particular oil and checking its purity is to ascertain the specific blend of components and to look at its chemical character.

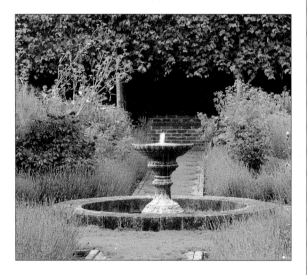

A herb garden with a chamomile path.
Most herbs grow in temperate climates, whereas
the majority of spices come from tropical climates.

Chemistry

In general, essential oils consist of chemical compounds that have hydrogen, carbon and oxygen as their building blocks. These can be subdivided into two groups: the hydrocarbons, which are made up almost exclusively of terpenes (monoterpenes, sesquiterpenes and diterpenes); and the oxygenated compounds, mainly esters, aldehydes, ketones, alcohols, phenols and oxides; acids, lactones, sulphur and nitrogen compounds are sometimes also present.

fresh longleaf pine

ALDEHYDES

Citral, citronellal and neural are important aldehydes found notably in lemon-scented oils such as melissa, lemongrass, lemon verbena, lemon-scented eucalyptus, citronella, etc. Aldehydes in general have a sedative effect; citral has been found to have specifically antiseptic properties. Other aldehydes include benzaldehyde, cinnamic aldehyde, cuminic aldehyde and perillaldehyde.

fresh pennyroyal

PHENOLS

These tend to have a bactericidal and strongly stimulating effect, but can be skin irritants. Common phenols include eugenol (found in clove and West Indian bay), thymol (found in thyme), carvacrol (found in oregano and savory); methyl eugenol, methyl chavicol, anethole, safrole, myristicin and apiol among others.

fresh summer savory

grapefruit peel, leaf and young fruit

TERPENES

Common terpene hydro-carbons include limonene (antiviral, found in **90 per cent** of citrus oils) and pinene (antiseptic, found in high proportions in pine and turpentine oils); also camphene, cadinene, caryophyllene, cedrene, dipentene, phellandrene, terpinene, sabinene, and myrcene among others. Some sesquiterpenes, such as chamazulene and farnesol (both found in chamomile oil), have been the object of great interest recently because of their outstanding anti-inflammatory and bactericidal properties.

ESTERS

Probably the most widespread group found in essential oils, which includes linalyl acetate (found in bergamot, clary sage and lavender), and geranyl acetate (found in sweet marjoram). They are characteristically fungicidal and sedative, often having a fruity aroma. Other esters include bornyl acetate, eugenyl acetate and lavendulyl acetate.

fresh spike lavender

KETONES

Some of the most common toxic constituents are ketones, such as thujone found in mugwort, tansy, sage and wormwood; and pulegone found in pennyroyal and buchu – but this does not mean that all ketones are dangerous. Non-toxic ketones include jasmone found in jasmine, and fenchone in fennel oil. Generally considered to ease congestion and aid the flow of mucus, ketones are often found in plants that are used for upper respiratory complaints, such as hyssop and sage. Other ketones include camphor, carvone, methone, methyl nonyl ketone and pinocamphone.

ALCOHOLS

One of the most useful groups of compounds, tending to have good antiseptic and antiviral properties with an uplifting quality; they are also generally non-toxic. Some of the most common terpene alcohols include linalol (found in rosewood, linaloe and lavender), citronellol (found in rose, lemon, eucalyptus and geranium) and geraniol (found in palmarosa); also borneol, methol, nerol, terpineol, farnesol, vetiverol, benzyl alcohol and cedrol among others.

fresh bay leaves

OXIDES

By far the most important oxide is cineol (or eucalyptol), which stands virtually in a class of its own. It has an expectorant effect, well known as the principal constituent of eucalyptus oil. It is also found in a wide range of other oils, especially those of a camphoraceous nature such as rosemary, bay laurel, tea tree and cajeput. Other oxides include linalol oxide found in hyssop (decumbent variety), ascaridol, bisabolol oxide and bisabolone oxide.

fresh rosemary

Methods of Extraction

In general, the term 'essential oil' is rather loosely applied to all aromatic products or extracts that are derived from natural sources. This is not strictly accurate, since many fragrance products, although they are used by the perfumery industry, are only partially composed of essential oils, and they are actually obtained by different methods of production.

For example, the terms 'concrete', 'absolute' and 'resinoid' should be used to denote a type of product which contains a mixture of volatile and non-volatile components, such as wax or resin. But in the market-place, rose maroc 'absolute' is often referred to simply as rose 'oil', while the vanilla-scented benzoin is commonly thought to be an essential oil, although it is actually a 'resinoid' or 'resin absolute'.

It is, however, always the essential oil content in a given product that accounts for its aromatic quality.

Some plant materials, especially flowers, are subject to deterioration and should be processed as soon as possible after harvesting; others, including seeds and roots, are either stored or transported for extraction, often to Europe or America. The method of extraction which is employed depends on the quality of the material which is being used, and also on the type of aromatic product that is required.

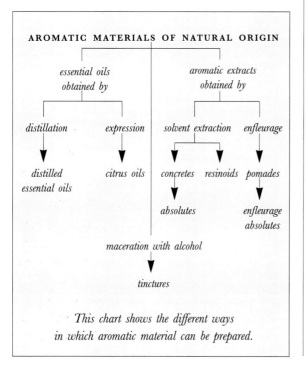

AROMATIC MATERIALS OF NATURAL ORIGIN

essential oils
obtained by

aromatic extracts
obtained by

distillation   expression   solvent extraction   enfleurage

distilled
essential oils   citrus oils   concretes   resinoids   pomades

absolutes   enfleurage
absolutes

maceration with alcohol

tinctures

*This chart shows the different ways
in which aromatic material can be prepared.*

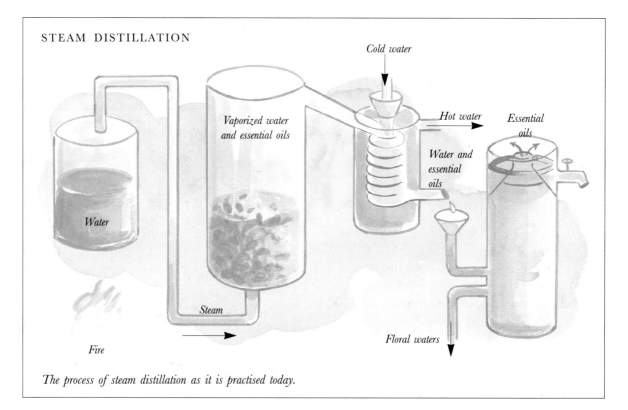

STEAM DISTILLATION

Cold water

Vaporized water
and essential oils

Hot water

Essential
oils

Water and
essential
oils

Water

Steam

Fire

Floral waters

The process of steam distillation as it is practised today.

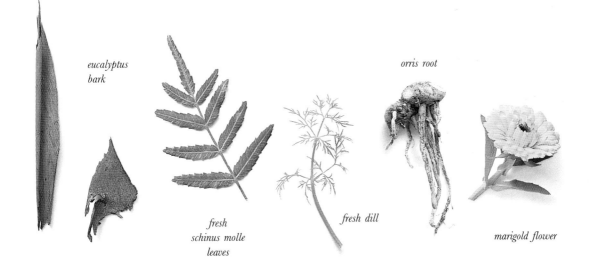

eucalyptus bark

orris root

fresh schinus molle leaves

fresh dill

marigold flower

Concretes are derived from five main sources: bark, leaves, herbs, roots and flowers.

Essential Oils

An essential oil is extracted from the plant material by two main methods: by simple expression or pressure, as is the case with most of the citrus oils including lemon and bergamot, or by steam, water or dry distillation. The majority of oils such as lavender, myrrh, sandalwood and cinnamon are produced by steam distillation. This process isolates only the volatile and water-insoluble parts of a plant – many other (often valuable) constituents, such as tannins, mucilage and bitters, are consequently excluded from the essential oil. Sometimes the resulting oil is redistilled or rectified to get rid of any remaining non-volatile matter; some essential oils are redistilled at different temperatures to obtain certain constituents and exclude others – as with camphor, which is split into three fractions, white, yellow and brown.

Essential oils are usually liquid, but can also be solid (orris) or semi-solid according to temperature (rose). They dissolve in pure alcohol, fats and oils but not in water and, unlike the so-called fixed plant oils (such as olive oil), they evaporate when exposed to air, leaving no oily residue behind.

Concretes

Concretes are prepared almost exclusively from raw materials of vegetable origin, such as the bark, flower, leaf, herb or root. The aromatic plant material is subjected to extraction by hydrocarbon-type solvents, rather than distillation or expression. This is necessary when the essential oil is adversely affected by hot water and steam, as is the case with jasmine; it also produces a more true-to-nature fragrance. Some plants, such as lavender and clary sage, are either steam distilled to produce an essential oil or used to produce a concrete by solvent extraction. The remaining residue is usually solid and of a waxy non-crystalline consistency.

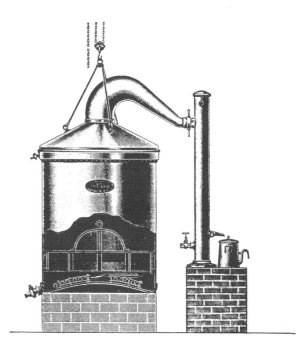

This type of apparatus, with a false bottom, was used for the distillation of plants such as peppermint and lavender.

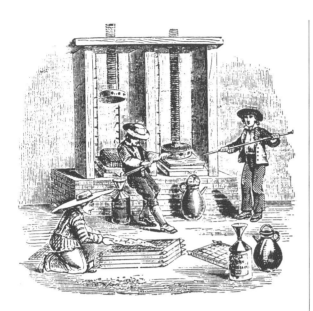

A traditional method of extracting oil involved subjecting the plants to extreme pressure.

Most concretes contain about 50 per cent wax, 50 per cent volatile oil, such as jasmine; in rare cases, as with ylang ylang, the concrete is liquid and contains about 80 per cent essential, 20 per cent wax. The advantage of concretes is that they are more stable and concentrated than pure essential oils.

Resinoids

Resinoids are prepared from natural resinous material by extraction with a hydrocarbon solvent, such as petroleum or hexane. In contradistinction to concretes, the resinoids are prepared from dead organic material, whereas concretes are derived from previously live tissue. Typical resinous materials are balsams (Peru balsam or benzoin), resins (mastic and amber), oleoresins (copaiba balsam and turpentine) and oleo gum resins (frankincense and myrrh). Resinoids can be viscous liquids, semi-solid or solid, but are usually homogeneous masses of non-crystalline character. Occasionally the alcohol-soluble fraction of a resinoid is called an absolute.

Some resinous materials like frankincense and myrrh are used either to make an essential oil by steam distillation or a resin absolute by alcohol extraction directly from the crude oleo gum resin. Benzoin, on the other hand, is insufficiently volatile to produce an essential oil by distillation: liquid benzoin is often simply a benzoin resinoid dissolved in a suitable solvent or plasticizing diluent.

Like concretes, resinoids are employed in perfumery as fixatives to prolong the effect of the fragrance.

Absolutes

An absolute is obtained from the concrete by a second process of solvent extraction, using pure alcohol (ethanol) in which the unwanted wax is only slightly soluble. An absolute is usually subjected to repeated treatment with alcohol; even so, as is the case with orange flower absolute, a small proportion of the wax remains. Absolutes can be further processed by molecular distillation, which removes every last trace of non-volatile matter. The alcohol is recovered by evaporation, which requires a gentle vacuum towards the end of the process. Some absolutes, however, will still retain traces of ethyl alcohol, at about 2 per cent or less, and these are not recommended for therapeutic work because of these remaining impurities.

Absolutes are usually highly concentrated viscous liquids, but they can in some cases be solid or semi-solid (clary sage absolute). In recent years, much research has been devoted to the extraction of essential oils and aromatic materials using liquid carbon dioxide; oils that are produced in this manner are of excellent odour quality and are entirely free of unwanted solvent residues or non-volatile matter.

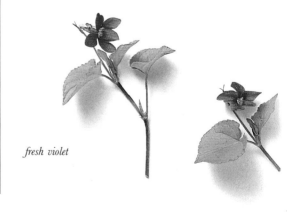

fresh violet

Pomades

True pomades are the products of a process known as enfleurage, which is virtually obsolete today.

This was once the principal method of obtaining aromatic materials from flowers that continued to produce perfume long after they were cut. A glass plate was covered in a thin coating of specially prepared and odourless fat, called a chassis. The freshly cut flowers, such as jasmine, or tuberose, were individually laid in the fat which became saturated with their volatile oils. The chassis would be frequently renewed with fresh material throughout the harvest. Eventually the fragrance-saturated fat, known as pomade, would be treated by extraction with alcohol to produce the pure absolute or perfume.

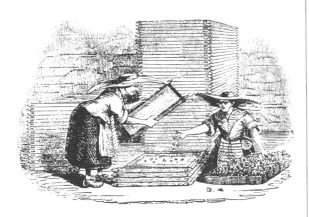

Enfleurage was a process of obtaining aromatic materials from cut flowers.

Natural versus 'Nature Identical'

Many perfumes or oils, once obtained from flowers such as carnations, gardenia and lilac, are nowadays produced almost entirely synthetically. In the pharmaceutical industry these chemically constructed products are called 'nature identical'. The perfumery and flavouring industries require continuity in their products and naturally occurring substances are always subject to change as the result of seasonal conditions. However, the so-called 'nature identical' products and the naturally occurring essential oils are of an

entirely different character, which is reflected in their relative costs – the synthetic types being much cheaper to produce than the genuine ones.

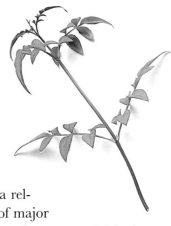

fresh jasmine

Many aromatic oils, such as lavender or geranium, contain a relatively small number of major constituents, several minor constituents and also a very large number of trace elements. To reconstruct such a complex combination of components including all the trace elements would be virtually impossible. Most 'nature identical' oils are said to be only about 96 per cent pure or accurate, yet it is the remaining 4 per cent, comprising the trace elements, that often really define a particular fragrance. Such is the case with galbanum oil where the pyrazines, present at rather less than 0.1 per cent, are responsible for the powerful green odour of the oil.

It is also the specific combination of constituents in a real essential oil, including the trace elements, which give it value therapeutically. The reason for this might be that these minute amounts of trace elements have a synergistic or controlling effect on the main ones. For example, there are over 300 different constituents in rose, some of which have not yet been identified, which is why synthetic rose oil is unconvincing. 'Nature identical' oils cannot be used therapeutically as substitutes for the naturally occurring aromatic materials, not only because the subtle balance of constituents is lost but also because they lack the vital 'life force' of oils of natural origin.

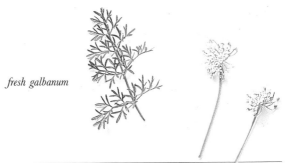

fresh galbanum

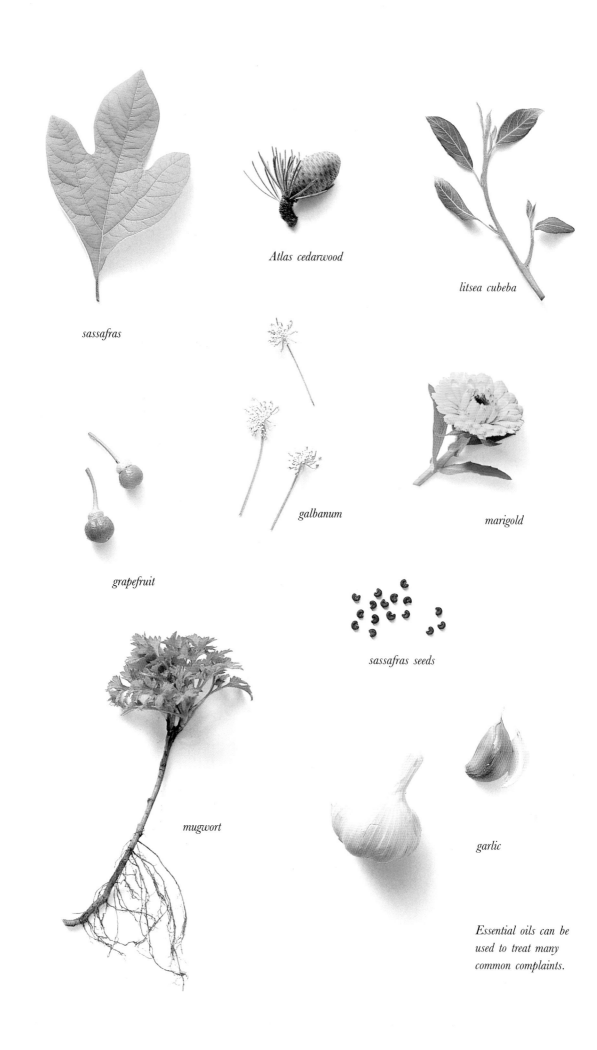

Atlas cedarwood

litsea cubeba

sassafras

galbanum

marigold

grapefruit

sassafras seeds

mugwort

garlic

Essential oils can be used to treat many common complaints.

Part II

THERAPEUTIC INDEX

Essential oils can be used to treat a wide range of common complaints, including those listed on the following pages. Special care must be taken regarding the use of oils that can cause irritation in concentration, and those oils known to be phototoxic, such as bergamot, lemon and orange. Before using a particular oil, the Safety Data information on the individual oils should be consulted, together with the general Safety Guidelines on pp. 26–7.

Many of the conditions mentioned here could benefit from combining an aromatherapy approach with other forms of treatment, such as dietary measures, exercise, herbal medicines, osteopathy or counselling, among others.

A guide to abbreviated terms of suggested application as outlined in the chapters 'How to Use Essential Oils at Home' (pp. 36–41) and 'Creative Blending' (pp. 43–7), is as follows:

B:	BATH	**I:**	INHALATION (STEAM)
C:	COMPRESS	**M:**	MASSAGE
D:	DOUCHE	**N:**	NEAT APPLICATION
F:	FLOWER WATER	**S:**	SKIN OIL/LOTION
H:	HAIR CARE	**V:**	VAPORIZATION

In the pages that follow common complaints are grouped according to different parts of the body: Skin Care; Circulation, Muscles and Joints; Respiratory System; Digestive System; Genito-urinary and Endocrine Systems; Immune System; Nervous System.

If, for example, you have been working long hours at a desk and have developed a painful cramp in your neck, you should turn to the section on Circulation, Muscles and Joints where you will find the heading 'Muscular Cramp and Stiffness'. Of the essential oils listed, those shown in italics are generally considered to be the most useful and/or readily available.

The choice of which oil to use depends on what is to hand, and on assessing the quality of each oil by consulting their entry in Part III of the book, where oils are listed in alphabetical order according to the Latin names of the plants from which they are derived. The Botanical Index at the back of the book (pp. 248–53) provides a useful cross-reference to both common and Latin plant names; the main entry for each oil is given there in bold type.

Skin Care

ACNE (M,S,F,B,I,N)

Bergamot, camphor (white), cananga, cedarwood (Atlas, Texas and Virginian), *chamomile (German and Roman)*, clove bud, galbanum, *geranium*, grapefruit, helichrysum, juniper, lavandin, *lavender (spike* and *true)*, *lemon*, lemongrass, lime, linaloe, litsea cubeba, mandarin, mint (peppermint and spearmint), myrtle, niaouli, *palmarosa*, patchouli, petitgrain, *rosemary*, rosewood, sage (clary and Spanish), sandalwood, *tea tree*, thyme, vetiver, violet, yarrow, ylang ylang.

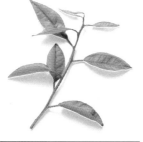

fresh bergamot

ALLERGIES (M,S,F,B,I)

Lemon balm, chamomile (German and *Roman)*, helichrysum, *true lavender*, spikenard.

ATHLETE'S FOOT (S)

Clove bud, eucalyptus, *lavender (spike* and *true)*, lemon, lemongrass, *myrrh*, patchouli, *tea tree*.

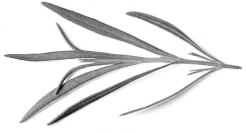

fresh spike lavender

BALDNESS AND HAIR CARE (S,H)

West Indian bay, white birch, cedarwood (Atlas, Texas and Virginian), *chamomile (German and Roman)*, grapefruit, juniper, patchouli, *rosemary*, sage (clary and Spanish), *yarrow*, ylang ylang.

BOILS, ABSCESSES AND BLISTERS (S,C,B)

Bergamot, chamomile (German and *Roman)*, eucalyptus blue gum, galbanum, helichrysum, lavandin, *lavender (spike* and *true)*, lemon, mastic, niaouli, clary sage, *tea tree*, thyme, turpentine.

BRUISES (S,C)

Arnica (cream), borneol, clove bud, *fennel*, geranium, *hyssop*, sweet marjoram, *lavender*, thyme.

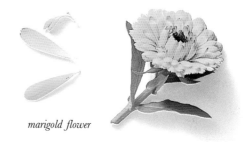

fresh lemon

BURNS (C,N)

Canadian balsam, chamomile (German and Roman), clove bud, eucalyptus blue gum, geranium, helichrysum, lavandin, *lavender (spike and true)*, marigold, niaouli, tea tree, yarrow.

marigold flower

CHAPPED AND CRACKED SKIN (S,F,B)

Peru balsam, *Tolu balsam, benzoin, myrrh, patchouli*, sandalwood.

CHILBLAINS (S,N)

Chamomile (German and Roman), *lemon*, lime, *sweet marjoram, black pepper.*

leaves and fruit peel of lime

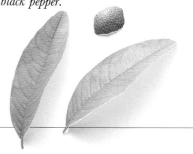

COLD SORES/HERPES (S)

Bergamot, eucalyptus blue gum, lemon, *tea tree*.

CONGESTED AND DULL SKIN (M,S,F,B,I)

Angelica, white birch, sweet fennel, *geranium*, *grapefruit*, lavandin, *lavender (spike and true)*, lemon, lime, mandarin, mint (peppermint and spearmint), myrtle, niaouli, orange (bitter and sweet), palmarosa, rose (cabbage and damask), *rosemary*, rosewood, ylang ylang.

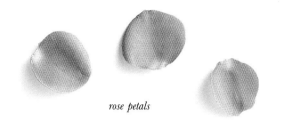

rose petals

CUTS/SORES (S,C)

Canadian balsam, benzoin, borneol, cabreuva, cade, *chamomile (German and Roman)*, clove bud, elemi, eucalyptus (blue gum, lemon and peppermint), galbanum, geranuium, helichrysum, hyssop, lavandin, *lavender (spike and true)*, lemon, lime, linaloe, *marigold*, mastic, myrrh, niaouli, Scotch pine, Spanish sage, Levant styrax, *tea tree*, thyme, turpentine, vetiver, *yarrow*.

fresh yarrow

DANDRUFF (S,H)

West Indian bay, cade, cedarwood (Atlas, Texas and Virginian), eucalyptus, *spike lavender*, lemon, patchouli, *rosemary*, sage (clary and Spanish), tea tree.

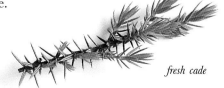

fresh cade

DERMATITIS (M,S,C,F,B)

White birch, cade, cananga, carrot seed, cedarwood (Atlas, Texas and Virginian), *chamomile (German and Roman)*, geranium, *helichrysum*, hops, hyssop, juniper, *true lavender*, linaloe, litsea cubeba, mint (peppermint and spearmint), *palmarosa*, patchouli, rosemary, sage (clary and Spanish), thyme.

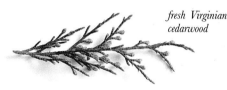

fresh Virginian cedarwood

DRY AND SENSITIVE SKIN (M,S,F,B)

Peru balsam, Tolu balsam, cassie, *chamomile (German and Roman)*, frankincense, *jasmine*, lavandin, lavender (spike and true), rosewood, *sandalwood*, violet.

fresh violet

ECZEMA (M,S,F,B)

Lemon balm, Peru balsam, Tolu balsam, *bergamot*, white birch, cade, carrot seed, cedarwood (Atlas, Texas and Virginian), *chamomile (German and Roman)*, geranium, *helichrysum*, hyssop, juniper, lavandin, *lavender (spike and true)*, marigold, myrrh, *patchouli, rose (cabbage and damask)*, rosemary, Spanish sage, thyme, violet, yarrow.

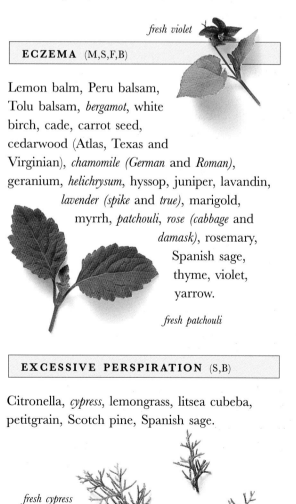

fresh patchouli

EXCESSIVE PERSPIRATION (S,B)

Citronella, *cypress*, lemongrass, litsea cubeba, petitgrain, Scotch pine, Spanish sage.

fresh cypress

Skin Care

GREASY OR OILY SKIN/SCALP (M,S,H,F,B)

West Indian bay, *bergamot*, cajeput, camphor (white), cananga, carrot seed, citronella, *cypress*, sweet fennel, *geranium*, jasmine, juniper, *lavender*, lemon, lemongrass, litsea cubeba, mandarin, marigold, mimosa, myrtle, niaouli, palmarosa, patchouli, petitgrain, rosemary, rosewood, *sandalwood*, clary sage, *tea tree*, thyme, vetiver, ylang ylang.

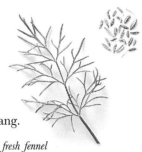

fresh fennel

HEMORRHOIDS/PILES (S,C,B)

Canadian balsam, copaiba balsam, coriander, cubeb, *cypress*, geranium, *juniper*, *myrrh*, myrtle, parsley, *yarrow*.

INSECT BITES (S,N)

Lemon balm, French basil, bergamot, cajeput, cananga, *chamomile (German* and *Roman)*, cinnamon leaf, blue gum eucalyptus, lavandin, *lavender (spike* and *true)*, lemon, marigold, niaouli, *tea tree*, thyme, ylang ylang.

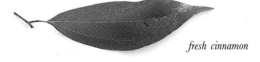

fresh cinnamon

INSECT REPELLENT (S,V)

Lemon balm, French basil, bergamot, borneol, camphor (white), *Virginian cedarwood*, *citronella*, clove bud, cypress, eucalyptus (blue gum and lemon-scented), geranium, *lavender*, lemongrass, litsea cubeba, mastic, patchouli, rosemary, turpentine.

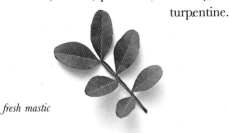

fresh mastic

IRRITATED AND INFLAMED SKIN (S,C,F,B)

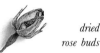

Angelica, benzoin, camphor (white), Atlas cedarwood, *chamomile (German* and *Roman)*, elemi, helichrysum, hyssop, jasmine, lavandin, *true lavender, marigold, myrrh, patchouli, rose (cabbage* and *damask)*, clary sage, spikenard, tea tree, yarrow.

dried rose buds

LICE (S,H)

Cinnamon leaf, blue gum eucalyptus, galbanum, geranium, lavandin, *spike lavender*, parsley, Scotch pine, rosemary, thyme, turpentine.

fresh common thyme

MOUTH AND GUM INFECTIONS/ULCERS (S,C)

Bergamot, cinnamon leaf, cypress, *sweet fennel*, lemon, mastic, *myrrh*, orange (bitter and sweet), sage (clary and Spanish), thyme.

PSORIASIS (M,S,F,B)

Angelica, bergamot, white birch, carrot seed, chamomile (German and Roman), *true lavender.*

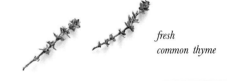

fresh bergamot

RASHES (M,S,C,F,B)

Peru balsam, *Tolu balsam*, carrot seed, *chamomile (German* and *Roman)*, hops, *true lavender, marigold,* sandalwood, spikenard, tea tree, yarrow.

RINGWORM (S,H)

Geranium, *spike lavender*, mastic, mint (peppermint and spearmint), *myrrh*, Levant styrax, *tea tree*, turpentine.

fresh spearmint

SCABIES (S)

Tolu balsam, bergamot, *cinnamon leaf*, lavandin, *lavender (spike* and *true)*, lemongrass, mastic, *mint (peppermint* and *spearmint)*, Scotch pine, rosemary, Levant styrax, thyme, turpentine.

SCARS AND STRETCH MARKS (M,S)

Cabreuva, elemi, *frankincense*, galbanum, *true lavender*, mandarin, *orange blossom*, palmarosa, patchouli, rosewood, *sandalwood*, spikenard, violet, yarrow.

true lavender leaves

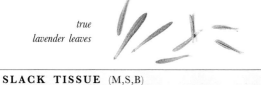

SLACK TISSUE (M,S,B)

Geranium, *grapefruit*, juniper, lemongrass, lime, mandarin, *sweet marjoram*, orange blossom, *black pepper*, petitgrain, rosemary, yarrow.

SPOTS (S,N)

Bergamot, cade, cajeput, camphor (white), lemon-eucalyptus, helichrysum, lavandin, *lavender (spike* and *true)*, *lemon*, lime, litsea cubeba, mandarin, niaouli, *tea tree*.

fresh mandarin leaves

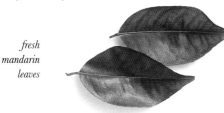

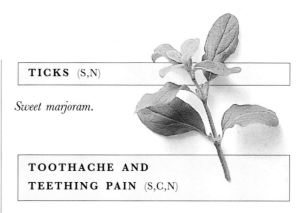

TICKS (S,N)

Sweet marjoram.

TOOTHACHE AND TEETHING PAIN (S,C,N)

Chamomile (German and *Roman)*, *clove bud*, mastic, mint (peppermint and spearmint), *myrrh*.

VARICOSE VEINS (S,C)

Cypress, lemon, lime, orange blossom, *yarrow.*

VERRUCAE (S,N)

Tagetes, tea tree.

leaves and peel of lime

WARTS AND CORNS (S,N)

Cinnamon leaf, *lemon*, lime, *tagetes*, tea tree.

WOUNDS (S,C,B)

Canadian balsam, Peru balsam, Tolu balsam, bergamot, cabreuva, *chamomile (German* and *Roman)*, clove bud, cypress, elemi, *eucalyptus (blue gum* and *lemon-scented)*, frankincense, galbanum, geranium, helichrysum, hyssop, juniper, lavandin, *lavender (spike* and *true)*, linaloe, marigold, mastic, *myrrh*, niaouli, patchouli, rosewood, Levant styrax, *tea tree*, turpentine, vetiver, *yarrow.*

WRINKLES AND MATURE SKIN (M,S,F,B)

Carrot seed, *elemi*, sweet fennel, *frankincense*, *galbanum*, geranium, jasmine, labdanum, true lavender, mandarin, mimosa, myrrh, *orange blossom*, palmarosa, patchouli, *rose (cabbage* and *damask)*, rosewood, clary sage, sandalwood, spikenard, ylang ylang.

Circulation, Muscles and Joints

ACCUMULATION OF TOXINS (M,S,B)

Angelica, white birch, carrot seed, celery seed, coriander, cumin, *sweet fennel, grapefruit, juniper,* lovage, parsley.

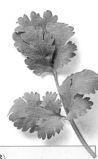

fresh coriander

ACHES AND PAINS (M,C,B)

Ambrette, star anise, aniseed, French basil, West Indian bay, cajeput, calamintha, camphor (white), *chamomile (German and Roman), coriander, eucalyptus (blue gum and peppermint),* silver fir, galbanum, *ginger,* helichrysum, lavandin, *lavender (spike and true),* lemongrass, *sweet marjoram,* mastic, mint (peppermint and spearmint), niaouli, nutmeg, *black pepper,* pine (longleaf and Scotch), *rosemary,* sage (clary and Spanish), hemlock spruce, thyme, turmeric, turpentine, vetiver.

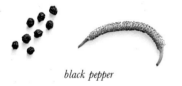

black pepper

ARTHRITIS (M,S,C,B)

Allspice, angelica, *benzoin,* white birch, cajeput, camphor (white), carrot seed, cedarwood (Atlas, Texas and Virginian), celery seed, *chamomile (German and Roman),* clove buds, coriander, *eucalyptus (blue gum and peppermint),* silver fir, *ginger,* guaiacwood, juniper, lemon, *sweet marjoram,* mastic, myrrh, nutmeg, parsley, *black pepper,* pine (longleaf and Scotch), *rosemary,* Spanish sage, thyme, turmeric, turpentine, vetiver, yarrow.

fresh turpentine

CELLULITIS (M,S,B)

White birch, cypress, *sweet fennel, geranium, grapefruit, juniper,* lemon, parsley, rosemary, thyme.

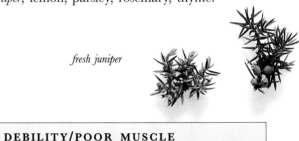

fresh juniper

DEBILITY/POOR MUSCLE TONE (M,S,B)

Allspice, ambrette, borneol, ginger, *grapefruit, sweet marjoram, black pepper,* pine (longleaf and Scotch), *rosemary,* Spanish sage.

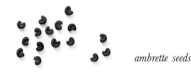

ambrette seeds

EDEMA AND WATER RETENTION (M,B)

Angelica, white birch, carrot seed, cypress, *sweet fennel,* geranium, *grapefruit,* juniper, *lovage,* mandarin, orange (bitter and sweet), rosemary, Spanish sage.

GOUT (M,S,B)

Angelica, French basil, *benzoin, carrot seed,* celery seed, coriander, guaiacwood, *juniper,* lovage, mastic, pine (longleaf and Scotch), *rosemary,* thyme, turpentine.

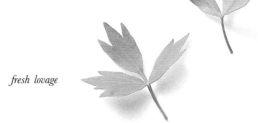

fresh lovage

HIGH BLOOD PRESSURE AND HYPERTENSION (M,B,V)

Lemon balm, cananga, *garlic*, *true lavender*, lemon, *sweet marjoram*, clary sage, *yarrow, ylang ylang.*

fresh lemon balm

MUSCULAR CRAMP AND STIFFNESS (M,C,B)

Allspice, ambrette, coriander, cypress, grapefruit, jasmine, lavandin, *lavender (spike* and *true)*, *sweet marjoram*, *black pepper*, pine (longleaf and Scotch), *rosemary*, thyme, vetiver.

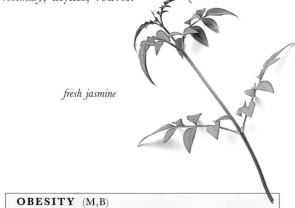

fresh jasmine

OBESITY (M,B)

White birch, sweet fennel, juniper, lemon, mandarin, orange (bitter and sweet).

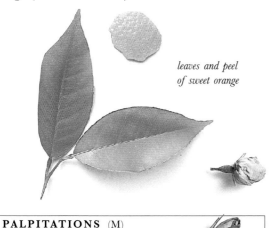

leaves and peel of sweet orange

PALPITATIONS (M)

Orange (bitter and sweet), orange blossom, rose (cabbage and damask), *ylang ylang.*

POOR CIRCULATION AND LOW BLOOD PRESSURE (M,B)

Ambrette, Peru balsam, West Indian bay, benzoin, white birch, borneol, cinnamon leaf, *coriander*, cumin, cypress, *blue gum eucalyptus*, galbanum, geranium, *ginger*, lemon, lemongrass, lovage, niaouli, nutmeg, orange blossom, *black pepper*, pine (longleaf and Scotch), rose (cabbage and damask), *rosemary, Spanish sage*, hemlock spruce, thyme, violet.

fresh hemlock spruce

RHEUMATISM (M,C,B)

Allspice, angelica, star anise, aniseed, Peru balsam, French basil, West Indian bay, benzoin, *white birch*, borneol, cajeput, calamintha, camphor (white), carrot seed, cedarwood (Atlas, Texas and Virginian), celery seed, *chamomile (German* and *Roman)*, cinnamon leaf, clove bud, coriander, *cypress, eucalyptus (blue gum* and *peppermint)*, sweet fennel, silver fir, galbanum, ginger, helichrysum, *juniper*, lavandin, *lavender (spike* and *true)*, lemon, lovage, *sweet marjoram*, mastic, niaouli, nutmeg, parsley, black pepper, *pine (longleaf* and *Scotch), rosemary*, Spanish sage, hemlock spruce, thyme, turmeric, turpentine, vetiver, violet, yarrow.

fresh Peru balsam

SPRAINS AND STRAINS (C)

West Indian bay, borneol, camphor (white), *chamomile (German* and *Roman)*, clove bud, eucalyptus (blue gum and peppermint), ginger, helichrysum, jasmine, lavandin, *lavender (spike* and *true)*, *sweet marjoram*, black pepper, pine (longleaf and Scotch), rosemary, thyme, turmeric, vetiver.

dried rose buds and petals

Respiratory System

ASTHMA (M,V,I)

Asafetida, lemon balm, Canadian balsam, Peru balsam, benzoin, cajeput, clove bud, costus, cypress, *elecampane*, eucalyptus (blue gum, lemon-scented and peppermint), *frankincense*, galbanum, helichrysum, hops, hyssop, lavandin, *lavender (spike* and *true)*, lemon, lime, sweet marjoram, *mint (peppermint* and *spearmint)*, myrrh, myrtle, niaouli, pine (longleaf and Scotch), rose (cabbage and damask), rosemary, *sage (clary* and *Spanish)*, hemlock spruce, tea tree, thyme.

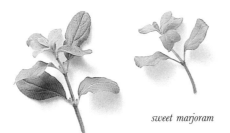

sweet marjoram

BRONCHITIS (M,V,I)

Angelica, star anise, aniseed, asafetida, lemon balm, *Canadian balsam*, copaiba balsam, Peru balsam, Tolu balsam, French basil, *benzoin, borneol*, cajeput, camphor (white), caraway, cascarilla bark, cedarwood (Atlas, Texas and Virginian), clove bud, costus, cubeb, cypress, *elecampane*, elemi, *eucalyptus (blue gum* and *peppermint)*, silver fir, *frankincense*, galbanum, helichrysum, hyssop, labdanum, lavandin, lavender (spike and true), lemon, *sweet marjoram*, mastic, mint (peppermint and spearmint), *myrrh, myrtle*, niaouli, orange (bitter and sweet), pine (longleaf and Scotch), rosemary, *sandalwood*, hemlock spruce, Levant styrax, tea tree, thyme, turpentine, violet.

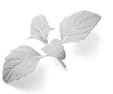

dried star anise

CATARRH (M,V,I)

Canadian balsam, Tolu balsam, cajeput, cedarwood (Atlas, Texas and Virginian), cubeb, elecampane, elemi, *eucalyptus (blue gum* and *peppermint)*, frankincense, galbanum, ginger,

hyssop, jasmine, lavandin, *lavender (spike* and *true)*, lemon, lime, mastic, *mint (peppermint* and *spearmint)*, myrrh, myrtle, niaouli, black pepper, *pine (longleaf* and *Scotch)*, sandalwood, Levant sytrax, *tea tree, thyme*, turpentine, violet.

fresh elecampane

CHILL (M,B)

fresh calamintha

Copaiba balsam, benzoin, cabreuva, calamintha, camphor (white), *cinnamon leaf, ginger*, grapefruit, orange (bitter and sweet), *black pepper*.

CHRONIC COUGHS (M,V,I)

Lemon balm, *Canadian balsam*, costus, cubeb, cypress, *elecampane*, elemi, *frankincense*, galbanum, helichrysum, hops, *hyssop*, jasmine, mint (peppermint and spearmint), myrrh, *myrtle*, sandalwood, Levant styrax.

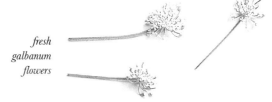

fresh galbanum flowers

COUGHS (M,V,I)

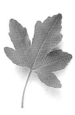

Levant styrax

Angelica, star anise, aniseed, *copaiba balsam, Peru balsam*, Tolu balsam, French basil, *benzoin*, borneol, cabreuva, cajeput, camphor (white), caraway, cascarilla bark, *Atlas cedarwood, eucalyptus (blue gum* and *peppermint)*, silver fir, ginger, *hyssop*, labdanum, *sweet marjoram*, myrrh, niaouli, black pepper, *pine (longleaf* and *Scotch)*, rose (cabbage and damask), rosemary, *sage (clary* and *Spanish)*, *hemlock spruce*, tea tree.

CROUP (M,I)

Tolu balsam.

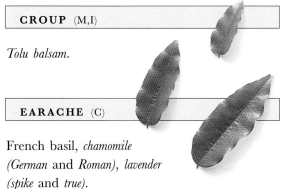

EARACHE (C)

French basil, *chamomile (German* and *Roman), lavender (spike* and *true).*

Tolu balsam

HALITOSIS/OFFENSIVE BREATH (S)

Bergamot, *cardomon, sweet fennel,* lavandin, lavender (spike and true), mint (peppermint and spearmint), *myrrh.*

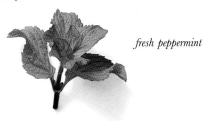

fresh peppermint

LARYNGITIS/HOARSENESS (I)

Tolu balsam, benzoin, caraway, cubeb, lemon-scented eucalyptus, frankincense, jasmine, lavandin, *lavender (spike* and *true),* myrrh, sage (clary and Spanish), *sandalwood, thyme.*

fresh Spanish sage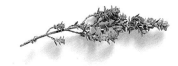

SINUSITIS (I)

French basil, cajeput, cubeb, *blue gum eucalyptus,* silver fir, ginger, labdanum, *peppermint,* niaouli, *pine (longleaf* and *Scotch), tea tree.*

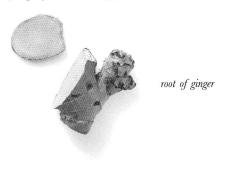

root of ginger

SORE THROAT AND THROAT INFECTIONS (V,I)

Canadian balsam, bergamot, cajeput, eucalyptus (blue gum, lemon-scented and peppermint), geranium, ginger, *hyssop,* lavandin, lavender (spike and true), myrrh, myrtle, niaouli, pine (longleaf and Scotch), *sage (clary* and *Spanish),* sandalwood, tea tree, *thyme,* violet.

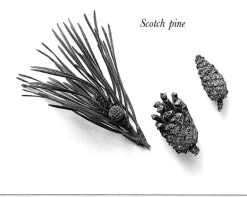

Scotch pine

TONSILLITIS (I)

Bay laurel, bergamot, geranium, hyssop, myrtle, sage (clary and Spanish), *thyme.*

fresh common thyme

WHOOPING COUGH (M,I)

Asafetida, helichrysum, hyssop, *true lavender,* mastic, *niaouli,* rosemary, sage (clary and Spanish), *tea tree,* turpentine.

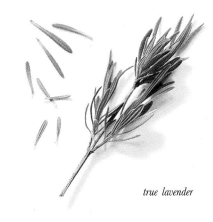

true lavender

Digestive System

COLIC (M)

Star anise, aniseed, lemon balm, calamintha, caraway, cardomon, carrot seed, *chamomile (German and Roman)*, clove bud, coriander, cumin, dill, sweet fennel, ginger, hyssop, lavandin, *lavender (spike and true)*, *sweet marjoram*, *mint (peppermint and spearmint)*, orange blossom, parsley, black pepper, rosemary, clary sage.

spike lavender

CONSTIPATION AND SLUGGISH DIGESTION (M,B)

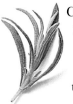

Cinnamon leaf, cubeb, sweet fennel, lovage, sweet marjoram, nutmeg, orange (bitter and sweet), palmarosa, *black pepper*, tarragon, turmeric, yarrow.

fresh tarragon

CRAMP/GASTRIC SPASM (M,C)

Allspice, star anise, aniseed, caraway, cardomon, cinnamon leaf, coriander, costus, cumin, galbanum, *ginger*, lavandin, *lavender (spike and true)*, lovage, mint (peppermint and spearmint), orange blossom, black pepper, *clary sage*, tarragon, lemon verbena, yarrow.

fresh yarrow

GRIPING PAINS (M)

Cardomon, dill, sweet fennel, parsley.

fresh parsley

HEARTBURN (M)

Cardomon, black pepper.

INDIGESTION/FLATULENCE (M)

Allspice, angelica, *star anise*, *aniseed*, lemon balm, French basil, bay laurel, calamintha, *caraway*,

cardomon, carrot seed, cascarilla bark, celery seed, *chamomile (German and Roman)*, cinnamon leaf, clove bud, coriander, costus, cubeb, cumin, dill, *sweet fennel*, galbanum, ginger, hops, hyssop, lavandin, *lavender (spike and true)*, lemongrass, linden, litsea cubeba, lovage, mandarin, *sweet marjoram, mint (peppermint and spearmint)*, myrrh, nutmeg, *orange (bitter and sweet)*, orange blossom, parsley, black pepper, petitgrain, rosemary, clary sage, tarragon, thyme, valerian, lemon verbena, yarrow.

fresh litsea cubeba

LIVER CONGESTION (M)

Carrot seed, celery seed, helichrysum, linden, rose (cabbage and damask), *rosemary*, Spanish sage, turmeric, lemon verbena.

fresh lemon verbena

LOSS OF APPETITE (M)

Bay laurel, *bergamot*, caraway, cardomon, ginger, myrrh, black pepper.

NAUSEA/VOMITING (M,V)

Allspice, lemon balm, French basil, cardomon, cascarilla bark, *chamomile (German and Roman)*, clove bud, coriander, *sweet fennel*, ginger, lavandin, *lavender (spike and true)*, *mint (peppermint and spearmint)*, nutmeg, black pepper, rose (cabbage and damask), rosewood, sandalwood.

fresh allspice

Genito-urinary/Endocrine Systems

AMENORRHEA/LACK OF MENSTRUATION (M,B)

French basil, bay laurel, carrot seed, celery seed, cinnamon leaf, dill, sweet fennel, hops, hyssop, juniper, lovage, *sweet marjoram, myrrh,* parsley, rose (cabbage and damask), *sage (clary* and *Spanish),* tarragon, yarrow.

fresh dill

CYSTITIS (C,B,D)

Canadian balsam, copaiba balsam, *bergamot,* cedarwood (Atlas, Texas and Virginian), celery seed, *chamomile (German* and *Roman),* cubeb, blue gum eucalyptus, frankincense, juniper, lavandin, *lavender (spike* and *true),* lovage, mastic, niaouli, parsley, Scotch pine, sandalwood, tea tree, thyme, turpentine, yarrow.

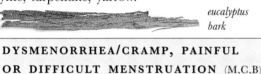

eucalyptus bark

DYSMENORRHEA/CRAMP, PAINFUL OR DIFFICULT MENSTRUATION (M,C,B)

Lemon balm, French basil, carrot seed, *chamomile (German* and *Roman),* cypress, frankincense, hops, jasmine, juniper, lavandin, *lavender (spike* and *true),* lovage, *sweet marjoram,* rose (cabbage and damask), rosemary, *sage (clary* and *Spanish),* tarragon, yarrow.

FRIGIDITY (M,S,B,V)

Cassie, cinnamon leaf, jasmine, nutmeg, *orange blossom,* parsley, *patchouli,* black pepper, *cabbage rose,* rosewood, clary sage, sandalwood, *ylang ylang.*

LABOUR PAIN AND CHILDBIRTH AID (M,C,B)

Cinnamon leaf, *jasmine, true lavender, nutmeg,* parsley, *rose (cabbage* and *damask), clary sage.*

LACK OF NURSING MILK (M)

Celery seed, dill, *sweet fennel,* hops.

LEUCORRHEA/WHITE DISCHARGE FROM THE VAGINA (B,D)

Bergamot, cedarwood (Atlas, Texas and Virginian), cinnamon leaf, cubeb, blue gum eucalyptus, frankincense, hyssop, lavandin, *lavender (spike* and *true),* sweet marjoram, mastic, *myrrh,* rosemary, clary sage, *sandalwood,* tea tree, turpentine.

MENOPAUSAL PROBLEMS (M,B,V)

Cypress, sweet fennel, *geranium,* jasmine, *rose (cabbage* and *damask).*

fresh cypress

MENORRHAGIA/EXCESSIVE MENSTRUATION (M,B)

Chamomile (German and Roman), *cypress, rose (cabbage* and *damask).*

PREMENSTRUAL TENSION/PMT (M,B,V)

Carrot seed, *chamomile (German* and *Roman),* geranium, *true lavender,* sweet marjoram, orange blossom, tarragon.

fresh true lavender

PRURITIS/ITCHING (D)

Bergamot, Atlas cedarwood, juniper, lavender, *myrrh, tea tree.*

fresh juniper

SEXUAL OVERACTIVITY (M,B)

Hops, *sweet marjoram.*

fresh sweet marjoram

THRUSH/CANDIDA (B,D)

Bergamot, geranium, myrrh, *tea tree.*

URETHRITIS (B,D)

Bergamot, cubeb, mastic, *tea tree,* turpentine.

Immune System

CHICKENPOX (C,S,B)

Bergamot, chamomile (German and Roman), eucalyptus (blue gum and lemon-scented), *true lavender*, tea tree.

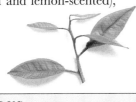

fresh bergamot

COLDS/FLU (M,B,V,I)

Angelica, star anise, aniseed, copaiba balsam, Peru balsam, French basil, bay laurel, West Indian bay, bergamot, *borneol*, cabreuva, cajeput, camphor (white), caraway, cinnamon leaf, citronella, clove bud, coriander, *eucalyptus (blue gum, lemon-scented and peppermint)*, silver fir, frankincense, ginger, grapefruit, helichrysum, juniper, lemon, lime, sweet marjoram, mastic, mint (peppermint and spearmint), myrtle, *niaouli*, orange (bitter and sweet), *pine (longleaf and Scotch)*, rosemary, rosewood, *Spanish sage*, hemlock spruce, *tea tree, thyme*, turpentine, yarrow.

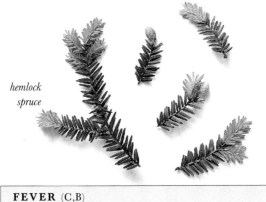

hemlock spruce

FEVER (C,B)

French basil, bergamot, borneol, camphor (white), *eucalyptus (blue gum, lemon-scented and peppermint)*, silver fir, ginger, helichrysum, juniper, lemon, lemongrass, lime, *mint (peppermint and spearmint)*, myrtle, niaouli, *rosemary*, rosewood, Spanish sage, hemlock spruce, *tea tree*, thyme, *yarrow*.

fresh niaouli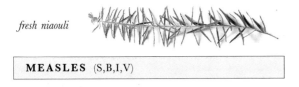

MEASLES (S,B,I,V)

Bergamot, *blue gum eucalyptus*, lavender (spike and true), *tea tree*.

Nervous System

ANXIETY (M,B,V)

Ambrette, *lemon balm*, French basil, *bergamot*, cananga, *frankincense*, hyssop, *jasmine*, juniper, *true lavender*, mimosa, orange blossom, hemlock spruce, Levant styrax, lemon verbena, *ylang ylang*.

Levant styrax

DEPRESSION (M,B,V)

Allspice, ambrette, lemon balm, Canadian balsam, French basil, *bergamot*, cassie, grapefruit, helichrysum, *jasmine, true lavender, orange blossom, rose (cabbage and damask)*, clary sage, *sandalwood*, hemlock spruce, vetiver, *ylang ylang*.

dried rose buds

HEADACHE (M,C,V)

Chamomile (German and Roman), citronella, cumin, eucalyptus (blue gum and peppermint), grapefruit, hops, lavandin, *lavender (spike and true)*, lemongrass, linden, sweet marjoram, *mint (peppermint and spearmint)*, rose (cabbage and damask), rosemary, rosewood, sage (clary and Spanish), thyme, violet.

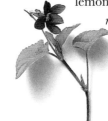

fresh violet

INSOMNIA (M,B,V)

Lemon balm, French basil, calamintha, *chamomile (German and Roman), hops, true lavender, linden*, mandarin, sweet marjoram, *orange blossom*, petitgrain, rose (cabbage and damask), sandalwood, thyme, *valerian*, lemon verbena, vetiver, violet, yarrow, ylang ylang.

MIGRAINE (C)

Angelica, lemon balm, French basil, chamomile (German and Roman), citronella, coriander, *true lavender*, linden, sweet marjoram, mint (peppermint and spearmint), clary sage, valerian, yarrow.

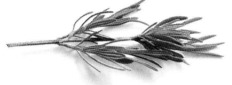

fresh true lavender

NERVOUS EXHAUSTION OR FATIGUE/DEBILITY (M,B,V)

Allspice, *angelica*, asafetida, *French basil*, *borneol*, cardomon, cassie, cinnamon leaf, citronella, coriander, costus, cumin, elemi, eucalyptus (blue gum and peppermint), ginger, grapefruit, helichrysum, hyacinth, hyssop, *jasmine*, lavandin, spike lavender, lemongrass, *mint (peppermint and spearmint)*, nutmeg, palmarosa, patchouli, petitgrain, Scotch pine, *rosemary*, *sage (clary and Spanish)*, thyme, *vetiver*, violet, ylang ylang.

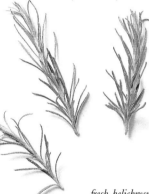

fresh helichrysum

NERVOUS TENSION AND STRESS (M,B,V)

Allspice, ambrette, angelica, asafetida, *lemon balm*, Canadian balsam, copaiba balsam, Peru balsam, French basil, *benzoin*, *bergamot*, borneol, calamintha, cananga, cardomon, cassie, *cedarwood (Atlas, Texas and Virginian)*, chamomile (German and Roman), cinnamon leaf, costus, cypress, elemi, *frankincense*, galbanum, geranium, helichrysum, *hops*, hyacinth, hyssop, *jasmine*, juniper, *true lavender*, lemongrass, linaloe, *linden*, mandarin, *sweet marjoram*, mimosa, mint (peppermint and

spearmint), orange (bitter and sweet), *orange blossom*, palmarosa, *patchouli*, petitgrain, Scotch pine, *rose (cabbage and damask)*, rosemary, rosewood, *clary sage*, *sandalwood*, hemlock spruce, thyme, valerian, lemon verbena, *vetiver*, violet, yarrow, *ylang ylang*.

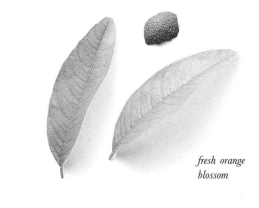

fresh linden

NEURALGIA/SCIATICA (M,B)

Allspice, West Indian bay, borneol, celery seed, *chamomile (German and Roman)*, citronella, coriander, eucalyptus (blue gum and peppermint), geranium, helichrysum, hops, *spike lavender*, *sweet marjoram*, mastic, mint (peppermint and spearmint), nutmeg, pine (longleaf and Scotch), *rosemary*, turpentine.

fresh spearmint

SHOCK (M,B,V)

Lemon balm, lavandin, lavender (spike and true), *orange blossom*.

fresh orange blossom

VERTIGO (V,I)

Lemon balm, lavandin, *lavender (spike and true)*, mint (peppermint and spearmint), violet.

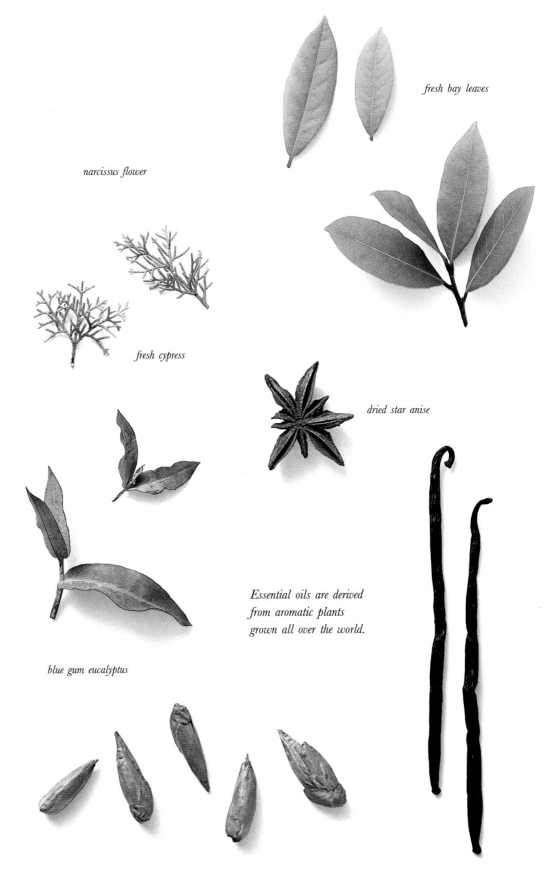

fresh bay leaves

narcissus flower

fresh cypress

dried star anise

blue gum eucalyptus

Essential oils are derived
from aromatic plants
grown all over the world.

Canadian balsam

vanilla pods

Part III

THE OILS

Part III is a systematic survey of 165 essential oils, shown in alphabetical order according to the Latin name of the plants from which they are derived. The oils covered in the following pages are all produced commercially, although some are little-known or in scarce demand. A number of the oils have been designated as unsuitable for therapeutic use, but have been included in this section for two reasons. First, to present a comprehensive picture of all the essential oils that are readily available, and second, to inform the reader about the possible dangers of such oils. Less common essential oils, such as blackcurrant (which is used mainly by the food industry), do not appear in this section, but are included in the Botanical Classification section under their common family name, in this case 'Grossulariaceae'.

Aromatic plants are found all over the world and essential oil production is an international industry, of which the 'aromatherapy market' plays a small but rapidly expanding part. Each year, more information is made available regarding the precise composition of individual essential oils, and each season the 'distribution' or place of cultivation of each plant is subject to change and development, due to political, climatic or economic influences. Demand for tea tree oil, for example, has led to new plantations being developed in California in recent years. Areas that are less subject to change are those such as the general description of the plant (illustrated in each case) and its herbal use or folk tradition. Detailed information on each essence also includes a botanical classification; methods of extraction; odour and colour characteristics; principal constituents; safety data; home and commercial uses.

Abelmoschus moschatus

Ambrette seed

FAMILY: MALVACEAE **SYNONYMS:** *HIBISCUS ABELMOSCHUS*, MUSK SEED, EGYPTIAN ALCEE, TARGET-LEAVED HIBISCUS, MUSKMALLOW

Herbal/Folk Tradition

Generally used as a stimulant and to ease indigestion, cramp and nervous dyspepsia. In Chinese medicine it is used to treat headache; in Egypt the seeds are used to sweeten the breath and are made into an emulsion with milk to be used for itch. The Arabs use the seed to mix with coffee. Widely used as a domestic spice in the East.

An evergreen shrub about 1.5m (5ft) high, bearing large single yellow flowers with purple centres. The capsules, in the form of five-cornered pyramids, contain greyish-brown kidney-shaped seeds that have a musky odour.

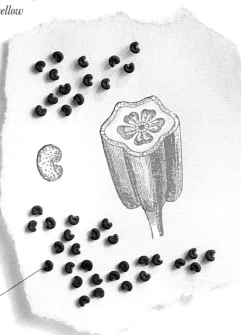

kidney-shaped
ambrette seed

AROMATHERAPY/ HOME USE

Circulation, Muscles and Joints: *Cramp, fatigue, muscular aches and pains, poor circulation.*
Nervous System: *Anxiety, depression, nervous tension and stress-related conditions.*

OTHER USES

Employed by the cosmetic and perfumery industries in oriental-type scents and for the adulteration of musk; also used as a musk substitute. Used for flavouring alcoholic and soft drinks as well as some foodstuffs, especially confectionery.

DISTRIBUTION

Indigenous to India; widely cultivated in tropical countries including Indonesia, Africa, Egypt, China, Madagascar, and the West Indies. Distillation of the oil is generally carried out in Europe and the USA.

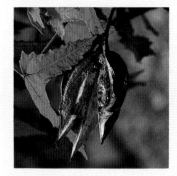

Abelmoschus moschatus

OTHER SPECIES

A variety, H. esculentus, is grown largely in Istanbul as a demulcent. Another variety is also found in Martinique, the seeds of which have a more delicate scent.

EXTRACTION
Essential oil by steam distillation of the seeds. Liquid ambrette seed oil should be allowed to age for several months before it is used. A concrete and absolute are also produced by solvent extraction.

CHARACTERISTICS
A pale yellowy-red liquid with a rich, sweet floral-musky odour, very tenacious. It blends well

with rose, orange blossom, sandalwood, clary sage, cypress, patchouli, oriental and 'sophisticated' bases.

ACTIONS
Antispasmodic, aphrodisiac, carminative, nervine, stimulant, stomachic.

PRINCIPAL CONSTITUENTS
Ambrettolide, ambrettolic acid, palmitic acid and farnesol.

Abies alba

Silver fir needle

FAMILY: PINACEAE SYNONYMS: *A. PECTINATA*, WHITESPRUCE, EUROPEAN SILVER FIR, EDELTANNE, WEISSTANNE, TEMPLIN (CONE OIL), STRASBURG OR VOSGES TURPENTINE (OIL), FIR NEEDLE (OIL)

Herbal/Folk Tradition

It is highly esteemed in Europe for its medicinal virtues and its fragrant scent. It is used mainly for respiratory complaints, fever, muscular and rheumatic pain.

A relatively small coniferous tree, with a regular pyramidal shape and a silvery white bark, grown chiefly for timber and as Christmas trees.

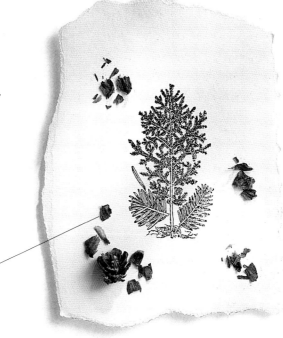

silver fir cone

EXTRACTION
Essential oil by steam distillation from the 1. needles and young twigs, and 2. fir cones, broken up pieces (templin oil).

CHARACTERISTICS
**1. A colourless or pale yellow liquid of pleasing, rich, sweet-balsamic odour.
2. Similar to the needle oil, but with a more orange-like fragrance. It blends well with galbanum, labdanum, lavender, rosemary, lemon, pine and marjoram.**

ACTIONS
Analgesic, antiseptic (pulmonary), antitussive, deodorant, expectorant, rubefacient, stimulant, tonic.

PRINCIPAL CONSTITUENTS
1. Santene, pinene, limonene, bornyl acetate, lauraldehyde among others. 2. Pinene, limonene, borneol, bornyl acetate, among others.

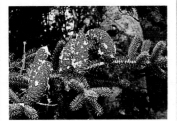

Abies alba

AROMATHERAPY/ HOME USE

Circulation, Muscles and Joints: *Arthritis, muscular aches and pains, rheumatism.*
Respiratory System: *Bronchitis, coughs, sinusitis, etc. Immune System: Colds, fever, flu.*

OTHER USES

Employed as an ingredient in some cough and cold remedies and rheumatic treatments. Used as a fragrance component in deodorants, room sprays, disinfectants, bath preparations, soaps and perfumes.

DISTRIBUTION

Native to North European mountainous regions; cultivated mainly in Switzerland, Poland, Germany, France, Austria and especially former Yugoslavia.

OTHER SPECIES

Oils that are distilled from the twigs and needles of various members of the coniferous families, Abies, Larix, Picea, Pinus *and* Tsuga *are all commonly called fir needle oil – it is therefore important to know the specific botanical name. There are many other members of the fir or* Abies *family, notably the Canadian balsam (*A. balsamea*) and the Siberian fir (*A. sibirica*), the most popular fir needle oil in Europe and the USA because of its fine fragrance. Others include the Japanese fir needle oil from* A. mayriana *or* A. sachalinensis. *See also entries in spruce, pines and the Botanical Classification section.*

Abies balsamea

Canadian balsam

SAFETY DATA *Generally non-toxic, non-irritant, non-sensitizing*

FAMILY: PINACEAE **SYNONYMS:** *A. BALSAMIFERA, PINUS BALSAAMEA,* BALSAM FIR, BALSAM TREE, AMERICAN SILVER FIR, BALM OF GILEAD FIR, CANADA TURPENTINE (OIL)

Herbal/Folk Tradition

The oleoresin is used extensively by Native Americans for ritual purposes and as an external treatment for burns, sores, cuts and to relieve heart and chest pains. It is also used internally for coughs.

A tall, graceful evergreen tree up to 20m (65ft) high, with a tapering trunk and numerous branches giving the tree an overall shape of a perfect cone. It forms blisters of oleoresin (the so-called balsam) on the trunk and branches, produced from special vesicles beneath the bark. The tree does not produce a 'true' balsam, since it does not contain benzoic or cinnamic acid in its esters; it is really an oleoresin, being a mixture of resin and essential oil.

dried
Canadian
balsam

EXTRACTION

1. The oleoresin is collected by puncturing vesicles in the bark.
2. An essential oil is produced by steam distillation from the oleoresin, known as Canada balsam or Canada turpentine. (An essential oil is also produced by steam distillation from the leaf or needles, known as fir needle oil.)

CHARACTERISTICS

1. The oleoresin is a thick pale yellow or green honey-like mass, which dries to crystal clear varnish, with a fresh sweet-balsamic, almost fruity odour. 2. A colourless mobile liquid with a sweet, soft-balsamic, pine-like scent. It blends well with pine, cedarwood, cypress, sandalwood, juniper, benzoin and other balsams.

ACTIONS

Antiseptic (genito-urinary, pulmonary), antitussive, astringent, cicatrizant, diuretic, expectorant, purgative, regulatory, sedative (nerve), tonic, vulnerary.

PRINCIPAL CONSTITUENTS

Consists almost entirely of monoterpenes, pinene, phellandrene, esters and alcohols.

AROMATHERAPY/HOME USE

Skin Care: *Burns, cuts, hemorrhoids, wounds.*
Respiratory System: *Asthma, bronchitis, catarrh, chronic coughs, sore throat.*
Genito-urinary System: *Cystitis, genito-urinary infections.*
Nervous System: *Depression, nervous tension, stress-related conditions – described as 'appeasing, sedative, elevating, grounding, opening'.[1]
'In large doses it is purgative and may cause nausea.' [2]*

OTHER USES

The oil from the oleoresin is used in certain ointments and creams as an antiseptic and treatment for hemorrhoids. Used in dentistry as an ingredient in root canal sealers. Also used as a fixative or fragrance component in soaps, detergents, cosmetics and perfumes. There is some low-level use in food products, alcoholic and soft drinks. The oleoresin is used as a medium in microscopy and as a cement in glassware.

DISTRIBUTION

Native to North America, particularly Quebec, Nova Scotia and Maine.

OTHER SPECIES

The hemlock spruce (Tsuga canadensis) also yields an exudation sold under the name of 'Canada balsam'. Many other species of fir produce oils from their needles – see entry on silver fir and Botanical Classification section. NB Not to be confused with the genuine balsam of Gilead (Commiphora opabalsamum).

Acacia dealbata

Mimosa

FAMILY: MIMOSACEAE **SYNONYMS:** *A. DECURRENS VAR. DEALBATA*, SYDNEY BLACK WATTLE

Herbal/Folk Tradition

The bark of mimosa, which is known as 'wattle bark', has a leather-like odour and astringent taste. It contains up to 42 per cent tannins (also gallic acid) and is used extensively by the tanning industry. It is employed medicinally in similar ways to oak bark, as a specific for diarrhea, and as an astringent gargle and ointment.

The extract of black catechu (*A. catechu*) is current in the British Herbal Pharmacopoeia as a specific for chronic diarrhea with colitis.

An attractive small tree up to 12m (39ft) high, having a greyish-brown bark with irregular longitudinal ridges, delicate foliage and clusters of ball-shaped fragrant yellow flowers.

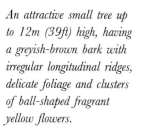

fresh
mimosa

EXTRACTION

A concrete and absolute by solvent extraction from the flowers and twig ends.

CHARACTERISTICS

**1. Concrete – a hard wax-like yellow mass with a sweet-woody, deep floral fragrance.
2. Absolute – an amber-coloured viscous liquid with a slightly green, woody-floral scent. It blends well with lavandin, lavender, ylang ylang, violet, styrax, citronella, Peru balsam, cassie, floral and spice oils.**

ACTIONS

Antiseptic, astringent.

PRINCIPAL CONSTITUENTS

Mainly hydrocarbons; palmic aldehyde, enanthic acid, anisic acid, acetic acid and phenols.

**AROMATHERAPY/
HOME USE**

Skin Care: *Oily, sensitive, general skin care.*
Nervous System: *Anxiety, nervous tension, over-sensitivity, stress.*

OTHER USES

Employed largely in soaps, due to its good fixative properties. Also in high-class perfumes, especially colognes, floral and oriental types.

DISTRIBUTION

Native to Australia; naturalized in
North and Central Africa. It was brought to Europe as an ornamental plant in the early nineteenth century, but it now grows wild. The concrete (and absolute) is produced mainly in southern France, and also Italy.

OTHER SPECIES

There are many varieties of Acacia, such as the East African type (A. arabica), which is very similar; the mimosa of the florist shop (A. floribunda); and the Brazilian mimosa or sensitive plant (Mimosa humilis), the

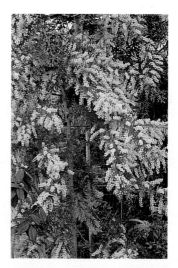

Acacia dealbata

homeopathic tincture of which is used for swelling of the ankles. It is also closely related to cassie.

Acacia farnesiana

Cassie

FAMILY: MIMOSACEAE **SYNONYMS:** *CASSIA ANCIENNE*, SWEET ACACIA, HUISACHE, POPINAC, OPOPANAX

Herbal/Folk Tradition

In India a local 'attar of cassie' is made as a perfume. The fresh flowers are used in baths for dry skin, and in the form of an infusion. In Venezuela the root is used for treating stomach cancer. In China it is used to treat rheumatoid arthritis and pulmonary tuberculosis.

There are many types of acacia employed in herbal medicine, notably the Senegal acacia which yields a gummy exudation from the trunk known as gum arabic or gum acacia, used mainly as a demulcent.

A bushy thorny shrub, much branched, up to 10m (33ft) high. It has a very delicate appearance, similar to mimosa, with fragrant fluffy yellow flowers.

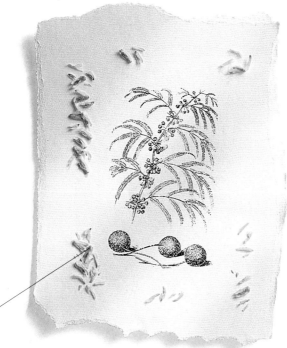

dried cassie flowers

AROMATHERAPY/ HOME USE

Use with care for:
Skin Care: *Dry, sensitive skin, perfume.*
Nervous System: *Depression, frigidity, nervous exhaustion, and stress-related conditions.*

OTHER USES

Used in high-class perfumes, especially oriental types. Used as a flavour ingredient in most food categories, especially fruit products, alcoholic and soft drinks.

DISTRIBUTION

Believed to be a native of the West Indies, now widely cultivated in tropical and semi-tropical regions throughout the world: mainly southern France and Egypt, also Lebanon, Morocco, Algeria and India.

OTHER SPECIES

*There are over 400 known species of acacia: other similar species are found in Central Africa, Zaire and Australia. It is closely related to mimosa (*A. dealbata*) and Roman cassie (*A. cavenia*), which are also used for the production of essential oils. Not to be confused with opopanax or bisabol myrrh (*Commiphora erythraea*), although they share a common name.*

EXTRACTION

An absolute by solvent extraction from the flowers.

CHARACTERISTICS

A dark yellow to brown viscous liquid with a warm, floral-spicy scent and rich balsamic undertone. It blends well with bergamot, costus, mimosa, frankincense, ylang ylang, orris and violet.

ACTIONS

Antirheumatic, antiseptic, antispasmodic, aphrodisiac, balsamic, insecticide.

PRINCIPAL CONSTITUENTS

The absolute contains about 25 per cent volatile constituents, mainly benzyl alcohol, methyl salicylate, farnesol, geraniol and linalol, among others.

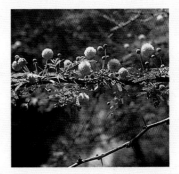

Acacia farnesiana

Achillea millefolium

Yarrow

FAMILY: ASTERACEAE (COMPOSITAE) **SYNONYMS:** MILFOIL, COMMON YARROW, NOSEBLEED, THOUSAND LEAF — AND MANY OTHER COUNTY NAMES

Herbal/Folk Tradition

An age-old herbal medicine used for a wide variety of complaints including fever, respiratory infections, digestive problems, nervous tension and externally for sores, rashes and wounds. Its use in the treatment of wounds is said to go back to Achilles who used it for injuries inflicted by iron weapons.

It is used in China mainly for menstrual problems and hemorrhoids. In Norway it is also used for rheumatism. The stalks are traditionally used for divination in the *I Ching*, the Chinese classic.

It is current in the British Herbal Pharmacopoeia as a specific for thrombotic conditions with hypertension.

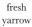

fresh
yarrow

EXTRACTION
Essential oil by steam distillation from the dried herb.

CHARACTERISTICS
A dark blue or greenish-olive liquid with a fresh, green, sweet-herbaceous, slightly camphoraceous odour. It blends well with cedarwood, pine, chamomile, valerian, vetiver and oakmoss.

ACTIONS
Anti-inflammatory, antipyretic, antirheumatic, antiseptic, antispasmodic, astringent, carminative, cicatrisant, diaphoretic, digestive, expectorant, hemostatic, hypotensive, stomachic, tonic.

PRINCIPAL CONSTITUENTS
Azulene (up to 51 per cent), pinenes, caryophyllene, borneol, terpineol, cineol, bornyl acetate, camphor, sabinene and thujone, among others. Constituents, especially azulene levels, vary according to source.

A perennial herb with a simple stem up to 1m (3ft) high, with finely dissected leaves giving a lacy appearance, bearing numerous pinky-white, dense flowerheads.

AROMATHERAPY/
HOME USE

Skin Care: *Acne, burns, cuts, eczema, hair rinse (promotes hair growth), inflammations, rashes, scars, tones the skin, varicose veins, wounds.*
Circulation, Muscles and Joints: *Arteriosclerosis, high blood pressure, rheumatoid artritis, thrombosis.*
Digestive System: *Constipation, cramp, flatulence, hemorrhoids, indigestion.*
Genito-urinary System: *Amenorrhea, dysmenorrhea, cystitis and other infections.*
Immune System: *Colds, fever, flu, etc.*
Nervous System: *Hypertension, insomnia, stress-related conditions.*

AROMATHERAPY/

OTHER USES
Limited use in pharmaceutical bath preparations for skin conditions, in perfumes and aftershaves. Also a flavour ingredient in vermouths and bitters.

DISTRIBUTION
Native to Eurasia; naturalized in North America. Now found in most temperate zones. The oil is distilled mainly in Germany, Hungary, France and former Yugoslavia, also USA and Africa.

OTHER SPECIES
A very extensive species. Varieties include the Ligurian yarrow (A. ligustica) and the musk yarrow or iva (A. moschata), which produces an oil containing cineol — used in preparing 'iva liquor', a medicinal aperitif.

Acorus calamus var. angustatus

Calamus

FAMILY: ARACEAE **SYNONYMS:** *CALAMUS AROMATICUS*, SWEET FLAG, SWEET SEDGE, SWEET ROOT, SWEET RUSH, SWEET CANE, SWEET MYRTLE, MYRTLE GRASS, MYRTLE SEDGE, CINNAMON SEDGE

Herbal/Folk Tradition

The properties of the herb are mainly due to the aromatic oil, contained largely in the root. It used to be highly esteemed as an aromatic stimulant and tonic for fever (typhoid), nervous complaints, vertigo, headaches, dysentery, etc. It is still current in the British Herbal Pharmacopoeia, for 'acute and chronic dyspepsia, gastritis, intestinal colic, anorexia, gastric ulcer'.[3] In Turkey and especially in India (where it is valued as a traditional medicine), it is sold as a candied rhizome for dyspepsia, bronchitis and coughs.

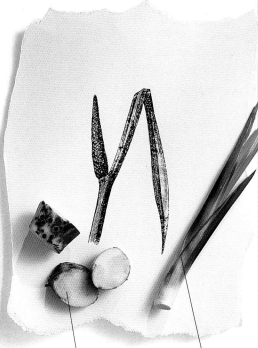

calamus root   fresh calamus

A reed-like aquatic plant about 1m (3ft) high, with sword-shaped leaves and small greenish-yellow flowers. It grows on the margins of lakes and streams with the long-branched rhizome immersed in the mud. The whole plant is aromatic.

EXTRACTION

Essential oil by steam distillation from the rhizomes (and sometimes the leaves).

CHARACTERISTICS

A thick, pale yellow liquid with a strong, warm, woody-spicy fragrance; poor-quality oils have a camphoraceous note. It blends well with cananga, cinnamon, labdanum, olibanum, patchouli, cedarwood, amyris, spice and oriental bases.

ACTIONS

Anticonvulsant, antiseptic, bactericidal, carminative, diaphoretic, expectorant, hypotensive, insecticide, spasmolytic, stimulant, stomachic, tonic, vermifuge.

PRINCIPAL CONSTITUENTS

Beta-asarone (amounts vary depending on source: the Indian oil contains up to 80 per cent, the Russian oil a maximum of 6 per cent), also calamene, calamol, calamenene, eugenol and shyobunones.

AROMATHERAPY/ HOME USE

None. 'Should not be used in therapy, whether internally or externally.'[4]

OTHER USES

Extensively used in cosmetic and perfumery work, in woody/ oriental/ leather perfumes and to scent hair powders and tooth powders in the same way as orris. Calamus and its derivatives (oil, extracts, etc.) are banned from use in foods.

DISTRIBUTION

Native to India; the oil is produced mainly in India and Russia and to a lesser extent in Europe (except Spain), Siberia, China, former Yugoslavia and Poland (Polish and Yugoslavian oils have a uniform lasting scent).

OTHER SPECIES

Not to be confused with the yellow flag iris, which it resembles in appearance; they are botanically unrelated. There are several other varieties of aromatic sedge, mostly in the East, for example, Calamus odoratus *used in India as a medicine and perfume.*

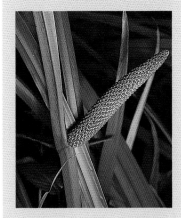

Acorus calamus var. angustatus

Agothosma betulina

Buchu

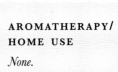

FAMILY: RUTACEAE **SYNONYMS:** *BAROSMA BETULINA*, SHORT BUCHU, MOUNTAIN BUCHU, BOOKOO, BUKU, BUCCO

Herbal/Folk Tradition

The leaves are used locally for antiseptic purposes and to ward off insects. In Western herbalism, the leaves are used for infections of the genito-urinary system, such as cystitis, urethritis and prostatitis. For inflammation of the bladder it is taken as an infusion. Current in the British Herbal Pharmacopoeia.

A small shrub with simple wrinkled leaves about 1–2cm (½in) long; other much smaller leaves are also present, which are bright green with finely serrated margins. It has delicate stems bearing five-petalled white flowers. The whole plant has a strong, aromatic, blackcurrant-like odour.

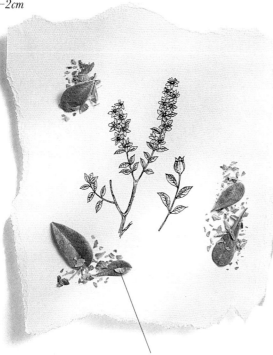

fresh and
dried buchu

AROMATHERAPY/ HOME USE

None.

OTHER USES

A tincture, extract and oleoresin are produced for pharmaceutical use. Limited use in blackcurrant flavour and fragrance work, for example, colognes and chyprè bases.

DISTRIBUTION

Native to the Cape of Good Hope in South Africa, it now grows wild all over South Africa. Dried leaves are exported to the Netherlands, Britain and the USA.

OTHER SPECIES

There are two main types of buchu leaf: 'round' or 'short' buchu is from A. betulina, while 'long' buchu is from A. crenulata. 'Round' buchu yields a higher proportion of volatile oil than 'long' buchu and they differ widely in their composition. However, an essential oil is extracted from both varieties using both wild and cultivated plants. There are more than twelve so-called Barosma species in South Africa – the 'true' buchus are B. crenulata (contains high amounts of pulegone, a toxic constituent), B. serratifolia and B. betulina.

EXTRACTION
Essential oil by steam distillation from the dried leaves.

CHARACTERISTICS
Dark yellowy-brown oil with a penetrating minty-camphoraceous odour.

ACTIONS
Antiseptic (especially urinary), carminative, diaphoretic, diuretic, insecticide, stimulant, tonic.

PRINCIPAL CONSTITUENTS
Diosphenol (25–40 per cent), limonene and methone, among others. The toxicity of buchu is unknown but since *B. betulina* yields oils high in diophenols, and *B. crenulata* yields oils high in pulegone, they should both be regarded as questionable at present.

Allium cepa

Onion

SAFETY DATA *Specific safety data unavailable at present – probably similar to garlic, i.e. generally non-toxic, non-irritant, possible sensitization*

FAMILY: LILIACEAE **SYNONYMS:** COMMON ONION, STRASBURG ONION

Herbal/Folk Tradition

Onion has an ancient reputation as a curative agent, highly extolled by the schools of Galen and Hippocrates. It is high in Vitamins A, B and C and shares many of the properties of garlic, to which it is closely related. Raw onion helps to keep colds and infections at bay, promotes strong bones and a good blood supply to all the tissues. It acts as an effective blood cleanser that, along with the sulphur it contains, helps to keep the skin clear and in good condition.

It has a sound reputation for correcting glandular imbalance and weight problems; it also improves lymphatic drainage, which is often responsible for edema and puffiness. It has long been used as a home 'simple' for a wide range of conditions.

A perennial or biennial herb up to 1.2m (4ft) high with hollow leaves and flowering stem, and a globe-like fleshy bulb.

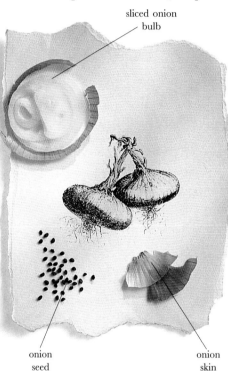

sliced onion bulb

onion seed

onion skin

AROMATHERAPY/ HOME USE

None, due to its offensive smell.

OTHER USES

Used in some pharmaceutical preparations for colds, coughs, etc. The oil is used extensively in most major food categories, especially meats, savouries, salad dressings, as well as alcoholic and soft drinks. It is not used in perfumery work.

DISTRIBUTION

Native of western Asia and the Middle East, it has a long history of cultivation all over the world, mainly for culinary use. The essential oil is produced mainly in France, Germany and Egypt from the 'red' onion.

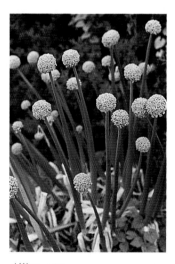

Allium cepa

OTHER SPECIES

Numerous species of onion have been developed, including the Spanish or silver-skinned onion, the Tripoli and the red onion. See also Botanical Classification.

EXTRACTION
Essential oil by steam distillation from the bulb. (An oleoresin is also produced in small quantities for flavouring use.)

CHARACTERISTICS
A pale yellow or brownish-yellow mobile liquid with strong, unpleasant, sulphur-aceous odour with a lachrymatory (tear-producing) effect.

ACTIONS
Anthelmintic, antimicrobial, antirheumatic, antiseptic, antisclerotic, antispasmodic, **antiviral, bactericidal, carminative, depurative, digestive, diuretic, expectorant, fungicidal, hypocholesterolemic, hypoglycemic, hypotensive, stomachic, tonic, vermifuge.**

PRINCIPAL
CONSTITUENTS
Mainly dipropyl disulphide, also methylpropyl disulphide, dipropyl trisulphide, methylpropyl trisulphide and allylpropyl disulphide, among others.

Allium sativum

Garlic

FAMILY: AMARYLLIDACEAE OR LILIACEAE **SYNONYMS:** COMMON GARLIC, ALLIUM, POOR MAN'S TREACLE!

Herbal/Folk Tradition

It has been used for thousands of years for its medicinal virtues: for respiratory and urinary tract infections; digestive disorders and infestations; skin eruptions; heart disease, high blood pressure and arteriosclerosis, as well as epidemics and fever. It was used in the First World War for preventing gangrene and sepsis.

It has a high reputation in the East: in China it is used for diarrhea, dysentery, tuberculosis, diphtheria, hepatitis, ringworm, typhoid and trachoma, among others. It is also held in high regard in the West: specific in the British Herbal Pharmacopoeia for chronic bronchitis. Its properties have been attested to by modern experimental and clinical research.

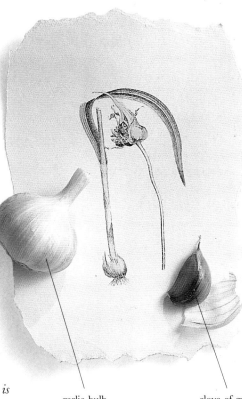

garlic bulb   clove of garlic

EXTRACTION
Essential oil by steam distillation from the fresh crushed bulbs.

CHARACTERISTICS
A colourless to pale yellow mobile liquid with a strong, unpleasant, familiar garlic-like odour.

ACTIONS
Amoebicidal, anthelmintic, antibiotic, antimicrobial, antiseptic, antitoxic, antitumour, antiviral, bactericidal, carminative, cholagogue, hypocholesterolemic, depurative, diaphoretic, diuretic, expectorant, febrifuge, fungicidal, hypoglycemic, hypotensive, insecticidal, larvicidal, promotes leucocytosis, stomachic, tonic.

PRINCIPAL CONSTITUENTS
Allicin, allylpropyl disulphide, diallyl disulphide, diallyl trisulphide, citral, geraniol, linalol, phellandrene, among others.

A strongly scented perennial herb up to 1.2m (4ft) high with long, flat, firm leaves and whitish flowering stems. The bulb is made up of several cloves pressed together within a thin white skin.

AROMATHERAPY/ HOME USE

Due to its unpleasant and pervasive smell, the oil is not often used externally. However, the capsules may be taken internally according to the instructions on the label for respiratory and gastro-intestinal infections, urinary tract infections such as cystitis, heart and circulatory problems, and to fight infectious diseases in general.

OTHER USES

The oil is made into capsules and also included in many health food products mainly to help reduce high blood pressure and protect against heart disease. Extensively employed as a flavour ingredient in most major food categories, especially savouries.

DISTRIBUTION

It is said to have originated in south-west Siberia and then spread to Europe and Central Asia. It is naturalized in North America and cultivated worldwide. Major oil-producing countries include Egypt, Bulgaria, France, China, Germany and Japan.

OTHER SPECIES

Closely related to the wild or wood garlic (A. ursinum) also known as 'ramsons'. There are also many other wild species with similar but less pronounced properties.

Aloysia triphylla

Lemon verbena

FAMILY: VERBENACEAE **SYNONYMS:** *A. CITRIODORA, VERBENA TRIPHYLLA, LIPPIA CITRIODORA, L. TRIPHYLLA*, VERBENA, HERB LOUISA

Herbal/Folk Tradition

'The uses of lemon verbena are similar to those of mint, orange flowers and melissa.'[5] It is indicated especially in nervous conditions that manifest as digestive complaints. The dried leaves are still used as a popular household tea especially in Europe, both as a refreshing, uplifting 'pick-me-up' and to help restore the liver after a hang-over.

A handsome deciduous perennial shrub up to 5m (16ft) high with a woody stem, very fragrant, delicate, pale green, lanceolate leaves arranged in threes, and small, pale purple flowers. Often grown as an ornamental bush in gardens.

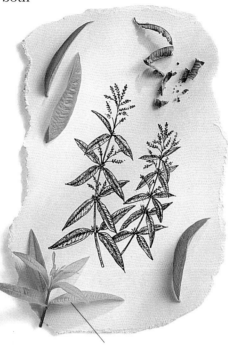

fresh lemon
verbena

EXTRACTION
Essential oil by steam distillation from the freshly harvested herb.

CHARACTERISTICS
A pale olive or yellow mobile liquid with a sweet, fresh, lemony, fruity-floral fragrance. It blends well with orange blossom, palmarosa, olibanum, Tolu balsam, elemi, lemon and other citrus oils.

ACTIONS
Antiseptic, antispasmodic, carminative, detoxifying, digestive, febrifuge, hepatobiliary stimulant, sedative (nervous), stomachic.

PRINCIPAL CONSTITUENTS
Citral (30–35 per cent), nerol and geraniol, among others.

X

AROMATHERAPY/ HOME USE

Digestive System: *Cramps, indigestion, liver congestion.*
Nervous System: *Anxiety, insomnia, nervous tension and stress-related conditions. True verbena oil is virtually non-existent. Most so-called verbena oil is either from the Spanish verbena (an inferior oil) or a mix of lemongrass, lemon, citronella, etc.*

OTHER USES

Used in perfumery and citrus colognes – 'eau de verveine' is still very popular in France, Europe and the USA.

DISTRIBUTION

Native of Chile and Argentina; cultivated (and found semi-wild) in the Mediterranean region – France, Tunisia, Algeria – as well as Kenya and China. The oil is produced mainly in southern France and North Africa.

OTHER SPECIES

Botanically related to the oregano family – see Botanical Classification section. Not to be mistaken for the so-called Spanish verbena or verbena oil (Spanish) (Thymus hiamalis), nor confused with the herb 'vervain' (Verbena officinalis). This is

further confused since the French name for verbena is verveine (Verveine citronelle, Verveine odorante).

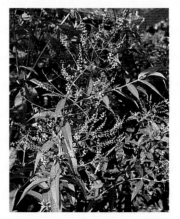

Aloysia triphylla

Alpinia officinarum

Galangal

FAMILY: ZINGIBERACEA SYNONYMS: *RADIX GALANGA MINORIS*, *LANGUAS OFFICINARUM*, GALANGA, SMALL GALANGAL, CHINESE GINGER, GINGER ROOT, COLIC ROOT, EAST INDIAN ROOT

Herbal/Folk Tradition

It is used as a local spice, especially in curries; in India it is employed in perfumery. The root is current in the British Herbal Pharmacopoeia, indicated for dyspepsia, flatulence, colic, nausea and vomiting.

EXTRACTION
Essential oil by steam distillation from the rhizomes. (An oleoresin is also produced by solvent extraction.)

CHARACTERISTICS
A greenish-yellow liquid with a fresh, spicy-camphoraceous odour. It blends well with chamomile maroc, sage, cinnamon, allspice, lavandin, pine needle, rosemary, patchouli, myrtle, opopanax and citrus oils.

ACTIONS
Antiseptic, bactericidal, carminative, diaphoretic, stimulant, stomachic.

PRINCIPAL CONSTITUENTS
Pinene, cineol, eugenol and sesquiterpenes.

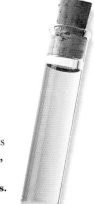

AROMATHERAPY/ HOME USE

(Possibly digestive upsets.)

OTHER USES

Employed as a flavour ingredient, especially in spice and meat products. Occasionally used in perfumery work.

DISTRIBUTION

Native to south-east China, especially the island of Hainan. Cultivated in China, Indonesia, Thailand and Japan.

OTHER SPECIES

Similar species grow in Malaysia, Java, India, etc. It is closely related to ginger (Zingiber officinale) and to the large galanga (Galanga officinalis). Not to be confused with the dried rhizomes of kaempferia galanga, known as 'kentjoer', which are used in Malaysia for medicinal purposes and for flavouring curry.

A reed-like plant reaching a height of about 1m (3ft), with irregularly branched rhizomes red or brown on the outside, light orange within.

galangal rhizome

dried galangal

Amyris balsamifera

Amyris

FAMILY: RUTACEAE **SYNONYMS:** *SCHIMMELIA OLEIFERA*, WEST INDIAN SANDALWOOD, WEST INDIAN ROSEWOOD

Herbal/Folk Tradition

The botanical origin of the tree yielding this oil remained obscure until 1886 when Kirkby and Holmes identified striking differences between this plant and true sandalwood by microscopic examination of the leaves. In recognition of this discovery the botanical name of amyris was changed from *Schimmerelia oleisera* to *Amyris balsamifera*. The locals call it 'candle wood' because of its high oil content; it burns like a candle. It is used as a torch by fishermen and traders. It also makes excellent furniture wood.

A small bushy tree with compound leaves and white flowers, which grows wild in thickets all over the island of Haiti.

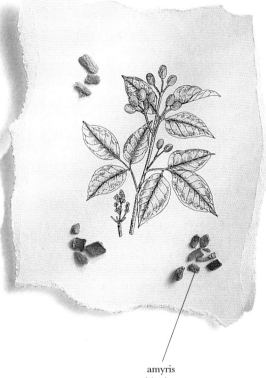

amyris
chippings

EXTRACTION
Essential oil by steam distillation from the broken-up wood and branches. Best if the wood is seasoned first. It provides a very plentiful yield.

CHARACTERISTICS
A pale yellow, slightly viscous liquid with a musty, faintly woody scent, quickly fading away. It blends well with lavandin, citronella, oakmoss, sassafras, cedarwood and other wood oils.

ACTIONS
Antiseptic, balsamic, sedative.

PRINCIPAL CONSTITUENTS
Caryphyllene, cadinene and cadinol.

AROMATHERAPY/
HOME USE
Perfume.

OTHER USES
As a cheap substitute for East Indian sandalwood in perfumes and cosmetics, although it does not have the same rich tenacity; chiefly employed as a fixative in soaps. Limited application in flavouring work, especially liqueurs.

DISTRIBUTION
Originally cultivated mainly in Haiti, it has now been introduced to tropical zones all over the world, e.g. Jamaica, South and Central America. The production of this oil has dropped with the passing of time due to adverse climatic conditions in Haiti.

OTHER SPECIES
Not to be confused with East Indian or Mysore sandalwood (Santalum album), to which it bears no relation.

Anethum graveolens

Dill

FAMILY: APIACEAE (UMBELLIFERAE) **SYNONYMS:** *PEUCEDANUM GRAVEOLENS, FRACTUS ANETHI,* EUROPEAN DILL, AMERICAN DILL

Herbal/Folk Tradition

Used since the earliest times as a medicinal and culinary herb. In Germany and Scandinavia especially, it is used with fish and cucumber, and the seeds baked in bread. In the West and East it is used as a soothing digestive aid for indigestion, wind, colic, etc., especially in children, for which it is still current in the British Herbal Pharmacopoeia.

Annual or biennial herb up to 1m (3ft) high with a smooth stem, feathery leaves and umbels of yellowish flowers followed by flat small seeds.

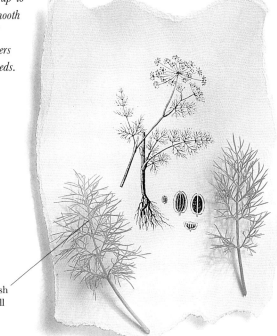

fresh
dill

AROMATHERAPY/ HOME USE

Digestive System: *Colic, dyspepsia, flatulence, indigestion.*
Genito-urinary and Endocrine Systems: *Lack of periods; promotes milk flow in nursing mothers.*

OTHER USES

Used in some pharmaceutical digestive preparations such as 'dill water'. The weed oil is used as a fragrance component in detergents, cosmetics, perfumes and especially soaps. Both oils are used extensively in alcoholic, soft drinks and foodstuffs, especially pickles and condiments.

DISTRIBUTION

Native to the Mediterranean and Black Sea regions; now cultivated worldwide, especially in Europe, USA, China and India. Dill seed oil is produced mainly in Europe (France, Hungary, Germany, Britain, Spain); dill weed oil in the USA.

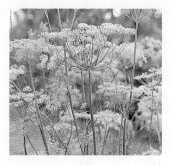

Anethum graveolens

EXTRACTION
Essential oil by steam (sometimes water) distillation from 1. fruit or seed, 2. herb or weed (fresh or partially dried).

CHARACTERISTICS
1. A colourless to pale yellow mobile liquid with a light fresh warm-spicy scent. 2. A colourless or pale yellow mobile liquid with a powerful sweet-spicy aroma. It blends well with elemi, mint, caraway, nutmeg, spice and citrus oils.

ACTIONS
Antispasmodic, bactericidal, carminative, digestive, emmenagogue, galactagogue, hypotensive, stimulant, stomachic.

PRINCIPAL CONSTITUENTS
1. Carvone (30–60 per cent), limonene, phellandrene, eugenol, pinene, among others. 2. Carvone (much less), limonene, pinene, etc., as well as terpinene. There are several different chemotypes of dill, for example, phellandrene is present in the English and Spanish oils but not in the German.

OTHER SPECIES

Indian dill or East Indian dill (A. sowa) is widely cultivated in the East, especially in India and Japan. A commercial oil produced from the seed has a different chemical composition and contains 'dill apiol'.

Angelica archangelica

Angelica

FAMILY: APIACEAE (UMBELLIFERAE) **SYNONYMS:** *A. OFFICINALIS,* EUROPEAN ANGELICA, GARDEN ANGELICA

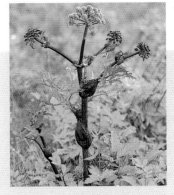

Angelica archangelica

Herbal/Folk Tradition

This herb has been praised for its virtues since antiquity. It strengthens the heart, stimulates the circulation and the immune system in general. It has been used for centuries in Europe for bronchial ailments, colds, coughs, indigestion, wind and to stimulate the appetite. As a urinary antiseptic it is helpful in cystitis and is also used for rheumatic inflammation. The Chinese employ at least ten kinds of angelica, well known for promoting fertility, fortifying the spirit and for treating female disorders generally; it has a reputation second only to ginseng. It is current in the British Herbal Pharmacopoeia as a specific for bronchitis associated with vascular deficiency. Candied angelica stalks are popular in France and Spain.

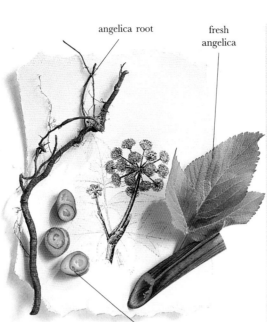

angelica root

fresh angelica

section of fresh stalk

A large hairy plant with ferny leaves and umbels of white flowers. It has a strong aromatic scent and a large rhizome.

AROMATHERAPY/ HOME USE

Skin Care: *Dull and congested skin, irritated conditions, psoriasis.*
Circulation, Muscles and Joints: *Accumulation of toxins, arthritis, gout, rheumatism, water retention.*
Respiratory System: *Bronchitis, coughs.*
Digestive System: *Anemia, anorexia, flatulence, indigestion.*
Nervous System: *Fatigue, migraine, nervous tension and stress-related disorders.*
Immune System: *Colds.*

OTHER USES

Highly valued as a fragrance component in soaps, lotions and perfumes especially colognes, oriental and heavy chyprès fragrances. It is employed in some cosmetics for its soothing effect on skin complaints. Used extensively as a flavouring agent in most food categories, and in alcoholic and soft drinks, especially liqueurs.

DISTRIBUTION

Native to Europe and Siberia, cultivated mainly in Belgium, Hungary and Germany.

OTHER SPECIES

There are over thirty different types of angelica but this is the most commonly used medicinally. See Botanical Classification section.

EXTRACTION
Essential oil produced by steam distillation from the
1. roots and rhizomes, and,
2. fruit or seed. An absolute is also produced on a small scale, from the roots.

CHARACTERISTICS
1. A colourless or pale yellow oil that turns yellowy-brown with age, with a rich herbaceous-earthy bodynote.
2. The seed oil is a colourless liquid with a fresher, spicy top note. It blends well with patchouli, opopanax, costus, clary sage, oakmoss, vetiver and with citrus oils.

ACTIONS
Antispasmodic, carminative, depurative, diaphoretic, digestive, diuretic, emmenagogue, expectorant, febrifuge, nervine, stimulant, stomachic, tonic. Reported to have bactericidal and fungicidal properties.

PRINCIPAL CONSTITUENTS
Root and seed oil contain phellandrene, pinene, limonene, linalol and borneol; rich in coumarins including osthol, angelicin, bergapten and imperatorin; also contains plant acids.

Aniba rosaeodora

Rosewood

FAMILY: LAURACEAE   SYNONYMS: *A. ROSAEODORA VAR. AMAZONICA*,
BOIS DE ROSE, BRAZILIAN ROSEWOOD

Herbal/Folk Tradition

Used for building, carving and French cabinet-making.
Nowadays, most rosewood goes to Japan for the
production of chopsticks.

EXTRACTION
**Essential oil by steam
distillation of the wood
chippings.**

CHARACTERISTICS
**Colourless to pale yellow
liquid with a very sweet,
woody-floral fragrance
with a spicy hint. Blends
well with most oils,
especially citrus, woods
and florals. It helps give
body and rounds off
sharp edges.**

ACTIONS
**Mildly analgesic, anti-
convulsant, antidepressant,
antimicrobial, antiseptic,
aphrodisiac, bactericidal,
cellular stimulant, cephalic,
deodorant, stimulant (immune
system), tissue regenerator,
tonic.**

PRINCIPAL CONSTITUENTS
**Linalol (90–97 per cent) in
cayenne rosewood; in the
Brazilian oil slightly less (80–90
per cent). Also cineol, terpineol,
geraniol, citronellal, limonene,
pinene, among others.**

AROMATHERAPY/ HOME USE

Skin Care: *Acne, dermatitis,
scars, wounds, wrinkles and
general skin care: sensitive, dry,
dull, combination oily/ dry, etc.
'Although it does not have any
dramatic curative power . . .
I find it very useful especially
for skin care. It is very mild
and safe to use.'*[6]
Immune System: *Colds,
coughs, fever, infections, stimulates
the immune system.*
Nervous System: *Frigidity,
headaches, nausea, nervous tension
and stress-related conditions.*

OTHER USES

*Once used extensively as a
source of natural linalol, now
increasingly replaced by the
synthetic form. Acetylated rosewood
oil is used extensively in perfumery
work — soaps, toiletries, cosmetics
and perfumes. The oil is employed
in most major food categories,
alcoholic and soft drinks.*

DISTRIBUTION

*Native to the Amazon region;
Brazil and Peru are the main
producers.*

OTHER SPECIES

*There are several species
of timber all known as
rosewood; however, the
essential oil is distilled only
from the above species. French
Guiana used to produce the
cayenne rosewood (Ocotea
caudata), which is superior
in quality to the Peruvian or
Brazilian type.*

*Medium-sized, tropical, evergreen tree with a reddish
bark and heartwood, bearing yellow flowers. Used
extensively for timber. NB: This is one of the trees
that is being extensively felled
in the clearing of the South
American rainforests; the
continual production of
rosewood oil is consequently
environmentally damaging.*

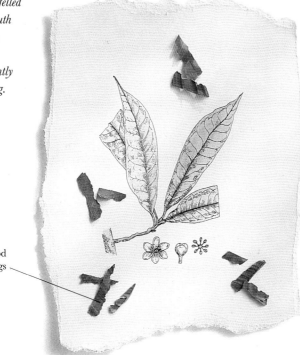

rosewood
chippings

Anthriscus cerefolium

Chervil

FAMILY: APIACEAE (UMBELLIFERAE)   **SYNONYMS:** *A. LONGIROSTRIS*, GARDEN CHERVIL, SALAD CHERVIL

Herbal/Folk Tradition

The name *chervil* comes from the Greek 'to rejoice', because of its delightful scent. The leaves are used as a domestic spice in salads, soups, omelettes, sauces and to flavour bread dough. In folk medicine it is used as a tea to 'tone up the blood and nerves. Good for poor memory and mental depression. Sweetens the entire digestive system.'[7]

The juice from the fresh herb is used to treat skin ailments such as eczema, abscesses and slow-healing wounds; also used for dropsy, arthritis and gout, among others.

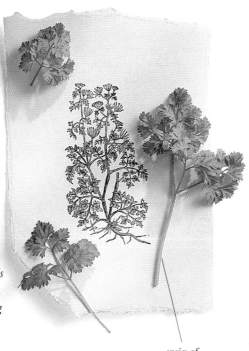

A delicate annual herb up to 30cm (12in) high, with a slender, much branched stem, bright green, finely-divided, fern-like leaves, umbels of flat white flowerheads and long smooth seeds or fruits. The whole plant has a pleasing aromatic scent when bruised.

sprig of
fresh chervil

EXTRACTION
Essential oil by steam distillation from seeds or fruit.

CHARACTERISTICS
A pale yellow liquid with a sweet-herbaceous, anisic odour.

ACTIONS
Aperitif, antiseptic, carminative, cicatrisant, depurative, diaphoretic, digestive, diuretic, nervine, restorative, stimulant (metabolism), stomachic, tonic.

PRINCIPAL CONSTITUENTS
Mainly methyl chavicol, also 1-allyl-2, 4-dimethoxy-benzene and anethole, among others.

AROMATHERAPY/ HOME USE
None.

OTHER USES
Extensively employed as a flavour ingredient by the food industry, especially in meat products, as well as in alcoholic and soft drinks. Methyl chavicol and anethole are known to have toxic and irritant effects; methyl chavicol is reported to have possible carcinogenic effects. Since these constitute the major proportion of the essential oil, it is best avoided for therapeutic use.

DISTRIBUTION
Native to Europe and western Asia; naturalized in the USA, Australia and New Zealand. Widely cultivated, especially in southern Europe and the USA.

OTHER SPECIES
*A cultivated form of its wild relative, the wild chervil or garden-beaked parsley (A. sylvestris), with which it shares similar properties and uses. Not to be confused with another common garden herb sweet cicely (*Myrrhis *odorata), also known as sweet or smooth chervil.*

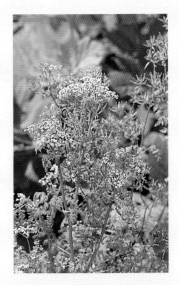

Anthriscus cerefolium

Apium graveolens

Celery seed

FAMILY: APIACEAE (UMBELLIFERAE) **SYNONYMS:** CELERY FRUIT

Herbal/Folk Tradition

Celery seed is widely used as a domestic spice. The seed is used in bladder and kidney complaints, digestive upsets and menstrual problems; the leaves are used in skin ailments. It is known to increase the elimination of uric acid and is useful for gout, neuralgia and rheumatoid arthritis. A remedy for hepatobiliary disorders, it has been found to have a regenerating effect on the liver.

Current in the British Herbal Pharmacopoeia as a specific for rheumatoid arthritis with mental depression.

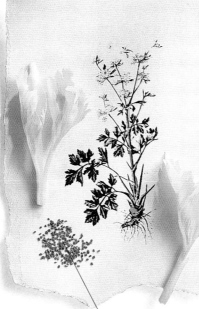

celery seed

A familiar biennial plant, 30–60cm (12–24in) high, with a grooved, fleshy, erect stalk, shiny pinnate leaves and umbels of white flowers.

AROMATHERAPY/ HOME USE

Circulation, Muscles and Joints: *Arthritis, build-up of toxins in the blood, gout, rheumatism.*
Digestive System: *Dyspepsia, flatulence, indigestion, liver congestion, jaundice.*
Genito-urinary and Endocrine Systems: *Amenorrhea, glandular problems, increases milk flow, cystitis.*
Nervous System: *Neuralgia, sciatica.*

OTHER USES

Used in tonic, sedative and carminative preparations, and as a fragrance component in soaps, detergents, cosmetics and perfumes. Extensively used as a flavouring agent in foods, especially by the spice industry, and in alcoholic and soft drinks.

DISTRIBUTION

Native to southern Europe; extensively cultivated as a domestic vegetable. The oil is produced principally in India, and also the Netherlands, China, Hungary and the USA.

OTHER SPECIES

There are many cultivated varieties, such as celeriac root (A. graveolens var. rapaceum) *and the salad vegetable (A.* graveolens var. dulce).

EXTRACTION
Essential oil by steam distillation from the whole or crushed seeds. (An oil from the whole herb, an oleoresin and extract are also produced in small quantities.)

CHARACTERISTICS
A pale yellow or orange oil with a spicy-warm, sweet, long-lasting odour. It blends well with lavender, pine, opopanax, lovage, tea tree, oakmoss, coriander and other spices.

ACTIONS
Anti-oxidative, antirheumatic, antiseptic (urinary), antispasmodic, aperitif, depurative, digestive, diuretic, carminative, cholagogue, emmenagogue, galactagogue, hepatic, nervine, sedative (nervous), stimulant (uterine), stomachic, tonic (digestive).

PRINCIPAL CONSTITUENTS
Limonene (60 per cent), apiol, selinene, santalol, sedanolide and sedanolic acid anhydride, among others.

Armoracia rusticana

Horseradish

FAMILY: BRASSICACEAE (CRUCIFERAE) **SYNONYMS:** *COCHLEARIA ARMORACIA, A. LAPATHIFOLIA,* RED COLE, RAIFORT

Herbal/Folk Tradition

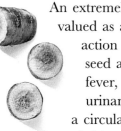

An extremely stimulating herb, once valued as a household remedy. Its action is similar to mustard seed and it was used for fever, digestive complaints, urinary infections and as a circulatory aid. Good for arthritis and rheumatism. It is still used as a condiment, especially in continental Europe.

A perennial plant with large leaves up to 50cm (20in) long, white flowers and a thick whitish tapering root, which is propagated easily.

horseradish root

section of root

EXTRACTION
Essential oil by water and steam distillation from broken roots that have been soaked in water. (A resinoid or concrete is also produced by solvent extraction.)

CHARACTERISTICS
A colourless or pale yellow mobile liquid with a sharp, potent odour and having a tear-producing effect.

ACTIONS
Antibiotic, antiseptic, diuretic, carminative, expectorant, laxative (mild), rubefacient, stimulant.

PRINCIPAL CONSTITUENTS
Allyl isothiocyanate (75 per cent), with phenylethyl isothiocyanate (which is produced only when the plant is bruised or crushed).

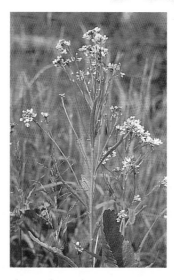

Armoracia rusticana

AROMATHERAPY/ HOME USE

None. 'This is one of the most hazardous of all essential oils. It should not be used in therapy either externally or internally.'[8]

OTHER USES

Used mainly in minute amounts in seasonings, ready-made salads, condiments and canned products.

DISTRIBUTION

Its origins are uncertain, but probably native to eastern Europe. It is now common throughout Russia, Europe and Scandinavia.

OTHER SPECIES

Possibly a cultivated form of Cochlearia macrocarpa, *a native of Hungary.*

Arnica montana

Arnica

FAMILY: ASTERACEAE (COMPOSITAE) SYNONYMS: *A. FULGENS*, *A. SORORIA*, LEOPARD'S BANE, WOLF'S BANE

Herbal/Folk Tradition

This herb stimulates the peripheral blood supply when applied externally, and is considered one of the best remedies for bruises and sprains. It helps relieve rheumatic pain and other painful or inflammatory skin conditions, as long as the skin is not broken! It is never used internally because of toxicity levels.

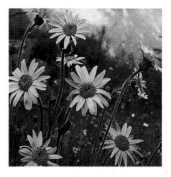

Arnica montana

EXTRACTION

Essential oil by steam distillation of 1. flowers, and 2. root. The yield of essential oil is very small. An absolute, tincture and resinoid are also produced.

CHARACTERISTICS

1. A yellowy-orange liquid with a greenish-blue hint and a strong bitter-spicy scent reminiscent of radish. 2. Dark yellow or butter-brown oil more viscous than the flower oil, with a strong bitter scent.

ACTIONS

Anti-inflammatory, stimulant, vulnerary.

PRINCIPAL CONSTITUENTS

Thymohydroquinone dimethyl ether (80 per cent approx.), isobutyric ester of phlorol (20 per cent approx.) and other minor traces.

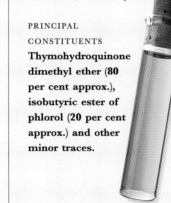

AROMATHERAPY/ HOME USE

None.

OTHER USES

The tincture is employed mainly in pharmaceutical skin products. The oil from the flowers finds occasional use in herbaceous-type perfumes. It is also used to flavour certain liqueurs.

DISTRIBUTION

Native to northern and central Europe; also found growing wild in Russia, Scandinavia and northern India. The oil is produced mainly in France, Belgium and Germany.

OTHER SPECIES

A related plant, A. cordifolia, and other species of arnica are used in the USA, where it is known as 'mountain tobacco'.

A perennial alpine herb with a creeping underground stem, giving rise to a rosette of pale oval leaves. The flowering, erect stem is up to 60cm (24in) high, bearing a single, bright yellow, daisy-like flower. The whole plant is very difficult to cultivate.

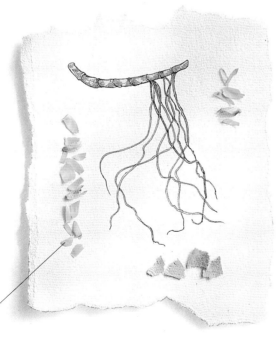

dried arnica petals

Artemisia absinthium

Wormwood

FAMILY: ASTERACEAE (COMPOSITAE)   **SYNONYMS:** COMMON WORMWOOD,
GREEN GINGER, ARMOISE, ABSINTHIUM (OIL)

Herbal/Folk Tradition

Used as an aromatic-bitter for anorexia, as a digestive
tonic and as a choleretic for liver and gall bladder
disorders, usually in the form of a dilute extract. It is
also used to promote menstruation, reduce fever and
expel worms. It was once used as a remedy for epilepsy
and as an aromatic strewing herb to banish fleas.

*A perennial herb
up to 1.5m (5ft)
high with a
whitish stem,
silvery-green,
divided leaves
covered in silky
fine hairs, and
pale yellow
flowers.*

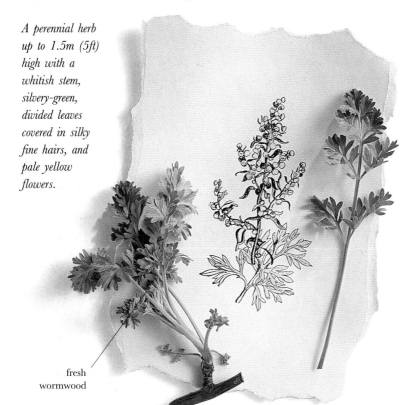

fresh
wormwood

EXTRACTION
**Essential oil by steam
distillation from the leaves
and flowering tops. (An
absolute is occasionally
produced by solvent
extraction.)**

CHARACTERISTICS
**A dark green or bluish oil with
a spicy, warm, bitter-green
odour and a sharp, fresh top
note. The 'de-thujonized' oil
blends well with oakmoss,
jasmine, orange blossom,
lavender and hyacinth.**

ACTIONS
**Anthelmintic,
choleretic,
deodorant,
emmenagogue,
febrifuge,
insect
repellant,
narcotic,
stimulant
(digestive), tonic,
vermifuge.**

PRINCIPAL CONSTITUENTS
**Thujone (up to 71 per
cent), azulenes, terpenes.**

AROMATHERAPY/ HOME USE
*None. 'Should not be used in
therapy either internally or
externally.'[9] Habitual use can
cause restlessness, nightmares,
convulsions, vomiting and, in
extreme cases, brain damage.
In 1915 the French banned
the production of the drink
Absinthe with this plant,
because of its narcotic and
habit forming properties.*

OTHER USES
*Occasionally used in rubefacient
pharmaceutical preparations and
as a fragrance component in
toiletries, cosmetics and perfumes.
Widely employed (at minute levels)
as a flavouring agent in alcoholic
bitters and vermouths; also to a
lesser extent in soft drinks and
some foods, especially confectionery
and desserts.*

DISTRIBUTION
*Native to Europe, North Africa,
and western Asia; naturalized in
North America. Extensively grown
in central and southern Europe,
Russia, North Africa and the USA,
where the oil is mainly produced.*

OTHER SPECIES
*There are many other Artemisia
species such as davana and the
Roman wormwood. See also entry
on mugwort (A. vulgaris).*

Artemisia dracunculus

Tarragon

FAMILY: ASTERCEAE (COMPOSITAE) **SYNONYMS:** ESTRAGON (OIL), LITTLE DRAGON, RUSSIAN TARRAGON

Herbal/Folk Tradition

The leaf is commonly used as a domestic herb, especially with chicken and fish, and to make tarragon vinegar. The name is thought to derive from an ancient use as an antidote to the bites of venomous creatures and 'madde dogges'. It was favoured by maharajahs of India who took it as a tisane, and in Persia it was used to induce appetite. 'The leaves, which are chiefly used, are heating and drying, and good for those that have the flux, or any prenatural discharge.'[10] The leaf was also formerly used for digestive and menstrual irregularities, while the root was employed as a remedy for toothache.

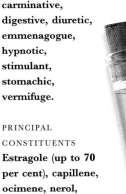

fresh tarragon

A perennial herb with smooth narrow leaves; an erect stem up to 1.2m (4ft) tall, and small yellowy-green, inconspicuous flowers.

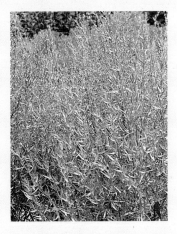

Artemisia dracunculus

AROMATHERAPY/ HOME USE

Digestive System: *Anorexia, dyspepsia, flatulence, hiccoughs, intestinal spasm, nervous indigestion, sluggish digestion.*
Genito-urinary System: *Amenorrhea, dysmenorrhea, PMT.*

OTHER USES

Used as a fragrance component in soaps, detergents, cosmetics and perfumes. Employed as a flavour ingredient in most major food categories, especially condiments and relishes, as well as alcoholic and soft drinks.

DISTRIBUTION

Native to Europe, southern Russia and western Asia. Now cultivated worldwide, especially in Europe and the USA. The oil is produced mainly in France, the Netherlands, Hungary and the USA.

OTHER SPECIES

The so-called French tarragon or 'sativa', which is cultivated as a garden herb, is a smaller plant with a sharper flavour than the Russian type and is a sterile derivative of the wild species.

EXTRACTION
Essential oil by steam distillation from the leaves.

CHARACTERISTICS
A colourless or pale yellow mobile liquid (turning yellow with age), with a sweet-anisic, spicy-green scent. It blends well with labdanum, galbanum, lavender, oakmoss, vanilla, pine and basil.

ACTIONS
Anthelmintic, antiseptic, antispasmodic, aperitif, carminative, digestive, diuretic, emmenagogue, hypnotic, stimulant, stomachic, vermifuge.

PRINCIPAL CONSTITUENTS
Estragole (up to 70 per cent), capillene, ocimene, nerol, phellandrene, thujone and cineol, among others.

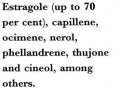

Artemisia vulgaris

Mugwort

FAMILY: ASTERACEAE (COMPOSITAE) **SYNONYMS:** ARMOISE, WILD WORMWOOD, FELON HERB, ST JOHN'S PLANT

Herbal/Folk Tradition

In Europe, the herb has been associated with superstition and witchcraft and was seen as a protective charm against evil and danger. It is said that St John the Baptist wore a girdle of the leaves in the wilderness. It was also seen as a woman's plant, used as a womb tonic, for painful or delayed menstruation and as a treatment for hysteria and epilepsy. It was also used to expel worms, control fever and as a digestive remedy.

In the East the white fluffy underside of the leaves is used for moxibustion, a process often combined with acupuncture, in which the compressed dried herb is burned over a certain point in the body to stimulate it with heat. Moxa was also used in Europe to relieve gout and rheumatism.

It is current in the British Herbal Pharmacopoeia as a specific for amenorrhea and dysmenorrhea.

An erect, much-branched, perennial herb up to 1.5m (5ft) high, with purplish stems, dark green divided leaves that are downy white beneath, and numerous small reddish-brown or yellow flowers.

dried mugwort leaves

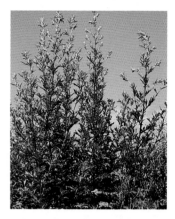

Artemisia vulgaris

AROMATHERAPY/ HOME USE

None. 'It should not be used in therapy either internally or externally.'[11]

OTHER USES

Used as a fragrance component in soaps, colognes and perfumes. Limited use in flavouring due to toxic levels of thujone.

DISTRIBUTION

Believed to have originated in eastern Europe and western Asia; now found in temperate zones all over the world. The oil is produced in southern France, Morocco, Germany, Hungary, India, China and Japan.

OTHER SPECIES

There are many different species in the Artemisia *group (see Botanical Classification), which includes wormwood and tarragon. There are also several different types of mugwort such as the great mugwort (A. arborescens) and the Chinese mugwort (A. moxa and A. sinensis), which are both used to make 'moxa' in Japan, containing mainly borneol.*

EXTRACTION
Essential oil by steam distillation from the leaves and flowering tops.

CHARACTERISTICS
A colourless or pale yellow liquid with a powerful camphoraceous, bitter-sweet, herbaceous odour. It blends well with oakmoss, patchouli, rosemary, lavandin, pine, sage, clary sage and cedarwood.

ACTIONS
Anthelmintic, antispasmodic, carminative, choleretic, diaphoretic, diuretic, emmenagogue, nervine, orexigenic, stimulant, stomachic, tonic (uterine, womb), vermifuge.

PRINCIPAL CONSTITUENTS
Thujone, cineol, pinenes and dihydromatricaria ester, among others.

Asarum canadense

Snakeroot

FAMILY: ARISTOLOCHIACEAE **SYNONYMS:** WILD GINGER, INDIAN GINGER

Herbal/Folk Tradition

This plant has been employed for centuries in folk medicine but is now little prescribed. It used to be used for chronic chest complaints, dropsy, rheumatism and painful bowel and stomach spasms. It was also considered a 'valuable stimulant in cases of amenorrhoea and colds' and for 'promoting a copious perspiration'.[12] The name (of the Virginian variety at least) derives from its use in aiding the body to combat nettle rash, poison ivy and some snake bites.

EXTRACTION
Essential oil by steam distillation from dried rhizomes and crushed roots.

CHARACTERISTICS
A brownish-yellow or amber liquid with a warm, woody-spicy, rich, ginger-like odour. It blends well with bergamot, costus, oakmoss, patchouli, pine needle, clary sage, mimosa, cassie and other florals.

ACTIONS
Anti-inflammatory, antispasmodic, carminative, diuretic, diaphoretic, emmenagogue, expectorant, febrifuge, stimulant, stomachic.

PRINCIPAL CONSTITUENTS
Pinene, linalol, borneol, terpineol, geraniol, eugenol and methyl eugenol, among others.

AROMATHERAPY/ HOME USE

May possibly be used for its antispasmodic qualities, for example, for period pains or indigestion.

OTHER USES

Occasionally used in perfumery work. Used mainly as a flavouring agent with other spicy materials, especially in confectionery.

DISTRIBUTION

Native to North America, especially North Carolina, Kansas and Canada. The oil is produced in the USA mainly from wild-growing plants.

OTHER SPECIES

It should not be confused with 'serpentaria oil' from the Virginian snakeroot (Aristolochia serpentaria), which belongs to the same botanical family but contains asarone and is considered toxic.

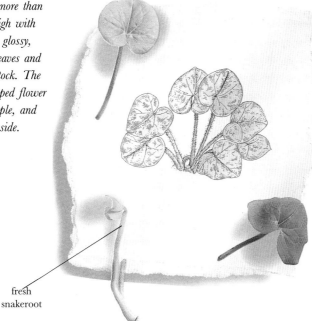

An inconspicuous but fragrant little plant not more than 35cm (14in) high with hairy stem, two glossy, kidney-shaped leaves and a creeping rootstock. The solitary bell-shaped flower is brownish purple, and creamy white inside.

fresh
snakeroot

Betula alba

White birch

FAMILY: BETULACEAE **SYNONYMS:** *B. ALBA VAR. PUBESCENS, B. ODORATA, B. PENDULA,* EUROPEAN WHITE BIRCH, SILVER BIRCH

Herbal/Folk Tradition

Birch buds were formerly used as a tonic in hair preparations. Birch tar is used in Europe for all types of chronic skin complaints: psoriasis, eczema, etc. In Scandinavia the young birch leaflets and twigs are used in the sauna to tone the skin and promote the circulation. The sap is also tapped and drunk as a tonic. Buds, leaves and bark are used for 'rheumatic and arthritic conditions, especially where kidney functions appear to need support . . . oedematous states; urinary infections and calculi.'[13]

Decorative tree, up to 15–20m (49–65ft) high, with slender branches, silvery-white bark broken into scales, and light green oval leaves. The male catkins are 2–5cm (1–2in) long, the female up to 15cm (6in) long.

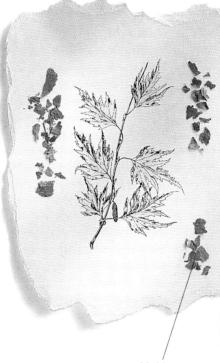

dried leaves

AROMATHERAPY/ HOME USE

Skin Care: *Dermatitis, dull or congested skin, eczema, hair care, psoriasis, etc.*

Circulation, Muscles and Joints: *Accumulation of toxins, arthritis, cellulitis, muscular pain, obesity, edema, poor circulation, rheumatism.*

OTHER USES

Birch bud oil is used primarily in hair tonics and shampoos, and in some cosmetics for its potential skin-healing effects. The crude tar is used in pharmaceutical preparations, ointments, lotions, etc., for dermatological diseases. It is also used in soap and leather manufacture – rectified birch tar oil provides the heart for many 'leather' type perfumes and aftershaves.

DISTRIBUTION

Native to the northern hemisphere; found throughout eastern Europe, Russia, Germany, Sweden, Finland, the Baltic coast, northern China and Japan.

OTHER SPECIES

Many cultivars exist of this species of birch. The paper birch (B. papyrifera) and B. verrucosa are also used for the production of birch oil and/ or birch tar.
NB. Should not be confused with the oil from the sweet birch (B. lenta), which is potentially toxic.

EXTRACTION
**1. Essential oil by steam distillation from the leaf-buds.
2. Crude birch tar is extracted by slow destructive distillation from the bark; this is subsequently steam-distilled to yield a rectified birch tar oil.**

CHARACTERISTICS
1. Pale yellow, viscous oil with a woody-green balsamic scent. It crystallizes at low temperatures. 2. The crude tar is an almost black, thick oily mass. The rectified oil is a brownish-yellow, clear oily liquid with a smoky, tar-like, 'Russian leather' odour. It blends well with other woody and balsamic oils.

ACTIONS
Anti-inflammatory, antiseptic, cholagogue, diaphoretic, diuretic, febrifuge, tonic.

PRINCIPAL CONSTITUENTS
1. Mainly betulenol and other sesquiterpenes. 2. In the tar oil: phenol, cresol, xylenol, guaiacol, creosol, pyrocatechol, pyrobetulin (which gives the 'leather' scent).

Betula lenta

Sweet birch

SAFETY DATA *Methyl salicylate, the major constituent, is not exactly toxic but very harmful in concentration*

FAMILY: BETULACEAE **SYNONYMS:** *B. CAPINEFOLIA*, CHERRY BIRCH, SOUTHERN BIRCH, MAHOGANY BIRCH, MOUNTAIN MAHOGANY

Herbal/Folk Tradition

The cambium (the layer directly under the bark) is eaten in the spring, cut into strips like vermicelli. The bark, in the form of an infusion, is used as a general stimulant and to promote sweating. As a decoction or syrup, it is used as a tonic for dysentery and is said to be useful in genito-urinary irritation. The flavour of wintergreen and birch bark, in the form of a tea, was popular with Native Americans and European settlers. More recently, this has been translated into a preference for 'root beer' flavourings.

A graceful tree about 25m (82ft) high, which has a pyramidal shape while young. It has bright green leaves and a dark reddish-brown aromatic bark, which is broken into plates or patches.

a sprig of
sweet birch

aromatic bark

EXTRACTION
Essential oil by steam distillation of the bark macerated in warm water.

CHARACTERISTICS
Colourless, pale yellow or reddish tinted liquid with an intense, sweet-woody, wintergreen-like scent.

ACTIONS
Analgesic, anti-inflammatory, antipyretic, antirheumatic, antiseptic, astringent, depurative, diuretic, rubefacient, tonic.

PRINCIPAL CONSTITUENTS
Almost entirely methyl salicylate (98 per cent), produced during the maceration process. It is almost identical in composition to wintergreen oil.

AROMATHERAPY/ HOME USE

None. 'It [Methyl salicylate] can be absorbed through the skin, and fatal poisoning via this route has been reported.'[14] It is also classed as an environmental hazard or marine pollutant.

OTHER USES

Limited use as a counter-irritant in anti-arthritic and antineuralgic ointments and analgesic balms. Limited use as a fragrance component in cosmetics and perfumes; extensively used as a flavouring agent, especially 'root beer', chewing gum, toothpaste, etc., (usually very low-level use).

DISTRIBUTION

Native to southern Canada and south-eastern USA; produced mainly in Pennsylvania.

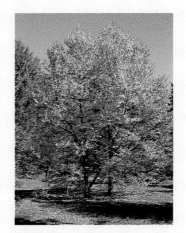

Betula lenta

OTHER SPECIES

There are numerous species of birch, spanning several continents, such as black birch (B. nigra) found in North America. Not to be confused with the European white birch (B. alba), which produced birch tar oil used in chronic skin diseases.

Boronia megastigma

Boronia

FAMILY: RUTACEAE **SYNONYMS:** BROWN BORONIA

Herbal/Folk Tradition

'A botanist in the Victorian era suggested this species would be suitable for graveyard planting because of its dark flowers!'[15]

A bushy evergreen shrub, up to 2m (6ft) high, which bears an abundance of fragrant, nodding flowers with an unusual colouring – the petals are brown on the outside, yellow on the inside. Often grown as an ornamental shrub in gardens.

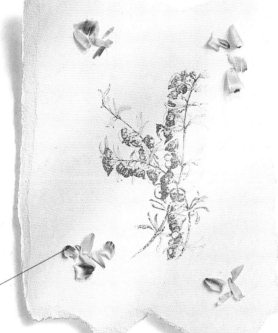

dried flowers

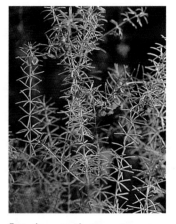

Boronia megastigma

AROMATHERAPY/ HOME USE

Perfume.

OTHER USES

The absolute is used in high-class perfumery work, especially florals. Used in specialized flavour work, especially rich fruit products.

DISTRIBUTION

Native to Western Australia; grows wild all over west and south-west Australia.

OTHER SPECIES

There are over fifteen species of boronia found in Western Australia; B. megastigma is one of the most common and the only one used for its perfume; other types smell of sarsaparilla, lemons or roses! Boronia is botanically related to the citrus tree.

EXTRACTION
A concrete and absolute by the enfleurage method or petroleum-ether extraction, from the flowers. An essential oil is also produced in small quantities by steam distillation.

CHARACTERISTICS
The concrete is a dark green butter-like mass with a beautiful warm, woody-sweet fragrance; the absolute is a green viscous liquid with a fresh, fruity-spicy scent and a rich, tenacious, floral undertone. It blends well with **clary sage, sandalwood, bergamot, violet, helichrysum, costus, mimosa and other florals.**

ACTIONS
Aromatic.

PRINCIPAL CONSTITUENTS
Notably ionone; also eugenol, triacontane, phenols, ethyl alcohol, and ethyl formate, among others.

Boswellia carteri

Frankincense

FAMILY: BURSERACEA **SYNONYMS:** OLIBANUM, GUM THUS

Herbal/Folk Tradition

Used since antiquity as an incense in India, China and in the West by the Catholic Church. In ancient Egypt it was used in rejuvenating face masks, cosmetics and perfumes. It has been used medicinally in the East and West for a wide range of conditions including syphilis, rheumatism, respiratory and urinary tract infections, skin diseases, as well as digestive and nervous complaints.

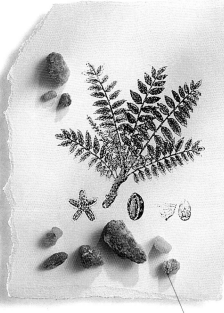

gum resin

A handsome small tree or shrub with abundant pinnate leaves and white or pale pink flowers. It yields a natural oleo gum resin.

AROMATHERAPY/ HOME USE

Skin Care: *Blemishes, dry and mature complexions, scars, wounds, wrinkles.*
Respiratory System: *Asthma, bronchitis, catarrh, coughs, laryngitis.*
Genito-urinary System: *Cystitis, dysmenorrhea, leucorrhea, metrorrhagia.*
Immune System: *Colds, flu.*
Nervous System: *Anxiety, nervous tension and stress-related conditions – 'Frankincense has, among its physical properties, the ability to slow down and deepen the breath ... which is very conducive to prayer and meditation.'[16]*

OTHER USES

The gum and oil are used as fixatives and fragrance components in soaps, cosmetics and perfumes,

especially oriental, spice and men's fragrances. Employed in some pharmaceuticals such as liniments and throat pastilles. Extensively used in the manufacture of incense. The oil is used in minute amounts in some foods (such as meat products), alcoholic and soft drinks.

DISTRIBUTION

Native to the Red Sea region; grows wild throughout north-east Africa. The gum is produced mainly in Somalia, Ethiopia, China and south Arabia, then distilled in Europe and India.

OTHER SPECIES

Other Boswellia *species also yield olibanum gum, such as the Indian variety* B. serrata. *Constituents vary according to type and locality. See also Botanical Classification section.*

EXTRACTION

Essential oil by steam distillation from selected oleo gum resin (approx. 3–10 per cent oil to 60–70 per cent resin). An absolute is also produced, for use mainly as a fixative.

CHARACTERISTICS

A pale yellow or greenish mobile liquid with a fresh, terpeney top note and a warm, rich, sweet-balsamic undertone. It blends well with sandalwood, pine, vetiver, geranium, lavender, mimosa, orange blossom, orange, bergamot, camphor, basil, pepper, cinnamon and other spices. It modifies the sweetness of citrus blends in an intriguing way.

ACTIONS

Anti-inflammatory, antiseptic, astringent, carminative, cicatrizant, cytophylactic, digestive, diuretic, emmenagogue, expectorant, sedative, tonic, uterine, vulnerary.

PRINCIPAL CONSTITUENTS

Mainly monoterpene hydrocarbons, notably pinene, dipentene, limonene, thujone, phellandrene, cymene, myrcene, terpinene; also octyl acetate, octanol, incensole, among others.

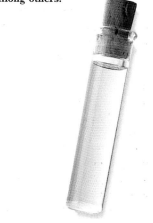

Brassica nigra

Mustard

SAFETY DATA *Oral toxin, dermal toxin, mucous membrane irritant.*
It is considered one of the most toxic of all essential oils

FAMILY: BRASSICACEAE (CRUCIFERAE) **SYNONYMS:** *SINAPSIS NIGRA*, *B. SINAPIOIDES*, BLACK MUSTARD

Herbal/Folk Tradition

The seeds are highly esteemed as a condiment and for their medicinal qualities. They have been used in the East and West to aid the digestion, warm the stomach and promote the appetite, and for cold, stiff or feverish conditions such as colds, chills, coughs, chilblains, rheumatism, arthritis, lumbago and general aches and pains.

EXTRACTION

Essential oil by steam (or water) distillation from the black mustard seeds, which have been macerated in warm water.

CHARACTERISTICS

A colourless or pale yellow liquid with a sharp, penetrating, acrid odour.

ACTIONS

Aperitif, antimicrobial, antiseptic, diuretic, emetic, febrifuge, rubefacient (produces blistering of the skin), stimulant.

PRINCIPAL CONSTITUENTS

Allyl isothiocyanate (99 per cent). NB: Black mustard seed or powder does not contain this constituent, which is formed only by contact with water during the production of the essential oil.

AROMATHERAPY/ HOME USE

None. 'It should not be used in therapy either externally or internally.'[17]

OTHER USES

Used in certain rubefacient or counter-irritant liniments. Used extensively by the food industry especially in pickles, seasonings and sauces. Little used as a fragrance component except in cat and dog repellents.

DISTRIBUTION

Common throughout south-eastern Europe, southern Siberia, Asia Minor and North Africa; naturalized in North and South America. Cultivated for its seed and oil in Britain, The Netherlands, Denmark, Germany and Italy.

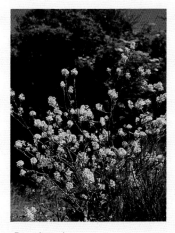

Brassica nigra

An erect annual up to 3m (10ft) high, with spear-shaped upper leaves, smooth flat pods containing about ten dark brown seeds, and bright yellow cabbage-like flowers.

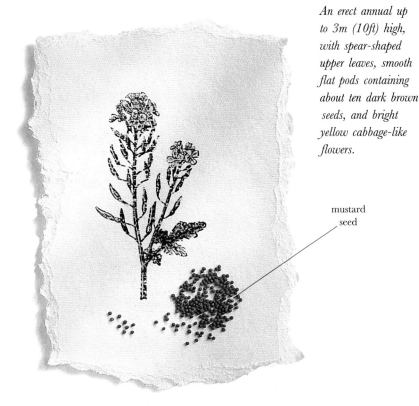

mustard seed

OTHER SPECIES

The Russian variety is known as brown mustard or 'sarepta' (B. juncea); the white mustard (B. alba) does not contain any essential oil. Also closely related is rape (B. napus) and other local species that are used in India and China.

Bulnesia sarmienti

Guaiacwood

SAFETY DATA *Non-toxic, non-irritant, non-sensitizing*

FAMILY: ZYGOPHYLLACEAE SYNONYMS: CHAMPACA WOOD (OIL), 'PALO SANTO',
PALO BALSAMO, PARAGUAY LIGNUM

Herbal/Folk Tradition

The wood is much used for ornamental carving. It was
formerly used for treating rheumatism and gout; guaiacum
is still current in the British Herbal Pharmacopoeia as
a specific for rheumatism and rheumatoid arthritis.
Valnet includes guaiacum in his 'elixirs' for gout,
venereal disease and in mouthwashes.

In recent years Guaiacwood oil has been
used in Bulgaria as a common adulterant for
rose oil, due to its tea rose-like odour. It can
be recognized, however, by the microscopic
examination of its principal consitutent, guaiol,
which forms sharp needle-like crystals that
separate from the oil on cooling. The addition
of guaiacwood oil to rose oil also raises the
congealing point of the oil and increases its
specific gravity so that its presence as an
adulterant may be quite easily detected.

*A small, wild tropical tree
up to 4m (13ft) high, with
a decorative hard wood.*

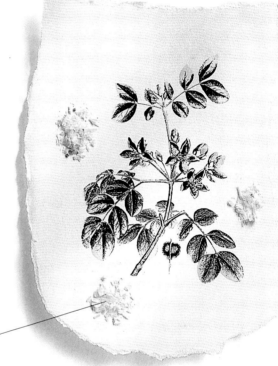

guaiacwood
sawdust

EXTRACTION
**Essential oil by steam
distillation from the broken
wood and sawdust.**

CHARACTERISTICS
**A yellow, amber or greenish,
soft or semi-solid mass with
a pleasant, tea rose-type
fragrance and sometimes an
unpleasant smoky undertone.
It blends well with geranium,
orange blossom, oakmoss,
rose, costus, sandalwood,
amyris, spice and
woody-floral bases.**

ACTIONS
**Anti-inflammatory,
anti-oxidant,
antirheumatic,
antiseptic,
diaphoretic, diuretic,
laxative.**

PRINCIPAL CONSTITUENTS
**Guaiol (42–72 per cent),
bulnesol, bulnesene,
guaiene, patchoulene,
guaioxide, among others.**

AROMATHERAPY/ HOME USE
**Circulation, muscles and
joints:** *Arthritis, gout, rheumatoid
arthritis.*

OTHER USES
*The fluid extract and tincture are
used in pharmacology, mainly as
a diagnostic reagent in blood tests.
Used as a fixative and fragrance
component in soaps, cosmetics
and perfumes. Guaiacwood oil is
used as a flavour component in
most categories of food product as
well as in drinks. It is also used
in food as an anti-oxidant.*

DISTRIBUTION
*Native to South America,
especially Paraguay and Argentina.
Some oil is distilled in Europe
and the USA.*

OTHER SPECIES
*Distinct from guaiac gum and
guaiac resin, known as guaiacum,
obtained from related trees
Guaiacum officinale and G.
sanctum. However, they are
somewhat similar products
and share common properties.*

Bursera glabrifolia

Linaloe

FAMILY: BURSERACEAE SYNONYMS: *B. DELPECHIANA*, MEXICAN LINALOE, 'COPAL LIMON'

Herbal/Folk Tradition

The seed oil is known in India as 'Indian lavender oil' and used chiefly as a local perfume ingredient and in soaps by the cosmetics industry of Mysore state. It is not much found outside India. In Mexico the wood oil is used in a similar fashion to rosewood, which contains similar constituents.

A tall, bushy tropical shrub or tree, with a smooth bark and bearing fleshy fruit. The wood is used only for distillation purposes when the tree is twenty or thirty years old. The oil is partially a pathological product since its production is stimulated by lacerating the trunk – which apparently must be wounded on the night of the full moon for the tree to produce any oil!

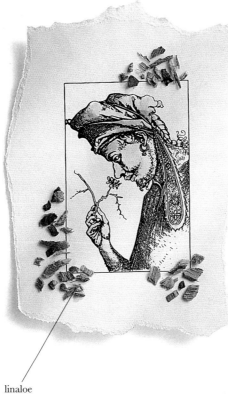

linaloe
chippings

EXTRACTION
Essential oil by steam distillation from the 1. wood, and 2. seed and husk. (An essential oil is also occasionally produced from the leaves and twigs.)

CHARACTERISTICS
1. A pale yellow liquid with a sweet-woody, floral scent, similar to rosewood. It blends well with rose, sandalwood, cedarwood, rosewood, frankincense, floral and woody fragrances. 2. A colourless liquid with a terpene-like odour, harsher than the wood oil.

ACTIONS
Anticonvulsant, anti-inflammatory, antiseptic, bactericidal, deodorant, gentle tonic.

PRINCIPAL CONSTITUENTS
1. Mainly linalol, some linalyl acetate. 2. Mainly linalyl acetate, some linalol.

AROMATHERAPY/ HOME USE

Skin Care: *Acne, cuts, dermatitis, wounds, etc., all skin types.*
Nervous System: *Nervous tension and stress-related conditions.*

OTHER USES

The wood oil is used in soaps, toiletries and perfumes. It is also used for the production of natural linalol, *although this is increasingly being replaced by synthetic linalol.*

DISTRIBUTION

Native to Central and South America, especially Mexico. It is cultivated in the Far East particularly in India (Mysore). The wood oil is produced mainly in Mexico; the seed (and husk) oil in India.

OTHER SPECIES

There are several species all known simply as linaloe: see Botanical Classification section. West Indian elemi (B. simaruba) is a close relative, as are myrrh and frankincense.

Calamintha officinalis

Calamintha

FAMILY: LAMIACEAE (LABIATAE)   **SYNONYMS:** *C. CLINOPODIUM, MELISSA CALAMINTA,* CALAMINT, COMMON CALAMINT, MILL MOUNTAIN, MOUNTAIN BALM, MOUNTAIN MINT, BASIL THYME, NEPETA (OIL), FRENCH MARJORAM (OIL), WILD BASIL (OIL), CATNIP (OIL)

Herbal/Folk Tradition

It has a long history of use as a herbal remedy mainly for nervous and digestive complaints, also menstrual pain, colds, chills and cramp. Catmint is current in the British Herbal Pharmacopoeia as a specific for flatulent colic in children and for the common cold.

An erect, bushy, perennial plant not more than 1m (3ft) high, with square stems, soft oval serrated leaves greyish-green beneath, and rather inconspicuous pale purple flowers. The whole plant has a strong aromatic scent, which is attractive to cats.

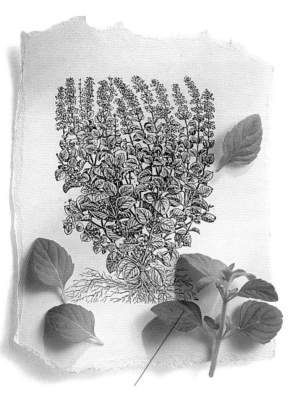

fresh
calamintha

AROMATHERAPY/ HOME USE

Circulation, Muscles and Joints: *Chills, cold in the joints, muscular aches and pains, rheumatism.*
Digestive System: *Colic, flatulence, nervous dyspepsia.*
Nervous System: *Insomnia, nervous tension and stress-related conditions.*

OTHER USES

Used as a wild cat lure in the USA. Occasionally used in perfumery work.

DISTRIBUTION

Native to Europe and parts of Asia (Himalayas), naturalized throughout North America and South Africa. Cultivated for its oil in the Mediterranean region, former Yugoslavia, Poland and in the USA.

OTHER SPECIES

There are numerous similar species found throughout the world, such as the lesser calamintha (C. nepeta), which has a stronger odour and is often used interchangeably with common calamint. It is also closely related to catmint or catnip (Nepeta cataria) also known as calamint, with which it shares similar properties. Not to be confused with winter and summer savory (Satureja montana and S. hortensis). (The Chinese shrub Actinidia poly-gama also contains metatabilacetone, which is responsible for its hallucinogenic and narcotic effects.)

EXTRACTION
Essential oil by steam distillation from the flowering tops.

CHARACTERISTICS
A pale yellow liquid with a herbaceous-woody, pungent odour, somewhat resembling pennyroyal.

ACTIONS
Anesthetic (local), antirheumatic, antispasmodic, astringent, carminative, diaphoretic, emmenagogue, febrifuge, nervine, sedative, tonic.

PRINCIPAL CONSTITUENTS
Citral, nerol, citronellol, limonene and geraniol, among others. The active ingredient that attracts cats is meta-tabilacetone (3–5 per cent). Constituents vary according to source.

Calamintha officinalis

Calendula officinalis

Marigold

FAMILY: ASTERACEAE (COMPOSITAE)   **SYNONYMS:** CALENDULA, MARYGOLD, MARYBUD, GOLD-BLOOM, POT MARIGOLD, HOLLYGOLD, COMMON MARIGOLD, POET'S MARIGOLD

Herbal/Folk Tradition

A herb of ancient medical repute, said to 'comfort the heart and spirits'. It was also used for skin complaints, menstrual irregularities, varicose veins, hemorrhoids, conjunctivitis and poor eyesight. The flowers are current in the British Herbal Pharmacopoeia, specific for enlarged or inflamed lymph nodes, sebaceous cysts, duodenal ulcers and inflammatory skin lesions.

The infused oil is useful for a wide range of skin problems including cracked and rough skin, nappy rash, grazes, cracked nipples, varicose veins and inflammations.

An annual herb up to 60cm (24in) high with soft, oval, pale green leaves and bright orange, daisy-like flowers.

marigold petals

flower head

EXTRACTION
An absolute by solvent extraction from the flowers. The real calendula absolute is produced only in small quantities and is difficult to get hold of.

CHARACTERISTICS
A dark greenish-brown viscous liquid with an intensely sharp, herbaceous odour. It blends well with oakmoss, hyacinth, floral and citrus oils.

ACTIONS
Antihemorrhagic, anti-inflammatory, antiseptic, antispasmodic, astringent, diaphoretic, cholagogue, cicatrizant, emmenagogue, febrifuge, fungicidal, styptic, tonic, vulnerary.

PRINCIPAL CONSTITUENTS
The absolute contains calendulin (a yellow resin), waxes and volatile oil.

AROMATHERAPY/ HOME USE

Skin Care: *Burns, cuts, eczema, greasy skin, inflammations, insect bites, rashes, wounds.*
NB: 'The infused oil is very valuable in Aromatherapy for its powerful skin-healing properties.'[18]

OTHER USES
Used in high-class perfumery.

DISTRIBUTION
Native to southern Europe and Egypt; naturalized throughout temperate regions of the world. Widely cultivated, especially in northern Europe for domestic and medicinal use. The absolute is produced only in France.

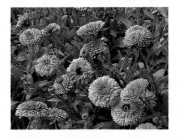

Calendula officinalis

OTHER SPECIES
There are several species of marigold, but the common marigold is the one generally used medicinally. It should not be confused with tagetes or taget from the Mexican marigold (Tagetes minuta) or the African marigold (T. erecta), the oil of which is also often called 'calendula'.

Cananga odorata

Cananga

FAMILY: ANNONACEAE **SYNONYMS:** *C. ODORATUM VAR. MACROPHYLLA*

Herbal/Folk Tradition

Used locally for infectious illnesses, for example, malaria. The beautiful flowers are also used for decorative purposes at festivals.

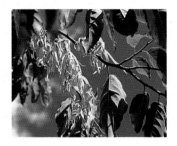

Cananga odorata

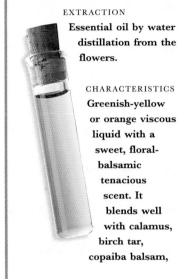

EXTRACTION
Essential oil by water distillation from the flowers.

CHARACTERISTICS
Greenish-yellow or orange viscous liquid with a sweet, floral-balsamic tenacious scent. It blends well with calamus, birch tar, copaiba balsam, labdanum, orange blossom, oakmoss, jasmine, guaiacwood and oriental-type bases.

ACTIONS
Antiseptic, antidepressant, aphrodisiac, hypotensive, nervine, sedative, tonic.

PRINCIPAL CONSTITUENTS
Caryophyllene, benzyl acetate, benzyl alcohol, farnesol, terpineol, borneol, geranyl acetate, safrol, linalol, limonene, methyl salicylate and over 100 minor components.

AROMATHERAPY/ HOME USE

Skin Care: *Insect bites, fragrance, general skin care.*
Nervous Systems: *Anxiety, depression, nervous tension and stress-related complaints.*

OTHER USES

Fragrance component in soaps, detergents, cosmetics and perfumes, especially men's fragrances. Limited use as a flavour ingredient in some food products, alcoholic and soft drinks.

DISTRIBUTION

Native to tropical Asia; Java, Malaysia, the Philippines, the Moluccas.

OTHER SPECIES

Very closely related to the tree that produces ylang ylang oil (C. odorate var. genuina). Cananga is considered an inferior product in perfumery work; being grown in different regions, the oil has a different quality, heavier and less delicate than ylang ylang. However, cananga is truly a 'complete' oil, whereas ylang ylang is made into several distillates.

A tall tropical tree, up to 30m (98ft) high, which flowers all year round. It bears large, fragrant, tender, yellow flowers that are virtually identical to those of the ylang ylang.

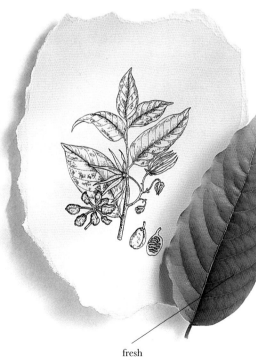

fresh
cananga
leaf

Cananga odorata var. genuina

Ylang ylang

FAMILY: ANNONACEAE **SYNONYMS:** *UNONA ODORANTISSIMUM,* FLOWER OF FLOWERS

Herbal/Folk Tradition

In Indonesia, the flowers are spread on the beds of newly married couples. In the Molucca Islands, an ointment is made from ylang ylang and cucuma flowers for cosmetic and hair care, skin diseases, to prevent fever and fight infections. In the Victorian age, the oil was used in the hair treatment Macassar oil. It was also used to soothe insect bites.

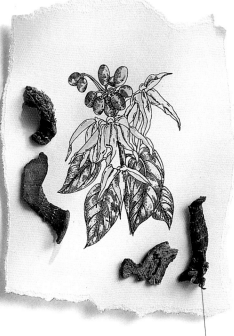

dried ylang ylang

A tall tropical tree up to 20m (65ft) high with large, tender, fragrant flowers, which can be pink, mauve or yellow. The yellow flowers are considered best for the extraction of essential oil.

AROMATHERAPY/ HOME USE

Skin Care: *Acne, hair growth, hair rinse, insect bites, irritated and oily skin, general skin care.*
Circulation, Muscles and Joints: *High blood pressure, hypernea (abnormally fast breathing), tachycardia, palpitations.*
Nervous System: *Depression, frigidity, impotence, insomnia, nervous tension and stress-related disorders – 'The writer, working with odorous materials for more than twenty years, long ago noticed that ... ylang ylang soothes and inhibits anger born of frustration.'[19]*

OTHER USES

Extensively used as a fragrance component and fixative in soaps, *cosmetics and perfumes; ylang ylang extra tends to be used in high-class perfumes, ylang ylang 3 in soaps, detergents, etc. Used as a flavour ingredient, mainly in alcoholic and soft drinks, fruit flavours and desserts.*

DISTRIBUTION

Native to tropical Asia, especially Indonesia and the Philippines. Major oil producers are Madagascar, Reunion and the Comoro Islands.

OTHER SPECIES

Very closely related to cananga (C. odoratum var. macrophylla), although the oil produced from the ylang ylang is considered for perfumery work, having a more refined quality.

EXTRACTION

Essential oil by water or steam distillation from the freshly picked flowers. The first distillate (about 40 per cent) is called ylang ylang extra, which is the top grade. Three further successive distillates are called Grades 1, 2 and 3. A 'complete' oil is also produced that represents the total or 'unfractionated' oil, but this is sometimes constructed by blending ylang ylang 1 and 2 together. (An absolute and concrete are also produced by solvent extraction for their long-lasting floral-balsamic effect.)

CHARACTERISTICS

Ylang ylang extra is a pale yellow, oily liquid with an intensely sweet, soft, floral-balsamic, slightly spicy scent – a good oil has a creamy rich top note. A very intriguing perfume oil in its own right, it also blends well with rosewood, jasmine, vetiver, opopanax, bergamot, mimosa, cassie, Peru balsam, rose, tuberose, costus and others. It is an excellent fixative. The other grades lack the depth and richness of the ylang ylang extra.

ACTIONS

Aphrodisiac, antidepressant, anti-infectious, antiseborrheic, antiseptic, euphoric, hypotensive, nervine, regulator, sedative (nervous), stimulant (circulatory), tonic.

PRINCIPAL CONSTITUENTS

Methyl benzoate, methyl salicylate, methyl paracretol, benzyl acetate, eugenol, geraniol, linalol and terpenes: pinene, cadinene, among others.

Canarium luzonicum

Elemi

SAFETY DATA *Non-toxic, non-irritant, non-sensitizing*

FAMILY: BURSERACEAE **SYNONYMS:** *C. COMMUNE*, MANILA ELEMI, ELEMI GUM, ELEMI RESIN, ELEMI (OLEORESIN)

Herbal/Folk Tradition

The gum or oleoresin is used locally for skin care, respiratory complaints and as a general stimulant. Elemi was one of the aromatics used by the ancient Egyptians for the embalming process.

A tropical tree up to 30m (98ft) high that yields a resinous pathological exudation with a pungent odour. Although it is called a gum, it is almost entirely made up of resin and essential oil.

elemi resin

EXTRACTION
Essential oil by steam distillation from the gum. (A resinoid and resin absolute are also produced in small quantities.)

CHARACTERISTICS
A colourless to pale yellow liquid with a light, fresh, balsamic-spicy, lemon-like odour. It blends well with myrrh, frankincense, labdanum, rosemary, lavender, lavandin, sage, cinnamon and other spices.

ACTIONS
Antiseptic, balsamic, cicatrizant, expectorant, fortifying, regulatory, stimulant, stomachic, tonic.

PRINCIPAL CONSTITUENTS
The gum contains about 10–25 per cent essential oil of mainly phellandrene, dipentene, elemol, elemicin, terpineol, carvone, and terpinolene, among others.

AROMATHERAPY/HOME USE

Skin Care: *Aged skin, infected cuts and wounds, inflammations, rejuvenation, wrinkles – 'signifies drying and preservation'.[20]*
Respiratory System: *Bronchitis, catarrhal conditions, unproductive coughs.*
Nervous System: *Nervous exhaustion and stress-related conditions.*

OTHER USES

Resinoid and oil are used primarily as fixatives but also as fragrance components in soaps, detergents, cosmetics and perfumes. Occasionally used as a flavouring ingredient in food products, alcoholic and soft drinks.

DISTRIBUTION

Native to the Philippine Islands and the Moluccas, where it is also cultivated. Distillation of the oil takes place at source.

OTHER SPECIES

There are several other species of Canarium *that grow wild or are cultivated in the Philippines and*

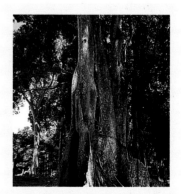

Canarium luzonicum

also yield a 'gum'. It is also closely related to the trees yielding myrrh, frankincense and opopanax.

Carphephorus odoratissimus

Deertongue

FAMILY: ASTERACEAE (COMPOSITAE) **SYNONYMS:** *TRILISA ODORATISSIMA, LIATRIS ODORATISSIMA, FRASERA SOECIOSA,* HOUND'S TONGUE, DEER'S TONGUE, CAROLINE VANILLA, VANILLA LEAF, WILD VANILLA, VANILLA TRILISA, WHART'S TONGUE, LIATRIX (OLEORESIN OR ABSOLUTE)

Herbal/Folk Tradition

The roots have been used for their diuretic effects, and applied locally for sore throats and gonorrhea. It has also been used as a tonic in treating malaria. In folklore the plant is associated with contraception and sterility in women. *Liatris squarrosa* is called 'the rattlesnake' because the roots are used to cure rattlesnake bites. *L. scariosa* is also used for snake bites in American folk medicine.

A herbaceous perennial plant distinguished by a naked receptacle and feathery pappus, with large, fleshy, dark green leaves, clasped at the base. When fresh, the leaves have little odour but when dried they acquire a vanilla-like odour, mainly because of the coumarin that can been seen in crystals on the upper sides of the leaves.

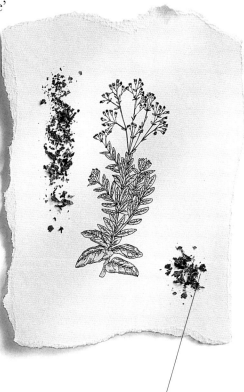

dried
deertongue
leaves

AROMATHERAPY/ HOME USE
None.

OTHER USES
The oleoresin is used as a fixative and fragrance component in soaps, detergents and perfumery work. Used for flavouring tobacco; also employed for the isolation of coumarin. Deertongue is also used to produce a charcoal de-colourized extract (Deertongue incolore), which has been reported to be non-irritating, non-sensitizing and non-phototoxic when applied to the skin of animals and humans. This product is used in perfumery.

DISTRIBUTION
Native to eastern USA; gathered on the savannah land between North Carolina and Florida.

OTHER SPECIES
There are several species of deertongue native to the USA, for example, blazing star or prairie pine (Liatris squarrosa), *and gayfeather* (L. spicata). *Not to be confused with the common vanilla* (Vanilla planifolia) *or with the European hound's tongue* (Cynoglossum officinale), *all of which have been used in herbal medicine.*

EXTRACTION
Oleoresin by solvent extraction from the dried leaves.

CHARACTERISTICS
A dark green, heavy, viscous liquid with a rich, herbaceous, new-mown hay scent. It blends well with oakmoss, labdanum, lavandin, frankincense, clove, patchouli and oriental-type fragrances.

ACTIONS
Antiseptic, demulcent, diaphoretic, diuretic, febrifuge, stimulant, tonic.

PRINCIPAL CONSTITUENTS
Mainly coumarin (1.6 per cent), with dihydrocoumarin and terpenes, aldehydes and ketones. Deertongue has a very complex chemical make-up totalling over 90 identified compounds.

Carum carvi

Caraway

FAMILY: APIACEAE (UMBELLIFERAE) **SYNONYMS:** *APIUM CARVI*, CARUM, CARAWAY FRUITS

Herbal/Folk Tradition

Used extensively as a domestic spice, especially in bread, cakes and cheeses. Traditional remedy for dyspepsia, intestinal colic, menstrual cramps, poor appetite, laryngitis and bronchitis. It promotes milk secretion and is considered specific for flatulent colic in children, according to the British Herbal Pharmacopoeia.

EXTRACTION

Essential oil by steam distillation from the dried ripe seed or fruit (approx. 2–8 per cent yield).

CHARACTERISTICS

Crude caraway oil is a pale yellowish-brown liquid with a harsh, spicy odour. The redistilled oil is colourless to pale yellow, with a strong, warm, sweet-spicy odour, like rye bread. It blends well with jasmine, cinnamon, cassia and other spices; however, it is very overpowering.

ACTIONS

Antihistaminic, antimicrobial, antiseptic, aperitif, astringent, carminative, diuretic, emmenagogue, expectorant, galactagogue, larvicidal, stimulant, spasmolytic, stomachic, tonic, vermifuge.

PRINCIPAL CONSTITUENTS

Mainly carvone (50–60 per cent) and limonene (40 per cent), with carveol, dihydrocarveol, dihydrocarvone, pinene, phellandrene, among others.

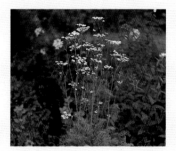

AROMATHERAPY/ HOME USE

Respiratory System: *Bronchitis, coughs, laryngitis.*
Digestive System: *Dyspepsia, colic, flatulence, gastric spasm, nervous indigestion, poor appetite. See also sweet fennel and dill.*
Immune System: *Colds.*

OTHER USES

Used in carminative, stomachic and laxative preparations and as a flavour ingredient in pharmaceuticals; also to mask unpleasant tastes and odours. Fragrance component in toothpaste, mouthwash products, cosmetics and perfumes. Extensively used as a flavour ingredient in most major food categories, especially condiments. The German brandy 'Kummel' is made from the seeds.

DISTRIBUTION

Native to Europe and western Asia, naturalized in North America. Now widely cultivated in Germany, the Netherlands, Scandinavia and Russia.

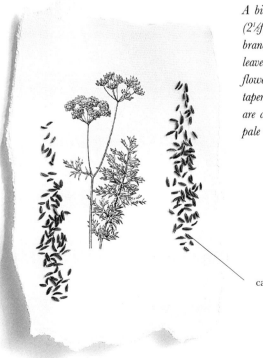

A biennial herb up to 75cm (2½ft) high with a much-branched stem, finely cut leaves and umbels of white flowers, with a thick and tapering root. The small seeds are curved, with five distinct pale ridges.

caraway seeds

Carum carvi

OTHER SPECIES

There are several varieties depending on origin – the English, Dutch and German types derive from Russia and are distinct from the Scandinavian variety. Those plants grown in northerly latitudes produce more oil.

Cedrus atlantica

Atlas cedarwood

FAMILY: PINACEAE **SYNONYMS:** ATLANTIC CEDAR, ATLAS CEDAR, AFRICAN CEDAR, MOROCCAN CEDARWOOD (OIL), LIBANOL (OIL)

Herbal/Folk Tradition

The oil from the Lebanon cedar was possibly the first to be extracted; it was used by the ancient Egyptians for embalming purposes, cosmetics and perfumery. The oil was one of the ingredients of 'mithridat', a renowned poison antidote that was used for centuries. The Lebanon cedar was prized as a building wood; its odour repelled ants, moths and other harmful insects, as does the oil from the Atlas cedar.

Traditionally, the oil was used in the East for bronchial and urinary tract infections, as a preservative and as an incense. It is still used as a temple incense by the Tibetans and is employed in their traditional medicine.

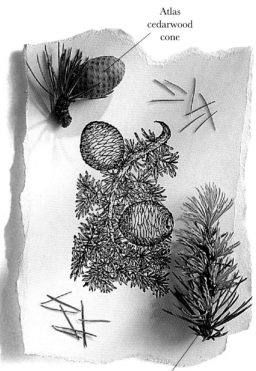

Atlas cedarwood cone

fresh cutting

Pyramid-shaped evergreen tree with a majestic stature, up to 40m (131ft) high. The wood itself is hard and strongly aromatic because of the high percentage of essential oil it contains.

EXTRACTION
Essential oil by steam distillation from the wood, stumps and sawdust. A resinoid and absolute are also produced in small quantities.

CHARACTERISTICS
A yellow, orange or deep amber viscous oil with a warm, camphoraceous top note and sweet tenacious, woody-balsamic undertone. It blends well with rosewood, bergamot, boronia, cypress, calamus, cassie, costus, jasmine, juniper, orange blossom, mimosa, labdanum, olibanum, clary sage, vetiver, rosemary, ylang ylang, oriental and floral bases.

ACTIONS
Antiseptic, antiputrescent, antiseborrheic, aphrodisiac, astringent, diuretic, expectorant, fungicidal, mucolytic, sedative (nervous), stimulant (circulatory), tonic.

PRINCIPAL CONSTITUENTS
Atlantone, caryophyllene, cedrol, cadinene, among others.

AROMATHERAPY/HOME USE

Skin Care: *Acne, dandruff, dermatitis, eczema, fungal infections, greasy skin, hair loss, skin eruptions, ulcers.*
Circulation, Muscles and Joints: *Arthritis, rheumatism.*
Respiratory System: *Bronchitis, catarrh, congestion, coughs.*
Genito-urinary System: *Cystitis, leucorrhea, pruritis.*
Nervous System: *Nervous tension and stress-related conditions.*

OTHER USES

Fragrance component and fixative in cosmetics and household products, soaps, detergents etc., as well as in perfumes, especially men's fragrances.

DISTRIBUTION

Native to the Atlas mountains of Algeria; the oil is produced mainly in Morocco.

OTHER SPECIES

Believed to have originated from the famous Lebanon cedars (C. libani), which grow wild in Lebanon and on the island of Cyprus. It is also a close botanical relation to the Himalayan deodar cedarwood (C. deodorate), which produces a very similar essential oil. (NB: the oil is quite different from the Texas or Virginian cedarwoods.)

Chamaemelum nobile

Roman chamomile

FAMILY: ASTERACEAE (COMPOSITAE) SYNONYMS: *ANTHEMIS NOBILIS*, CAMOMILE, ENGLISH CHAMOMILE, GARDEN CHAMOMILE, SWEET CHAMOMILE, TRUE CHAMOMILE

Herbal/Folk Tradition

This herb has had a medical reputation in Europe and especially in the Mediterranean region for over 2,000 years, and it is still in widespread use. It was employed by the ancient Egyptians and the Moors, and it was one of the Saxons' nine sacred herbs, which they called 'maythen'. It was also held to be the 'plant's physician', since it promoted the health of plants nearby.

It is current in the British Herbal Pharmacopoeia for the treatment of dyspepsia, nausea, anorexia, vomiting in pregnancy, dysmenorrhea and specifically flatulent dyspepsia associated with mental stress.

dried Roman chamomile

fresh pinnate leaves

A small, stocky, perennial herb, up to 25cm (10in) high, with a much-branched hairy stem, half spreading or creeping. It has feathery pinnate leaves and daisy-like white flowers that are larger than those of the German chamomile. The whole plant has an apple-like scent.

AROMATHERAPY/ HOME USE

Skin Care: *Acne, allergies, boils, burns, cuts, chilblains, dermatitis, earache, eczema, hair care, inflammations, insect bites, rashes, sensitive skin, teething pain, toothache, wounds.*
Circulation, Muscles and Joints: *Arthritis, inflamed joints, muscular pain, neuralgia, rheumatism, sprains.*
Digestive System: *Dyspepsia, colic, indigestion, nausea.*
Genito-urinary System: *Dysmenorrhea, menopausal problems, menorrhagia.*
Nervous System: *Headache, insomnia, nervous tension, migraine and stress-related complaints.*

OTHER USES

Used in pharmaceutical antiseptic ointments and in carminative, antispasmodic and tonic preparations. Extensively used in cosmetics, soaps, detergents, high-class perfumes and hair and bath products. Used as a flavour ingredient in most major food categories, including alcoholic and soft drinks.

DISTRIBUTION

Native to southern and western Europe; naturalized in North America. Cultivated in Britain, Belgium, Hungary, the USA, Italy and France.

OTHER SPECIES

There are a great many varieties of chamomile found throughout the world, four of which are native to the British Isles, but the only one of these used therapeutically is the Roman chamomile (C. nobile).

EXTRACTION
Essential oil by steam distillation of the flower heads.

CHARACTERISTICS
A pale blue liquid (turning yellow on keeping) with a warm, sweet, fruity-herbaceous scent. It blends well with bergamot, clary sage, oakmoss, jasmine, labdanum, orange blossom, rose, geranium and lavender.

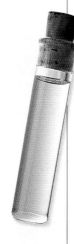

ACTIONS
Analgesic, anti-anemic, antineuralgic, antiphlogistic, antiseptic, antispasmodic, bactericidal, carminative, cholagogue, cicatrizant, digestive, emmenagogue, febrifuge, hepatic, hypnotic, nerve sedative, stomachic, sudorific, tonic, vermifuge, vulnerary.

PRINCIPAL CONSTITUENTS
Mainly esters of angelic and tiglic acids (approx. 85 per cent), with pinene, farnesol, nerolidol, chamazulene, pinacar-vone, cineol, among others.

Chenopodium ambrosioides var. anthelminticum

Wormseed

SAFETY DATA *A very toxic oil*

FAMILY: CHENOPODIACEAE **SYNONYMS:** *C. ANTHELMINTICUM*, AMERICAN WORMSEED, CHENOPDIUM, CALIFORNIAN SPEARMINT, JESUIT'S TEA, MEXICAN TEA, HERB SANTI MARIAE, BALTIMORE (OIL)

Herbal/Folk Tradition

'Used for many years by the local Indians as an effective anthelmintic . . . several Indian tribes of the eastern part of the United States use the whole of the herb decocted to help ease painful menstruation and other female complaints.'[22]

Apart from being used to expel roundworm, hookworm and dwarf tapeworm, the herb has also been employed for asthma, catarrh and other chest complaints, and to treat nervous disease. In China it is used to treat articular rheumatism. Causes dizziness and vomiting in concentration.

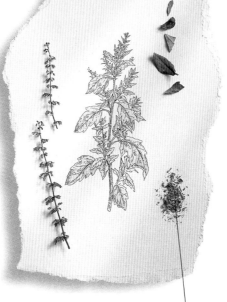

dried flowers

A hairy, coarse, perennial wayside herb up to 1m (3ft) high with stout, erect stem, oblong-lanceolate leaves and numerous greenish-yellow flowers, the same colour as the leaves.

EXTRACTION
Essential oil by steam distillation from the whole herb, especially the fruit or seeds.

CHARACTERISTICS
A colourless or pale yellow oil with a sweet-woody, camphoraceous, heavy and nauseating odour.

ACTIONS
Anthelmintic, antirheumatic, antispasmodic, expectorant, hypotensive.

PRINCIPAL CONSTITUENTS
Ascaridole (60–80 per cent), cymene, limonene, terpinene, myrcene.

AROMATHERAPY/ HOME USE

None. 'Should not be used in therapy either internally or externally. One of the most toxic essential oils.'[23] Cases of fatal poisoning have been reported even in low doses. Effects can be cumulative. Due to high ascaridole content, the oil may explode when heated or treated with acids.

OTHER USES

In pharmaceuticals its anthelmintic applications have been replaced by synthetics. Used as a fragrance component in soaps, detergents,

cosmetics and perfumes. Its use is not permitted in foods.

DISTRIBUTION

Native to South America; cultivated mainly in east and south-east USA, also India, Hungary and Russia.

OTHER SPECIES

The parent plant, C. ambrosioides, is also used to produce an essential oil with similar properties. There are many different members on the Chenopodium or Goosefoot family, such as Good King Henry (C. bonus-henricus),

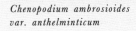

Chenopodium ambrosioides var. anthelminticum

a European variety whose leaves were eaten like spinach. See also Botanical Classification section. The so-called Russian wormseed oil or wormseed Levant (Artemisia cana) is quite different from the American type, although it is also used as an anthelmintic and is extremely toxic, containing mainly cineol.

Cinnamomum camphora

Camphor

FAMILY: LAURACEAE **SYNONYMS:** *LAURUS CAMPHORA*, TRUE CAMPHOR, HON-SHO, LAUREL CAMPHOR, GUM CAMPHOR, JAPANESE CAMPHOR, FORMOSA CAMPHOR

Herbal/Folk Tradition

A long-standing traditional preventative of infectious disease; a lump of camphor would be worn around the neck as a protection. In addition it was used for nervous and respiratory diseases in general, and for heart failure! However, in its crude form it is very poisonous in large doses and has been removed from the British Herbal Pharmacopoeia.

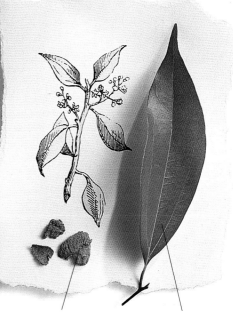

A tall, handsome, evergreen tree, up to 30m (98ft) high, not unlike the linden. It has many branches bearing clusters of small white flowers followed by red berries. It produces a white crystalline substance, the crude camphor, from the wood of mature trees over fifty years old.

camphor bark   fresh camphor

EXTRACTION
Crude camphor is collected from the trees in crystalline form. The essential oil is produced by steam distillation from the wood, root stumps and branches and then rectified under vacuum and filter pressed to produce three fractions, known as white, brown and yellow camphor.

CHARACTERISTICS
White camphor is the lightest (lowest boiling) fraction, a colourless to pale yellow liquid with a sharp, pungent camphoraceous odour. Brown camphor is the middle fraction. Yellow camphor, a blue-green or yellowish liquid, is the heaviest.

ACTIONS
Anti-inflammatory, antiseptic, antiviral, bactericidal, counter-irritant, diuretic, expectorant, stimulant, rubefacient, vermifuge.

PRINCIPAL CONSTITUENTS
1. White camphor contains mainly cineol, with pinene, terpineol, menthol, thymol and no safrol. 2. Brown camphor contains up to 80 per cent safrol and some terpineol. 3. Yellow camphor contains mainly safrol, sesquiterpenes and sesquiterpene alcohols.

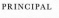

AROMATHERAPY/ HOME USE
Brown and yellow camphor 'should not be used in therapy, either internally or externally'.[24] White camphor may be used with care for:
Skin Care: *Acne, inflammation, oily conditions, spots; also for insect prevention (flies, moths, etc.).*
Circulation, Muscles and Joints: *Arthritis, muscular aches and pains, rheumatism, sprains, etc.*
Respiratory System: *Bronchitis, chills, coughs.*
Immune System: *Colds, fever, flu, infectious diseases.*

OTHER USES
White and brown camphor are used as the starting material for the isolation of many perfumery chemicals, for example safrol and cineol. White camphor is used as a solvent in the paint and lacquer industry, and for the production of celluloid. Fractions of white oil are used as fragrance and masking agents in detergents, soaps, disinfectants and household products. It is, however, an environmental hazard or marine pollutant.

DISTRIBUTION
Native to Japan and Taiwan principally, also China; cultivated in India, Sri Lanka, Egypt, Madagascar, southern Europe and the USA.

OTHER SPECIES
There are many species of camphor: the ho-sho variety produces ho leaf and ho wood oil; the Chinese variety produces apopin oil; the Japan and Taiwan type, known as hon-sho or true camphor, produces two chemotypes: camphor-safrol (Japan) and camphor-linalol (Taiwan). All these are to be distinguished from the Borneo camphor or borneol, which is of different botanical origin.

Cinnamomum cassia

Cassia

SAFETY DATA *Dermal toxin, dermal irritant, dermal sensitizer, mucous membrane irritant*

FAMILY: LAURACEAE **SYNONYMS:** *C. AROMATICUM*, *LAURUS CASSIA*, CHINESE CINNAMON, FALSE CINNAMON, CASSIA CINNAMON, CASSIA LIGNEA

Herbal/Folk Tradition

Extensively used as local domestic spice. It is used medicinally in much the same way as Ceylon cinnamon, mainly for digestive complaints such as flatulent dyspepsia, colic, diarrhea and nausea, as well as the common cold, rheumatism, kidney and reproductive complaints. In Chinese medicine it is used particularly for vascular disorders. A great deal of research has been carried out in recent years regarding the pharmacological actions of cassia. The volatile oil has been shown to be carminative and antiseptic, while the main constituent, cinnamic aldehyde, is a weak central nervous system stimulant at low doses and a depressant at high doses. Cassia has also shown promising results as a radiation protective agent when used experimentally in China.

The powdered bark is current in the British Herbal Pharmacopoeia as a specific for flatulent dyspepsia or colic with nausea.

AROMATHERAPY/ HOME USE

None. 'Should never be used on the skin (one of the most hazardous oils).'[25]

OTHER USES

Some pharmaceutical applications due to bactericidal properties, such as mouthwashes, toothpastes, gargles; also tonic and carminative preparations. Extensively used in food flavouring, including alcoholic and soft drinks. Little used in perfumes and cosmetics, because of its dark colour.

DISTRIBUTION

Native to the south-eastern parts of China; found to a lesser extent in Vietnam and India (Cochin).

OTHER SPECIES

Not to be confused with the Ceylon cinnamon bark (C. verum), which is from a related species. There are also several other varieties from different regions used for essential oil production. See Botanical Classification section.

EXTRACTION
Essential oil 1. by steam distillation from the leaves, and 2. by water distillation from the bark, leaves, twigs and stalks.

CHARACTERISTICS
1. Leaf oil is brownish-yellow (the rectified oil is pale yellow), with a sweet woody-spicy tenacious odour.

2. Bark oil is a dark brown liquid with a strong, spicy-warm, resinous odour.

ACTIONS
Antidiarrheal, anti-emetic, antimicrobial, astringent, carminative, spasmolytic.

PRINCIPAL CONSTITUENTS
Leaf and bark oil contain mainly cinnamic aldehyde (75–90 per cent) with some methyl eugenol, salicylaldehyde and methylsalicylaldehyde.

A slender, evergreen tree up to 20m (65ft) high, with leathery leaves and small white flowers. It is usually cut back to form bushes for commercial production. The fruit is approximately the size of a small olive. The bark may be easily distinguished from that of cinnamon, with which it is often confused, as it is thicker, darker and coarser — the flavour being more pungent and less sweet.

dried cassia stalks

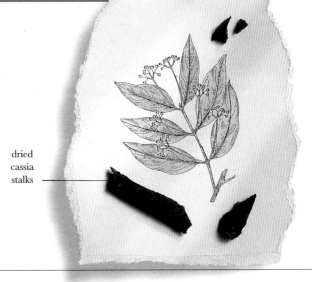

Cinnamon

Cinnamomum zeylanicum

FAMILY: LAURACEAE SYNONYMS: *C. VERUM, LAURUS CINNAMOMUM,* CEYLON CINNAMON, SEYCHELLES CINNAMON, MADAGASCAR CINNAMON, TRUE CINNAMON, CINNAMON LEAF (OIL), CINNAMON BARK (OIL)

Herbal/Folk Tradition

The inner bark of the new shoots from the cinnamon tree are gathered every two years and used in the form of sticks as a domestic spice. It has been used for thousands of years in the East for a variety of complaints, including colds, flu, digestive and menstrual problems, rheumatism, kidney troubles and as a general stimulant. Current in the British Herbal Pharmacopoeia as a specific for flatulent colic and dyspepsia with nausea.

A tropical evergreen up to 15m (49ft) high, with strong branches and thick scabrous bark with young shoots speckled greeny-orange. It has shiny green, leathery leaves, small white flowers and oval bluish-white berries. The leaves have a spicy smell when bruised.

crushed cinnamon

sticks of cinnamon

EXTRACTION
Essential oil by water or steam distillation from the 1. leaves and twigs, and 2. dried inner bark.

CHARACTERISTICS
1. A yellow to brownish liquid with a warm-spicy, somewhat harsh odour. 2. A pale to dark yellow liquid with a sweet, warm-spicy, dry, tenacious odour. It blends well with olibanum, ylang ylang, orange, mandarin, benzoin, Peru balsam and in oriental-type mixtures.

ACTIONS
Anthelmintic, antidiarrheal, antidote (to poison), antimicrobial, antiseptic, antispasmodic, antiputrescent, aphrodisiac, astringent, carminative, digestive, emmenagogue, hemostatic, orexigenic, parasiticide, refrigerant, spasmolytic, stimulant (circulatory, cardiac, respiratory), stomachic, vermifuge.

PRINCIPAL CONSTITUENTS
1. Leaf – eugenol (80–96 per cent), eugenol acetate, cinnamaldehyde (3 per cent), benzyl benzoate, linalol, safrol among others. 2. Bark – cinnamaldehyde (40–50 per cent), eugenol (4–10 per cent), benzaldehyde, cuminaldehyde, pinene, cineol, phellandrene, furfurol, cymene, linalol, among others.

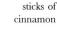

AROMATHERAPY/HOME USE
Cinnamon bark oil – none. 'Should never by used on the skin (one of the most hazardous oils).'[26] Cinnamon leaf oil:
Skin Care: *Lice, scabies, tooth and gum care, warts, wasp stings.*
Circulation, Muscles and Joints: *Poor circulation, rheumatism.*
Digestive System: *Anorexia, colitis, diarrhea, dyspepsia, intestinal infection, sluggish digestion, spasm.*
Genito-urinary System: *Childbirth (stimulates contractions), frigidity, leucorrhea, metrorrhagia, scanty periods.*
Immune System: *Chills, colds, flu, infectious diseases.*
Nervous System: *Debility, nervous exhaustion and stress-related conditions.*

OTHER USES
Both bark and leaf oils are used for their fragrance and therapeutic actions in nasal sprays, cough syrups and dental preparations. The leaf oil is used in soaps, cosmetics, toiletries and perfumes. Both are used in food flavouring, especially alcoholic and soft drinks.

DISTRIBUTION
Native to Sri Lanka, Madagascar, the Comoro Islands, south India, Burma and Indochina. It is also cultivated in India, Jamaica and Africa – each region tending to have its own particular species.

OTHER SPECIES
Madagascar cinnamon is considered superior to the various other types, such as the Saigon cinnamon (C. loureirii) and the Batavia cinnamon (C. burmanii). See also Botanical Classification section.

Cistus ladanifer

Labdanum

FAMILY: CISTACEAE **SYNONYMS:** CISTUS (OIL), GUM CISTUS, CISTE, CYSTE (ABSOLUTE), LABDANUM GUM, AMBREINE, EUROPEAN ROCK ROSE

Herbal/Folk Tradition

One of the early aromatic substances of the ancient world. The gum was used formerly for catarrh, diarrhea, dysentery and to promote menstruation; externally it was used in plasters. The oil from the closely related plant frostwort *(Helianthemum canadense)*, also known as cistus, also has many medicinal qualities and is said to be useful for scrofulous skin conditions, ulcers and tumours, including cancer.

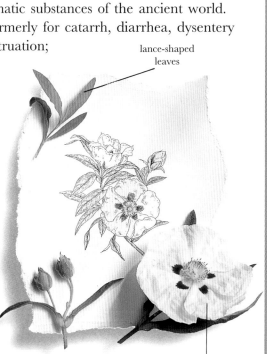

lance-shaped leaves

fresh flower

A small sticky shrub up to 3m (10ft) high with lance-shaped leaves that are white and furry on the underside, and fragrant white flowers. Labdanum gum, a dark brown solid mass, is a natural oleoresin obtained by boiling the plant material in water.

EXTRACTION

1. A resinoid or resin concrete and absolute by solvent extraction from the crude gum. **2. An essential oil** by steam distillation from the crude gum, the absolute, or from the leaves and twigs of the plant directly.

CHARACTERISTICS

1. Absolute – a semi-solid green or amber mass with a rich, sweet, herbaceous-balsamic odour. **2. Oil** – a dark yellow or amber viscous liquid with a warm, sweet, dry-herbaceous musky scent. It blends well with oakmoss, clary sage, pine, juniper, calamus, opopanax, lavender, lavandin, bergamot, cypress, vetiver, sandalwood, patchouli, olibanum, maroc chamomile and oriental bases.

ACTIONS

Antimicrobial, antiseptic, antitussive, astringent, balsamic, emmenagogue, expectorant, tonic.

PRINCIPAL CONSTITUENTS

It contains over **170 pinenes,** including camphene, sabinene, myrcene, phellandrene, limonene, cymene, cineol, borneol, nerol, geraniol, fenchone, etc. Exact constituents vary according to source.

AROMATHERAPY/ HOME USE

Skin Care: *Mature skin, wrinkles.*
Respiratory System: *Coughs, bronchitis, rhinitis, etc.*
Immune System: *Colds.*

OTHER USES

Used as a fixative and fragrance component in lotions, powders, soaps, detergents, colognes and perfumes, especially oriental perfumes and aftershaves. Employed in most major food categories, particularly meat products, as well as alcoholic and soft drinks.

DISTRIBUTION

Native to the Mediterranean mountainous regions and the Middle East. Now found throughout the Mediterranean region, especially southern France, Spain, Portugal, Greece, Morocco, Cyprus and former Yugoslavia. The oil is produced mainly in Spain.

OTHER SPECIES

Labdanum gum is also obtained from other Cistus *species, notably* C. incanus, *and other subspecies: see Botanical Classification section.*

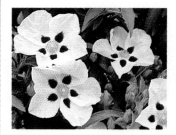

Cistus ladanifer

Citrus aurantifolia

Lime

FAMILY: RUTACEAE **SYNONYMS:** *C. MEDICA VAR. ACIDA, C. LATIFOLIA,* MEXICAN LIME, WEST INDIAN LIME, SOUR LIME

Herbal/Folk Tradition

The fruit is often used indiscriminately in place of lemon with which it shares many qualities. It is used for similar purposes including fever, infections, sore throat, colds, etc. In the past was used as a remedy for dyspepsia with glycerin of pepsin.

EXTRACTION

Essential oil by 1. cold expression of the peel of the unripe fruit; the expressed oil is preferred in perfumery work, and 2. steam distillation of the whole ripe crushed fruit (a by-product of the juice industry).

CHARACTERISTICS

1. A pale yellow or olive-green liquid with a fresh, sweet, citrus-peel odour. 2. A water-white or pale yellow liquid with a fresh, sharp, fruity-citrus scent. It blends well with orange blossom, citronella, lavender, lavandin, rosemary, clary sage and other citrus oils.

ACTIONS

Antirheumatic, antiscorbutic, antiseptic, antiviral, aperitif, bactericidal, febrifuge, restorative, tonic.

PRINCIPAL CONSTITUENTS

Limonene, pinenes, camphene, sabinene, citral, cymene, cineols and linalol, among others. The expressed 'peel' oil, but not the 'whole fruit' oil, also contains coumarins.

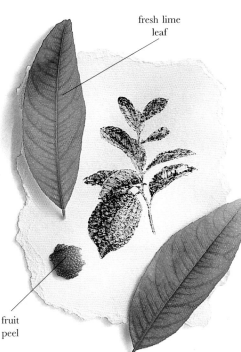

A small evergreen tree up to 4.5m (15ft) high, with stiff sharp spines, smooth ovate leaves and small white flowers. The bitter fruit is a pale green colour, about half the size of a lemon.

fresh lime leaf

fruit peel

AROMATHERAPY/ HOME USE

Skin Care: *Acne, anemia, brittle nails, boils, chilblains, corns, cuts, greasy skin, herpes, insect bites, mouth ulcers, spots, varicose veins, warts.*

Circulation, Muscles and Joints: *Arthritis, cellulitis, high blood pressure, nosebleeds, obesity (congestion), poor circulation, rheumatism.*

Respiratory System: *Asthma, throat infections, bronchitis, catarrh.*

Digestive System: *Dyspepsia.*

Immune System: *Colds, flu, fever and infections.*

OTHER USES

Both oils, but mainly the expressed, are used as fragrance components in soaps, detergents, cosmetics and perfumes. Mainly the distilled oil, but also the terpeneless oil, is used by the food industry, especially in soft drinks – 'lemon and lime' flavour. The juice is used for the production of citric acid.

DISTRIBUTION

Probably native to south Asia; naturalized in many tropical and subtropical regions of the world. It is cultivated mainly in south Florida, the West Indies (Cuba), Central America (Mexico) and Italy.

OTHER SPECIES

There are several species of lime such as the Italian lime (C. limetta), which is used to produce an oil called 'limette'; and the leech-lime (C. hystrix), occasionally used to produce an essential oil called combava.

Citrus aurantium var. amara

Bitter orange

FAMILY: RUTACEAE **SYNONYMS:** *C. VULGARIS, C. BIGARADIA*, SEVILLE ORANGE, SOUR ORANGE BIGARADE (OIL)

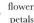

SAFETY DATA *Phototoxic; otherwise generally non-toxic, non-irritant and non-sensitizing. Limonene has been reported to cause contact dermatitis in some individuals*

'Oranges and lemons strengthen the heart, are good for diminishing the coagubility of the blood, and are beneficial for palpitation, scurvy, jaundice, bleedings, heartburn, relaxed throat, etc. They are powerfully anti-scorbutic, either internally or externally applied.'[27] The dried bitter orange peel is used as a tonic and carminative in treating dyspepsia.

In Chinese medicine the dried bitter orange and occasionally its peel are used in treating prolapse of the uterus and of the anus, diarrhea, and blood in the feces. Ingestion of large amounts of orange peel in children, however, has been reported to cause toxic effects.

flower petals

outer peel of fruit

fresh bitter orange

EXTRACTION

An essential oil by cold expression (hand or machine pressing) from the outer peel of the almost ripe fruit. (A terpeneless oil is also produced.) The leaves are used for the production of petitgrain oil; the blossom for neroli oil.

CHARACTERISTICS

A dark yellow or brownish-yellow mobile liquid with a fresh, dry, almost floral odour with a rich, sweet undertone.

ACTIONS

Anti-inflammatory, antiseptic, astringent, bactericidal, carminative, choleretic, fungicidal, sedative (mild), stomachic, tonic.

PRINCIPAL CONSTITUENTS

Over 90 per cent monoterpenes: mainly limonene, myrcene, camphene, pinene, ocimene, cymene, and small amounts of alcohols, aldehydes and ketones.

An evergreen tree up to 10m (33ft) high with dark green, glossy, oval leaves, paler beneath, with long but not very sharp spines. It has a smooth greyish trunk and branches, and very fragrant white flowers. The fruits are smaller and darker than the sweet orange. It is well known for its resistance to disease and is often used as root stock for other citrus trees, including the sweet orange.

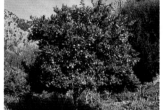

Citrus aurantium var. amara

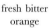

AROMATHERAPY/ HOME USE

See sweet orange.

OTHER USES

Used in certain stomachic, laxative and carminative preparations. Employed as a fragrance component in soaps, detergents, cosmetics, colognes and perfumes. Extensively used as a flavouring material, especially in liqueurs and soft drinks. Also utilized as a starting material for the isolation of natural limonene.

DISTRIBUTION

Native to the Far East, especially India and China, but has become well adapted to the Mediterranean climate. It also grows abundantly in the USA (California), Israel and South America. Main producers of the oil include Spain, Guinea, the West Indies, Italy, Brazil and the USA.

OTHER SPECIES

There are numerous different species according to location – oils from Spain and Guinea are said to be of superior quality.

Citrus aurantium var. amara

Orange blossom

FAMILY: RUTACEAE SYNONYMS: *C. VULGARIS, C. BIGARADIA*, ORANGE FLOWER, NEROLI, NEROLI BIGARADE

Herbal/Folk Tradition

This oil was named after a princess of Nerola in Italy, who wore it as a perfume. Orange flowers have many folk associations. They were used in bridal bouquets: to calm nervous apprehension before the couple retired to the marriage bed.

In Europe an infusion of dried flowers is used as a mild stimulant of the nervous system, and as a blood cleanser. The distillation water, known as orange flower water, is a popular cosmetic and household article.

An evergreen tree up to 10m (33ft) high with glossy dark green leaves and fragrant white flowers.

flower petal

orange blossom leaves

AROMATHERAPY/ HOME USE

Skin Care: *Scars, stretch marks, thread veins, mature and sensitive skin, tones the complexion, wrinkles.*
Circulation, Muscles and Joints: *Palpitations, poor circulation.*
Digestive system: *Diarrhea (chronic), colic, flatulence, spasm, nervous dyspepsia.*
Nervous system: *Anxiety, depression, nervous tension, PMT, shock, stress-related conditions – 'I find that by far the most important uses of neroli are in helping with problems of emotional origin.'*[28]

OTHER USES

Neroli oil and orange flower water are used to flavour pharmaceuticals. The absolute is used extensively in high-class perfumery work, especially oriental, floral and citrus blends; also as a fixative. The oil is used in eau-de-cologne and toilet waters (traditionally with lavender, lemon, rosemary and bergamot). Limited use as a flavour ingredient in foods, alcoholic and soft drinks.

DISTRIBUTION

Native to the Far East, but well adapted to the Mediterranean climate. Major producers include Italy, Tunisia, Morocco, Egypt, the USA and especially France.

OTHER SPECIES

The sweet orange (C. aurantium var. dulcis) is also used to make an absolute and oil called neroli Portugal or neroli petalae; however, it is less fragrant and considered of inferior quality.

EXTRACTION

1. A concrete and absolute are produced by solvent extraction from the freshly picked flowers. **2.** An essential oil is produced by steam distillation from the freshly picked flowers. An orange flower water and an absolute are produced as a by-product of the distillation process.

CHARACTERISTICS

1. The absolute is a dark brown or orange viscous liquid with a fresh, delicate yet rich, warm sweet-floral fragrance; very true to nature. It blends well with jasmine, benzoin, myrrh and all citrus oils. **2.** The oil is a pale yellow mobile liquid (darkening with age) with a light, sweet-floral fragrance and terpeney top note. Blends well with virtually all oils: chamomile, coriander, geranium, benzoin, clary sage, jasmine, lavender, rose, ylang ylang, lemon and other citrus oils.

ACTIONS

Antidepressant, antiseptic, antispasmodic, aphrodisiac, bactericidal, carminative, cicatrizant, cordial, deodorant, digestive, fungicidal, hypnotic (mild), stimulant (nervous), tonic (cardiac, circulatory).

PRINCIPAL CONSTITUENTS

Linalol (34 per cent approx.), linalyl acetate (6–17 per cent), limonene (15 per cent approx.), pinene, nerolidol, geraniol, nerol, methyl anthranilate, indole, citral, jasmone, among others.

Citrus aurantium var. amara

Petitgrain

FAMILY: RUTACEAE **SYNONYMS:** *C. BIGARADIA*, PETITGRAIN BIGARADE (OIL), PETITGRAIN PARAGUAY (OIL). SEE ALSO BITTER ORANGE

Herbal/folk tradition

At one time the oil used to be extracted from the green unripe oranges when they were still the size of cherries – hence the name petitgrains or 'little grains'. One of the classic ingredients of eau-de-cologne.

The oil of petitgrain is produced from the leaves and twigs of the same tree that produces bitter orange oil and orange blossom oil: see bitter orange and orange blossom.

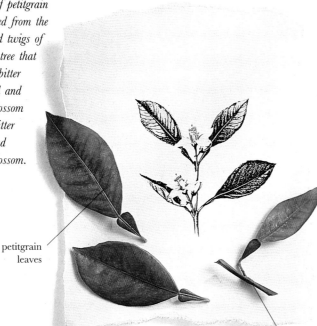

petitgrain
leaves

fresh
petitgrain

EXTRACTION
Essential oil by steam distillation from the leaves and twigs. An orange 'leaf and flower' water absolute is also produced, known as *petitgrain sur fleurs*.

CHARACTERISTICS
A pale yellow to amber liquid with a fresh-floral citrus scent and a woody-herbaceous undertone. It blends well with rosemary, lavender, geranium, bergamot, bitter orange, orange blossom, labdanum, oakmoss, clary sage, jasmine, benzoin, palmarosa, clove and balsams.

ACTIONS
Antiseptic, antispasmodic, deodorant, digestive, nervine, stimulant (digestive, nervous), stomachic, tonic.

PRINCIPAL CONSTITUENTS
40–80 per cent esters: mainly linalyl acetate and geranyl acetate, as well as linalol, nerol, terpineol, geraniol, nerolidol, farnesol, limonene, among others.

AROMATHERAPY/ HOME USE

Skin Care: *Acne, excessive perspiration, greasy skin and hair, toning.*
Digestive System: *Dyspepsia, flatulence.*
Nervous System: *Convalescence, insomnia, nervous exhaustion and stress-related conditions.*

OTHER USES

Extensively used as a fragrance component in soaps, detergents, cosmetics and perfumes, especially colognes (sometimes used to replace orange blossom). Employed as a flavour component in many foods, especially confectionery, as well as alcoholic and soft drinks.

DISTRIBUTION

Native to southern China and north-east India. The best-quality petitgrain oil comes from France but a good-quality oil is also produced in North Africa, Paraguay and Haiti from semi-wild trees.

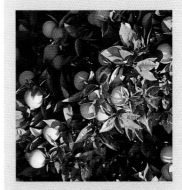

Citrus aurantium var. amara

OTHER SPECIES

A type of petitgrain is also produced in small quantities from the leaves, twigs and small unripe fruit of the lemon, sweet orange, mandarin and bergamot trees.

Citrus bergamia

Bergamot

FAMILY: RUTACEAE
SYNONYMS: *CITRUS AURANTIUM SUBSP. BERGAMIA*

Herbal/Folk Tradition

Named after the Italian city of Bergamot in Lombardy, where the oil was first sold. The oil has been used in Italian folk medicine for many years, primarily for fever (including malaria) and worms. Recent research in Italy has shown that bergamot oil has a wide spectrum of applications, being particularly useful for mouth, skin, respiratory and urinary tract infections.

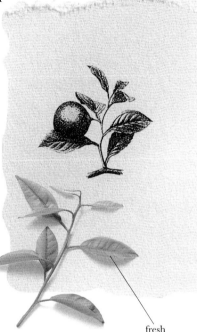

A small tree, about 4.5m (15ft) high with smooth oval leaves, bearing small round fruit that ripen from green to yellow, much like a miniature orange in appearance.

fresh bergamot

EXTRACTION
Essential oil by cold expression of the peel of the nearly ripe fruit. (A rectified or terpeneless oil is produced by vacuum distillation or solvent extraction.)

CHARACTERISTICS
A light greenish-yellow liquid with a fresh sweet-fruity, slightly spicy-balsamic undertone. On aging it turns a brownish-olive colour. It blends well with lavender, orange blossom, jasmine, cypress, geranium, lemon, chamomile, juniper, coriander and violet.

ACTIONS
Analgesic, anthelmintic, antidepressant, antiseptic (pulmonary, genito-urinary), antispasmodic, antitoxic, carminative, digestive, diuretic, deodorant, febrifuge, laxative, parasiticide, rubefacient, stimulant, stomachic, tonic, vermifuge, vulnerary.

PRINCIPAL CONSTITUENTS
Known to have about 300 compounds present in the expressed oil; mainly linalyl acetate (30–60 per cent), linalol (11–22 per cent) and other alcohols, sesquiterpenes, terpenes, alkanes and furocoumarins (including bergapten, 0.30–0.39 per cent).

AROMATHERAPY/ HOME USE

Skin Care: *Acne, boils, cold sores, eczema, insect repellent and insect bites, oily complexion, psoriasis, scabies, spots, varicose ulcers, wounds.*
Respiratory System: *Halitosis, mouth infections, sore throat, tonsillitis.*
Digestive System: *Flatulence, loss of appetite.*
Genito-urinary System: *Cystitis, leucorrhea, pruritis, thrush.*
Immune System: *Colds, fever, flu, infectious diseases.*
Nervous System: *Anxiety, depression and stress-related conditions, having a refreshing and uplifting quality.*

OTHER USES
Extensively used as a fragrance and, to a degree, a fixative in cosmetics, toiletries, suntan lotions and perfumes – it is a classic ingredient of eau-de-cologne. Widely used in most major food categories and beverages, notably Earl Grey tea.

DISTRIBUTION
Native to tropical Asia. Extensively cultivated in Calabria in southern Italy and also grown commercially on the Ivory Coast.

OTHER SPECIES
Not to be confused with the herb bergamot or bee balm (Monarda didyma).

Citrus limon

Lemon

> **SAFETY DATA** *Non-toxic; may cause dermal irritation or sensitization reactions in some individuals – apply in moderation. Phototoxic – do not use on skin exposed to direct sunlight*

FAMILY: RUTACEAE **SYNONYMS:** *C. LIMONUM*, CEDRO OIL

Herbal/Folk Tradition

The juice and peel are widely used as a domestic seasoning. It is very nutritious, being high in vitamins A, B and C. In Spain and other European countries, lemon is something of a 'cure-all', especially with regard to infectious illness. It was used for fever, such as malaria and typhoid, and employed specifically for scurvy on English ships at sea.

Taken internally, the juice is considered invaluable for acidic disorders, such as arthritis and rheumatism, and of great benefit in dysentery and liver congestion.

A small evergreen tree up to 6m (20ft) high with serrated oval leaves, stiff thorns and very fragrant flowers. The fruit turns from green to yellow on ripening.

fresh lemon

outer peel of fruit

AROMATHERAPY/ HOME USE

See Lime.

OTHER USES

Used as a flavouring agent in pharmaceuticals. Extensively used as a fragrance component in soaps, detergents, cosmetics, toilet waters and perfumes. Extensively employed by the food industry in most types of product, including alcoholic and soft drinks.

DISTRIBUTION

Native to Asia, probably east India; it now grows wild in the Mediterranean region especially in Spain and Portugal. It is cultivated extensively worldwide in Italy, Sicily, Cyprus, Guinea, Israel, South and North America (California and Florida).

OTHER SPECIES

There are about forty-seven varieties that are said to have been developed in cultivation, such as the Java lemon (C. javanica). The lemon is also closely related to the lime, cedrat (or citron) and bergamot.

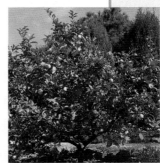

Citrus limon

EXTRACTION

Essential oil by cold expression from the outer part of the fresh peel. A terpeneless oil is also produced on a large scale (cedro oil).

CHARACTERISTICS

A pale greeny-yellow liquid (turning brown with age), with a light, fresh, citrus scent. It blends well with lavender, orange blossom, ylang ylang, rose, sandalwood, olibanum, chamomile, benzoin, fennel, geranium, eucalyptus, juniper, oakmoss, lavandin, elemi, labdanum and other citrus oils.

ACTIONS

Anti-anemic, antimicrobial, antirheumatic, antisclerotic, antiscorbutic, antiseptic, antispasmodic, antitoxic, astringent, bactericidal, carminative, cicatrizant, depurative, diaphoretic, diuretic, febrifuge, hemostatic, hypotensive, insecticidal, rubefacient, stimulates white corpuscles, tonic, vermifuge.

PRINCIPAL CONSTITUENTS

Limonene (approx. 70 per cent), terpinene, pinenes, sabinene, myrcene, citral, linalol, geraniol, octanol, nonanol, citronellal, bergamotene, among others.

Citrus reticulata

Mandarin

FAMILY: RUTACEAE **SYNONYMS:** *C. NOBILIS, C. MADURENSIS, C. UNSHIU, C. DELICIOSA,* EUROPEAN MANDARIN, TRUE MANDARIN, TANGERINE, SATSUMA

Herbal/Folk Tradition

The name comes from the fruit that was a traditional gift to the Mandarins of China. In France it is regarded as a safe children's remedy for indigestion, hiccoughs, etc., and for the elderly since it helps strengthen the digestive function and liver.

EXTRACTION

Essential oil by cold expression from the outer peel. A mandarin petitgrain oil is also produced in small quantities by steam distillation from the leaves and twigs.

CHARACTERISTICS

Mandarin oil is a yellowy-orange mobile liquid with a blue-violet hint, having an intensely sweet, almost floral citrus scent. It blends well with other citrus oils, especially orange blossom, and spice oils such as nutmeg, cinnamon and clove. Tangerine oil is an orange mobile liquid with

a fresh, sweet, orange-like aroma. It has less body than mandarin and is little used in perfumery work.

ACTIONS

Antiseptic, antispasmodic, carminative, digestive, diuretic (mild), laxative (mild), sedative, stimulant (digestive and lymphatic), tonic.

PRINCIPAL CONSTITUENTS

Limonene, methyl methyl-anthranilate, geraniol, citral, citronellal, among others.

A small evergreen tree up to 6m (20ft) high with glossy leaves, fragrant flowers and bearing fleshy fruit. The tangerine is larger than the mandarin and rounder, with a yellower skin, more like the original Chinese type.

AROMATHERAPY/ HOME USE

Skin Care: *Acne, congested and oily skin, scars, spots, stretch marks, toner.*
Circulation, Muscles and Joints: *Fluid retention, obesity.*
Digestive System: *Digestive problems, dyspepsia, hiccoughs, intestinal problems.*
Nervous System: *Insomnia, nervous tension, restlessness. It is often used for children and pregnant women and is recommended in synergistic combinations with other citrus oils.*

OTHER USES

Mandarin oil is used in soaps, cosmetics and perfumes, especially colognes. It is employed as a flavouring agent especially in confectionery, soft drinks and liqueurs.

DISTRIBUTION

Native to southern China and the Far East. Brought to Europe in 1805 and to the USA forty years later, where it was renamed the tangerine. The mandarin is produced mainly in Italy, Spain, Algeria, Cyprus, Greece, the Middle East and Brazil; the tangerine in Texas, Florida, California and Guinea.

OTHER SPECIES

There are many cultivars within this species: the terms tangerine (C. reticulata) and mandarin are used somewhat interchangeably, as is the word satsuma. They could be said to represent different chemotypes since the oils are quite different; see the Botanical Classification section.

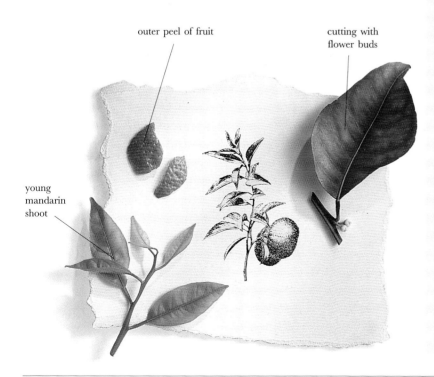

outer peel of fruit

cutting with flower buds

young mandarin shoot

Citrus sinensis

Sweet orange

FAMILY: RUTACEAE **SYNONYMS:** *C. AURANTIUM VAR. DULCIS, C. AURANTIUM VAR. SINENSIS,* CHINA ORANGE, PORTUGAL ORANGE

Herbal/folk tradition

A very nutritious fruit, containing vitamins A, B and C. In Chinese medicine the dried sweet orange peel is used to treat coughs, colds, anorexia and malignant breast sores. Li Shih-chên says: 'The fruits of all the different species and varieties of citrus are considered by the Chinese to be cooling. The sweet varieties increase bronchial secretion and the sour promote expectoration. They all quench thirst, and are stomachic and carminative.'[29]

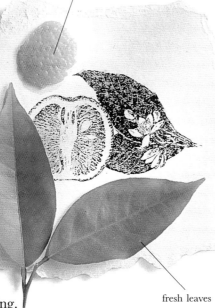

fruit peel

fresh leaves

An evergreen tree, smaller than the bitter variety, less hardy with fewer or no spines. The fruit has a sweet pulp and non-bitter membranes.

EXTRACTION

1. Essential oil by cold expression (hand or machine) of the fresh ripe or almost ripe outer peel. 2. Essential oil by steam distillation of the fresh ripe or almost ripe outer peel. An oil of inferior quality is also produced by distillation from the essences recovered as a byproduct of orange juice manufacture. Distilled sweet orange oil oxidizes very quickly, and anti-oxidant agents are often added at the place of production. (An oil from the flowers is also produced occasionally called neroli Portugal or neroli petalae; an oil from the leaves is also produced in small quantities.)

CHARACTERISTICS

1. A yellowy-orange or dark orange mobile liquid with a sweet, fresh-fruity scent, richer than the distilled oil. It blends well with lavender, orange blossom, lemon, clary sage, myrrh and spice oils such as nutmeg, cinnamon and clove. 2. A pale yellow or colourless mobile liquid with a sweet, light-fruity scent, but little tenacity.

ACTIONS

Antidepressant, anti-inflammatory, antiseptic, bactericidal, carminative, choleretic, digestive, fungicidal, hypotensive, sedative (nervous), stimulant (digestive and lymphatic), stomachic, tonic.

PRINCIPAL CONSTITUENTS

Over 90 per cent monoterpenes, mainly limonene. The cold expressed oil also contains bergapten, auraptenol and acids.

AROMATHERAPY/ HOME USE

Distilled orange oil is phototoxic: its use on the skin should be avoided if there is danger of exposure to direct sunlight. However, there is no evidence to show that expressed sweet orange oil is phototoxic although it too contains coumarins.
Skin Care: *Dull and oily complexions, mouth ulcers.*
Circulation, Muscles and Joints: *Obesity, palpitations, water retention.*
Respiratory System: *Bronchitis, chills.*
Digestive System: *Constipation, dyspepsia, spasm.*
Immune System: *Colds, flu.*
Nervous System: *Nervous tension and stress-related conditions.*

OTHER USES

Sweet orange peel tincture is used to flavour pharmaceuticals. Extensively used as a fragrance component in soaps, detergents, cosmetics and perfumes, and in the food and drinks industry.

DISTRIBUTION

Native to China; extensively cultivated in the USA (California and Florida) and round the Mediterranean (France, Spain, Italy). The expressed oil comes mainly from Israel, Cyprus, Brazil and North America; the distilled oil mainly from the Mediterranean and North America.

OTHER SPECIES

Numerous cultivated varieties of sweet orange, e.g. Jaffa, Navel and Valencia. Many other subspecies such as the Japanese orange (C. aurantium var. natsudaidai). See also bitter orange.

Citrus x paradisi

Grapefruit

FAMILY: RUTACEAE **SYNONYMS:** *C. RACEMOSA, C. MAXIMA VAR. RACEMOSE,* SHADDOCK (OIL)

Herbal/Folk Tradition

It shares the nutritional qualities of other citrus species, being high in Vitamin C and a valuable protection against infectious illness.

A cultivated tree, often over 10m (33ft) high with glossy leaves and large yellow fruits, believed to have derived from the shaddock (C. grandis).

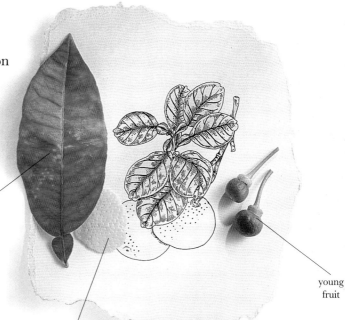

fresh leaf

fruit peel

young fruit

EXTRACTION

Essential oil by cold expression from the fresh peel. (Some oil is distilled from the peel and remains of the fruit after the juice has been utilized, but this is of inferior quality.)

CHARACTERISTICS

A yellow or greenish mobile liquid with a fresh, sweet citrus aroma. It blends well with lemon, palmarosa, bergamot, orange blossom, rosemary, cypress, lavender, geranium, cardomon and other spice oils.

ACTIONS

Antiseptic, antitoxic, astringent, bactericidal, diuretic, depurative, stimulant (lymphatic, digestive), tonic.

PRINCIPAL CONSTITUENTS

Limonene (90 per cent), cadinene, paradisiol, neral, geraniol, citronellal, sinensal, as well as esters, coumarins and furocoumarins.

AROMATHERAPY/ HOME USE

Skin Care: *Acne, congested and oily skin, promotes hair growth, tones the skin and tissues.*
Circulation, Muscles and Joints: *Cellulitis, exercise preparation, muscle fatigue, obesity, stiffness, water retention.*
Immune System: *Chills, colds, flu.*
Nervous System: *Depression, headaches, nervous exhaustion, performance stress.*

OTHER USES

Employed as a fragrance component in soaps, detergents, cosmetics and perfumes. Extensively used in desserts, soft drinks and alcoholic beverages.

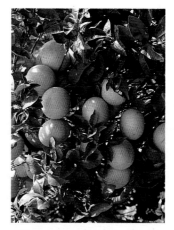

Citrus x paradisi

DISTRIBUTION

Native to tropical Asia and the West Indies: cultivated in California, Florida, Brazil and Israel. The oil is produced mainly in California.

OTHER SPECIES

C. paradisi *is a recent hybrid of* C. maxima *and* C. sinesis. *There are many different cultivars; for example, 'Duncan' is standard in Florida.*

Commiphora erythraea

Opopanax

FAMILY: BURSERACEAE   **SYNONYMS:** *C. ERYTHRAEA VAR. GLABRASCENS,* BISABOL MYRRH, SWEET MYRRH

Herbal/Folk Tradition

Opopanax derived from *Opopanax chironium* is described as having antispasmodic, expectorant, emmenagogue and antiseptic properties, which used to be employed in asthma, hysteria and visceral afflictions. In the Far East the bisabol myrrh is used extensively as an ingredient in incense.

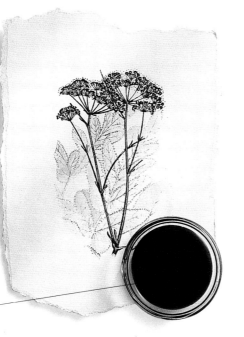

A tall tropical tree, similar to myrrh (to which it is closely related), which contains a natural oleo gum resin in tubular vessels between the bark and wood of the trunk. The locals make incisions in the trunk of the tree to increase the yield. The crude gum dries to form dark reddish-brown tear-shaped lumps with a sweet-woody, root-like odour.

opopanax gum

AROMATHERAPY/ HOME USE

Possibly similar uses to myrrh.

OTHER USES

Used as a fixative and fragrance component in high-class perfumery. Used in liqueurs to lend body and add wine-like notes.

DISTRIBUTION

Native to East Africa (Somalia) and eastern Ethiopia (Harrar Province) where it grows wild. The essential oil production is generally carried out in the USA and Europe from the crude oleo gum resin.

OTHER SPECIES

The original or 'true' opopanax used in perfumery was derived from a large plant Opopanax chironium *or* Pastinaca opopanax, *a plant similar to the parsnip of the Umbelliferae family and native to the Levant region, Sudan and Arabia. The oleo gum resin was obtained by cutting into the stem at the base, which then produces reddish-yellow tears of a strong root-like, parsnip or celery-type smell. This type of opopanax is now unavailable and has been replaced by a similar type of oil known as 'bisabol myrrh'. Not to be confused with cassie (Acacia farnesiana), which is also known as 'opopanax'.*

Commiphora erythraea

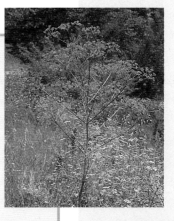

EXTRACTION

**1. Essential oil by steam (or water) distillation from the crude oleo gum resin.
2. A resinoid by solvent extraction from the crude oleo gum resin.**

CHARACTERISTICS

**1. An orange, yellow or olive liquid with a sweet-balsamic, spicy, warm, animal-like odour (it does not contain a medicinal note like myrrh). It resinifies on exposure to air.
2. A solid dark mass with a warm, powdery, sweet-balsamic, rooty odour.**

It blends well with clary sage, coriander, labdanum, bergamot, myrrh, frankincense, vetiver, sandalwood, patchouli, mimosa, fir needle and orange blossom.

ACTIONS

Antiseptic, antispasmodic, balsamic, expectorant.

PRINCIPAL CONSTITUENTS

The crude contains resins, gums (50–80 per cent) and essential oils (10–20 per cent), notably the sesquiterpene 'bisabolene' and sesquiterpene alcohols.

Commiphora myrrha

Myrrh

SAFETY DATA *Non-irritant, non-sensitizing, possibly toxic in high concentration. Not to be used during pregnancy*

FAMILY: BURSERACEAE **SYNONYMS:** *BALSAMODENDROM MYRRHA,* GUM MYRRH, COMMON MYRRH, HIRABOL MYRRH, MYRRHA

Herbal/Folk Tradition

In China it is used for arthritis, menstrual problems, sores and hemorrhoids. In the West it is considered to have an 'opening, heating, drying nature' (Joseph Miller), good for asthma, coughs, common cold, catarrh, sore throat, weak gums and teeth, ulcers and sores. It has also been used to treat leprosy. Current in the British Herbal Pharmacopoeia as a specific for mouth ulcers, gingivitis and pharyngitis.

The Commiphora species that yield myrrh are shrubs or small trees up to 10m (33ft) high, with knotted branches, trifolate aromatic leaves and white flowers.

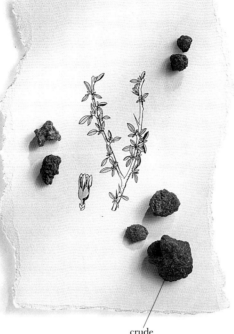

crude myrrh

AROMATHERAPY/ HOME USE

Skin Care: *Athlete's foot, chapped and cracked skin, eczema, mature complexions, ringworm, wounds, wrinkles.*
Circulation, Muscles and Joints: *Arthritis.*
Respiratory System: *Asthma, bronchitis, catarrh, coughs, gum infections, gingivitis, mouth ulcers, sore throat, voice loss.*
Digestive System: *Diarrhea, dyspepsia, flatulence, hemorrhoids, loss of appetite.*
Genito-urinary System: *Amenorrhea, leucorrhea, pruritis, thrush.*
Immune System: *Colds.*

OTHER USES

The oil, resinoid and tincture are used in pharmaceutical products, including mouthwashes, gargles and toothpaste; also used in dentistry. The oil and resinoid are used as fixatives and fragrance components in soaps, detergents, cosmetics and perfumes, especially oriental types and heavy florals. Used as flavour ingredients in most major food categories, alcoholic and soft drinks.

DISTRIBUTION

The Commiphora species are native to north-east Africa and south-west Asia, especially the Red Sea region (Somalia, Yemen and Ethiopia).

OTHER SPECIES

There are several C. *species that yield myrrh oleoresin: African or Somali myrrh (*C. molmol*) and Arabian or Yemen myrrh (*C. abyssinica*). Bisabol myrrh or opopanax (*C. erythraea*) also belongs to the same family.*

EXTRACTION

**1. Resinoid (and resin absolute) by solvent extraction of the crude myrrh.
2. Essential oil by steam distillation of the crude myrrh.**

CHARACTERISTICS

1. The resinoid is a dark reddish-brown viscous mass, with a warm, rich, spicy-balsamic odour. It is not pourable at room temperature so a solvent, such as diethyl phthalate, is sometimes added. 2. The essential oil is a pale yellow to amber oily liquid with a warm, sweet-balsamic, slightly spicy-medicinal odour. It blends well with frankincense, sandalwood, benzoin, oakmoss, cypress, juniper, mandarin, geranium, patchouli, thyme, mints, lavender, pine and spices.

ACTIONS

Anticatarrhal, anti-inflammatory, antimicrobial, antiphlogistic, antiseptic, astringent, balsamic, carminative, cicatrizant, emmenagogue, expectorant, fungicidal, revitalizing, sedative, stimulant (digestive, pulmonary), stomachic, tonic, uterine, vulnerary.

PRINCIPAL CONSTITUENTS

The crude contains resins, gum and about 8 per cent essential oil composed mainly of heerabolene, limonene, dipentene, pinene, eugenol, cinnamaldehyde, cuminaldehyde, cadinene, among others.

Copaifera officinalis

Copaiba balsam

FAMILY: FABACEAE (LEGUMINOSAE) **SYNONYMS:** COPAHU BALSAM, COPAIBA, COPAIVA, JESUIT'S BALSAM, MARACAIBO BALSAM, PARA BALSAM

Herbal/Folk Tradition

Used for centuries in Europe in the treatment of chronic cystitis and bronchitis; also for treating piles, chronic diarrhea and intestinal problems.

EXTRACTION

1. The crude balsam is collected by drilling holes into the tree trunks; it is one of the most plentiful naturally occurring perfume materials. 2. An essential oil is obtained by dry distillation from the crude balsam. It is mainly the 'para balsams' with a high oil content (**60–80 per cent**) that are used for distillation.

CHARACTERISTICS

1. The crude balsam is a viscous, yellowy-brown or greenish-grey liquid that hardens upon exposure to air with a mild, woody, slightly spicy odour. It blends well with styrax, amyris, lavandin, cedarwood, lavender, oakmoss, woods and spices. 2. The oil is a pale yellow or greenish mobile liquid with a mild, sweet, balsamic-peppery odour. It blends well with cananga, ylang ylang, vanilla, jasmine, violet and other florals.

ACTIONS

Bactericidal, balsamic, disinfectant, diuretic, expectorant, stimulant.

PRINCIPAL CONSTITUENTS

Mainly caryophyllene.

AROMATHERAPY/HOME USE

Digestive System:
Intestinal infections, piles.
Respiratory System:
Bronchitis, chills, colds, coughs, etc.
Genito-urinary System:
Cystitis.
Nervous System:
Stress-related conditions.

OTHER USES

The oleoresin is used in pharmaceutical products especially cough medicines and diuretics. The oil and crude balsam are extensively used as a fixative and fragrance component in all types of perfumes, soaps, cosmetics and detergents. The crude is also used in porcelain painting.

DISTRIBUTION

Native to north-east and central South America. Produced mainly in Brazil; also Venezuela, Guyana, Surinam and Colombia.

OTHER SPECIES

Several Copaifera *species yield an oleoresin: the Venezuelan type 'Maracaibo balsam' has a low oil content; the Brazilian type 'para balsam' has a high oil content. See also Botanical Classification section.*

Wild-growing tropical tree up to 18m (59ft) high, with thick foliage and many branches. The natural oleoresin occurs as a physiological product from various Copaifera *species. Not a 'true' balsam.*

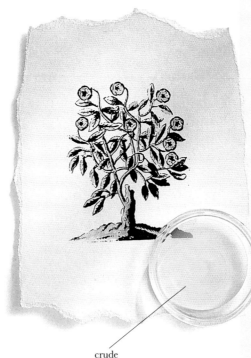

crude
copaiba balsam

Coriandrum sativum

Coriander

FAMILY: APIACEAE (UMBELLIFERAE)   **SYNONYMS:** CORIANDER SEED, CHINESE PARSLEY

Herbal/Folk Tradition

A herb with a long history of use; the seeds were found in the ancient Egyptian tomb of Rameses II. The seeds and leaves are widely used as a garnish and domestic spice, especially in curries. It has been used therapeutically, mainly in the form of an infusion for children's diarrhea, digestive upsets, griping pains, anorexia and flatulence.

In Chinese medicine the whole herb is used for dysentery, piles, measles, nausea, toothache and for painful hernia.

A strongly aromatic annual herb about 1m (3ft) high with bright green delicate leaves, umbels of lace-like white flowers, followed by a mass of green (turning brown) round seeds.

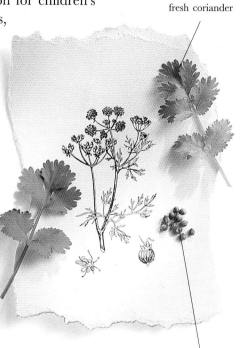

fresh coriander

coriander seeds

EXTRACTION

Essential oil by steam distillation from the crushed ripe seeds. (An essential oil is also produced by stem distillation from the fresh and dried leaves, which contains a high proportion of decylaldehyde.)

CHARACTERISTICS

A colourless to pale yellow liquid with a sweet, woody-spicy, slightly musky fragrance. It blends well with clary sage, bergamot, jasmine, olibanum, orange blossom, petitgrain, citronella, sandalwood, cypress, pine, ginger, cinnamon and other spice oils.

ACTIONS

Analgesic, aperitif, aphrodisiac, anti-oxidant, anti-rheumatic, antispasmodic, bactericidal, depurative, digestive, carminative, cytotoxic, fungicidal, larvicidal, lipolytic, revitalizing, stimulant (cardiac, circulatory, nervous system), stomachic.

PRINCIPAL CONSTITUENTS

Mainly linalol (55–75 per cent), decylaldehyde, borneol, geraniol, carvone, anethole, among others; constituents vary according to source.

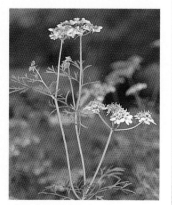

Coriandrum sativum

AROMATHERAPY/ HOME USE

Circulation, Muscles and Joints: *Accumulation of fluids and toxins, arthritis, gout, muscular aches and pains, poor circulation, rheumatism, stiffness.*
Digestive System: *Anorexia, colic, diarrhea, dyspepsia, flatulence, nausea, piles, spasm.*
Immune System: *Colds, flu, infections (general), measles.*
Nervous System: *Debility, migraine, neuralgia, nervous exhaustion.*

OTHER USES

Used as a flavouring agent in pharmaceutical preparations, especially digestive remedies.

Used as a fragrance component in soaps, toiletries and perfumes. Employed by the food industry especially in meat products and to flavour liqueurs such as Chartreuse and Benedictine; also used for flavouring tobacco.

DISTRIBUTION

Native to Europe and western Asia; naturalized in North America. Cultivated throughout the world, the oil is produced mainly in Russia, former Yugoslavia and Romania.

OTHER SPECIES

Various chemotypes of the same species are found according to geographical location.

Croton eleuteria

Cascarilla bark

FAMILY: EUPHORBIACEAE **SYNONYMS:** CASCARILLA, SWEETWOOD BARK, SWEET BARK, BAHAMA CASCARILLA, AROMATIC QUINQUINA, FALSE QUINQUINA

Herbal/Folk Tradition

The bark is used as an aromatic bitter and tonic for dyspepsia, diarrhea, dysentery, fever, debility, nausea, flatulence, vomiting and chronic bronchitis. The leaves are used as a digestive tea and for flavouring tobacco. The bark also yields a good black dye.

A large shrub or small tree up to 12m (39ft) high, with ovate silver-bronze leaves, pale yellowish-brown bark and small white fragrant flowers. It bears fruits and flowers all year round.

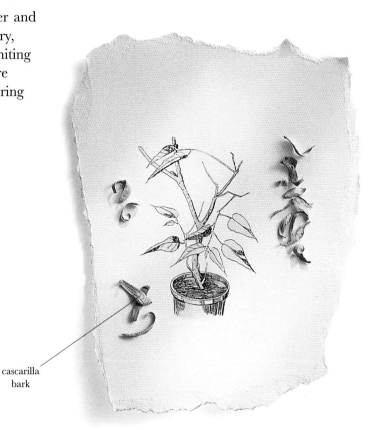

cascarilla
bark

EXTRACTION
Essential oil by steam distillation from the dried bark (1.5–3 per cent yield).

CHARACTERISTICS
A pale yellow, greenish or dark amber liquid with a spicy, aromatic, warm-woody odour. It blends well with nutmeg, pepper, pimento, sage, oakmoss, oriental and spicy bases.

ACTIONS
Astringent, antimicrobial, antiseptic, carminative, digestive, expectorant, stomachic, tonic.

PRINCIPAL CONSTITUENTS
Cymene, diterpene, limonene, caryophyllene, terpineol and eugenol, among others.

AROMATHERAPY/HOME USE

Respiratory System: *Bronchitis, coughs.*
Digestive System: *Dyspepsia, flatulence, nausea.*
Immune System: *flu.*

OTHER USES

Fragrance component in soaps, detergents, cosmetics and perfumes, especially men's fragrances.
Flavour ingredient in most major food categories, soft drinks and alcoholic beverages, especially vermouths and bitters.

DISTRIBUTION

Native to the West Indies, probably the Bahama Islands; found growing wild in Mexico, Colombia and Ecuador. The oil is produced mainly on the Bahamas and Cuba; some distillation takes place in the USA, France and Britain from the imported bark.

OTHER SPECIES

An essential oil is also distilled locally from other Croton *species. White, red and black cascarillas are also found in commerce.*

Cuminum cyminum

Cumin

FAMILY: APIACEAE (UMBELLIFERAE) **SYNONYMS:** *C. ODORUM*, CUMMIN, ROMAN CARAWAY

Herbal/Folk Tradition

A traditional Middle Eastern spice, and one of the main ingredients of curry. Although it has gone out of use in Western herbalism it is still largely used in traditional Ayurvedic medicine, principally as a general stimulant but especially for digestive complaints such as colic, sluggish digestion and dyspepsia.

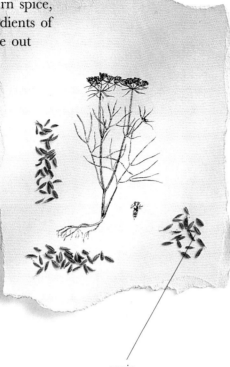

cumin
seed

A small, delicate, annual herb about 50cm (20in) high with a slender stem, dark green feathery leaves and small pink or white flowers followed by small oblong seeds.

AROMATHERAPY/ HOME USE

Circulation, Muscles and Joints: *Accumulation of fluids or toxins, poor circulation.*
Digestive System: *Colic, dyspepsia, flatulence, indigestion, spasm.*
Nervous System: *Debility, headaches, migraine, nervous exhaustion.*

OTHER USES

Used in veterinary medicine in digestive preparations. As a fragrance component in cosmetics and perfumes, and a flavour ingredient in many foods and drinks, especially meat products and condiments.

DISTRIBUTION

Native to upper Egypt, but from the earliest times cultivated in the Mediterranean region, especially Spain, France and Morocco; also in India and Russia. The oil is produced mainly in India, Spain and France.

OTHER SPECIES

Closely related to coriander (Coriandrum sativum), with which it shares many properties.

EXTRACTION
Essential oil by steam distillation from the ripe seeds.

CHARACTERISTICS
A pale yellow or greenish liquid with a warm, soft, spicy-musky scent. It blends well with lavender, lavandin, rosemary, galbanum, rosewood, cardomon and oriental-type fragrances.

ACTIONS
Anti-oxidant, antiseptic, antispasmodic, antitoxic, aphrodisiac, bactericidal, carminative, depurative, digestive, diuretic, emmenagogue, larvicidal, nervine, stimulant, tonic.

PRINCIPAL CONSTITUENTS
Mainly aldehydes (up to 60 per cent), including cuminaldehyde; monoterpene hydrocarbons (up to 52 per cent), including pinenes, terpinenes, cymene, phellandrene, myrcene and limonene; also farnesene and caryophyllene, among others.

Cupressus sempervirens

Cypress

FAMILY: CUPRESSACEAE **SYNONYMS:** ITALIAN CYPRESS, MEDITERRANEAN CYPRESS

Herbal/Folk Tradition

It was highly valued as a medicine and as an incense by ancient civilizations and it is still used as a purification incense by the Tibetans. It benefits the urinary system and is considered useful where there is excessive loss of fluid, such as heavy perspiration or menstrual loss and diarrhea: 'The cones are . . . very drying and binding, good to stop fluxes of all kinds.'[30]

The Chinese consider the nuts very nutritious, beneficial for the liver and respiratory system and to check profuse perspiration.

A tall evergreen tree with slender branches and a statuesque conical shape. It bears small flowers and round, brownish-grey cones or nuts.

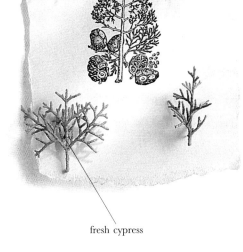

fresh cypress

EXTRACTION

Essential oil by steam distillation from the needles and twigs. An oil from the cones is available occasionally. (A concrete and absolute are also produced in small quantities.)

CHARACTERISTICS

A pale yellow to greenish-olive mobile liquid with a smoky, sweet-balsamic tenacious odour. It blends well with cedarwood, pine, lavender, mandarin, clary sage, lemon, cardomon, Maroc chamomile, ambrette seed, labdanum, juniper, benzoin, bergamot, orange, marjoram and sandalwood.

ACTIONS

Antirheumatic, antiseptic, antispasmodic, astringent, deodorant, diuretic, hepatic, styptic, sudorific, tonic, vasoconstrictive.

PRINCIPAL CONSTITUENTS

Pinene, camphene, sylvestrene, cymene, sabinol, among others.

AROMATHERAPY/ HOME USE

Skin Care: *Hemorrhoids, oily and overhydrated skin, excessive perspiration, insect repellent, pyorrhea (bleeding of the gums), varicose veins, wounds.*
Circulation, Muscles and Joints: *Cellulitis, muscular cramp, edema, poor circulation, rheumatism.*
Respiratory System: *Asthma, bronchitis, spasmodic coughing.*
Genito-urinary System: *Dysmenorrhea, menopausal problems, menorrhagia.*
Nervous System: *Nervous tension and stress-related conditions.*

OTHER USES

Employed in some pharmaceutical products; used as a fragrance component in colognes, aftershaves and perfumes.

DISTRIBUTION

Native to the eastern Mediterranean; now grows wild in France, Italy, Corsica, Sardinia, Sicily, Spain, Portugal, North Africa, Britain and, to a lesser degree, the Balkan countries. Cultivation and distillation usually take place in France, also Spain and Morocco.

OTHER SPECIES

There are many other species of cypress found throughout the world that are used to produce an essential oil, such as C. lusitanica. With regard to oil quality, C. sempervirens is considered superior.

Curcuma longa

Turmeric

FAMILY: ZINGIBERACEAE **SYNONYMS:** *C. DOMESTICA, AMOMOUM CURCUMA,* CURCUMA, INDIAN SAFFRON, INDIAN YELLOW ROOT, CURMUMA (OIL)

Herbal/Folk Tradition

A common household spice, especially for curry powder. It is high in minerals and vitamins, especially vitamin C. It is also used extensively as a local home medicine.

In Chinese herbalism it is used for bruises, sores, ringworm, toothache, chest pains, colic and menstrual problems, usually in combination with other remedies. It was once used as a cure for jaundice.

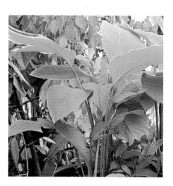

Curcuma longa

EXTRACTION
Essential oil by steam distillation from the 'cured' rhizome – boiled, cleaned and sun-dried. (An oleoresin, absolute and concrete are also produced by solvent extraction.)

CHARACTERISTICS
A yellowy-orange liquid with a faint blue fluorescence and a fresh spicy-woody odour. It blends well with cananga, labdanum, elecampane, ginger, orris, cassie, clary sage and mimosa.

ACTIONS
Analgesic, anti-arthritic, anti-inflammatory, anti-oxidant, bactericidal, cholagogue, digestive, diuretic, hypotensive, insecticidal, laxative, rubefacient, stimulant.

PRINCIPAL CONSTITUENTS
Mainly tumerone (60 per cent), with ar-tumerone, atlantones, zingiberene, cineol, borneol, sabinene and phellandrene, among others.

AROMATHERAPY/ HOME USE

Circulation, Muscles and Joints: *Arthritis, muscular aches and pains, rheumatism.*
Digestive System: *Anorexia, sluggish digestion, liver congestion. 'The essential oil of turmeric must be used in moderation and with care for a fairly limited period.'*[31]

OTHER USES

Employed in perfumery work, for oriental and fantasy-type fragrances. The oleoresin is used as a flavour ingredient in some foods, mainly curries, meat products and condiments.

DISTRIBUTION

Native in southern Asia; extensivley cultivated in India, China, Indonesia, Jamaica and Haiti. The oil is distilled mainly in India, China and Japan. Some roots are imported to Europe and the USA for distillation.

OTHER SPECIES

Closely related to the common ginger (Zingiber officinale). *Not to be confused with the Indian turmeric or American yellow root* (Hydrastis canadensis).

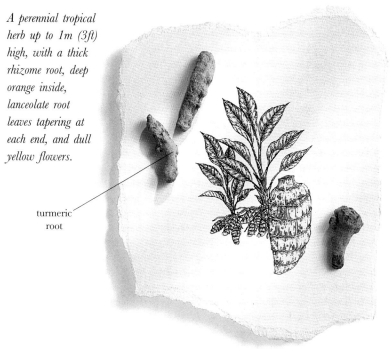

A perennial tropical herb up to 1m (3ft) high, with a thick rhizome root, deep orange inside, lanceolate root leaves tapering at each end, and dull yellow flowers.

turmeric root

Cymbopogon citratus

Lemongrass

FAMILY: POACEAE (GRAMINEAE) SYNONYMS: 1. *ANDROPOGON CITRATUS, A. SCHOENATHUS*, WEST INDIAN LEMONGRASS, MADAGASCAR LEMONGRASS, GUATEMALA LEMONGRASS 2. *ANDROPOGON FLEXUOSUS, CYMBOPOGON FLEXUOSUS*, EAST INDIAN LEMONGRASS, COCHIN LEMONGRASS, NATIVE LEMONGRASS, BRITISH INDIA LEMONGRASS, 'VERVAINE INDIENNE' OR FRANCE INDIAN VERBENA

Herbal/Folk Tradition

Employed in traditional Indian medicine for infectious illness and fever; modern research carried out in India shows that it also acts as a sedative on the central nervous system. It is also used as an insecticide and for flavouring food. After the distillation process, the exhausted grass is used locally to feed cattle.

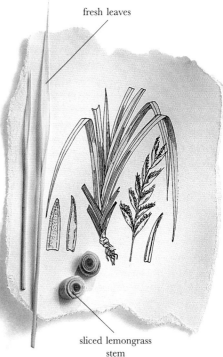

fresh leaves

sliced lemongrass stem

EXTRACTION
Essential oil by steam distillation from the fresh and partially dried leaves (grass), finely chopped.

A fast-growing, tall, aromatic perennial grass up to 1.5m (5ft) high, producing a network of roots and rootlets that rapidly exhaust the soil.

CHARACTERISTICS
1. A yellow, amber or reddish-brown liquid with a fresh, grassy-citrus scent and an earthy undertone. 2. A yellow or amber liquid with a fresh, grassy-lemony scent, generally lighter than the West Indian type.

ACTIONS
Analgesic, antidepressant, antimicrobial, anti-oxidant, antipyretic, antiseptic, astringent, bactericidal, carminative, deodorant, febrifuge, fungicidal, galactagogue, insecticidal, nervine, sedative (nervous), tonic.

PRINCIPAL CONSTITUENTS
1. Citral (65–85 per cent), myrcene (12–25 per cent), dipentene, methylheptenone, linalol, geraniol, nerol, citronellol and farnesol, among others. 2. Citral (up to 85 per cent), geraniol, methyl-eugenol, borneol, dipentene; constituents vary according to type.

AROMATHERAPY/ HOME USE

Skin Care: *Acne, athlete's foot, excessive perspiration, insect repellent (fleas, lice, ticks), open pores, pediculosis, scabies, tissue toner.*
Circulation, Muscles and Joints: *Muscular pain, poor circulation and muscle tone, slack tissue.*
Digestive System: *Colitis, indigestion, gastro-enteritis.*
Immune System: *Fevers, infectious disease.*
Nervous System: *Headaches, nervous exhaustion and stress-related conditions.*

OTHER USES

Extensively used as a fragrance component in soaps, detergents, cosmetics and perfumes. Employed as a flavour ingredient in most major food categories including alcoholic and soft drinks. Also used for the isolation of citral and for the adulteration of more costly oils such as verbena or melissa.

DISTRIBUTION

Native to Asia, there are two main types: 1. The West Indian lemongrass, which is probably native to Sri Lanka, now cultivated mainly in the West Indies, Africa and tropical Asia. Main oil producers include Guatemala and India. 2. The East Indian lemongrass, which is native to eastern India (Travancore, etc.), now cultivated mainly in western India!

OTHER SPECIES

There are several varieties of lemongrass of which the East Indian and the West Indian types are the most common. Chemotypes within each variety are also quite pronounced.

Cymbopogon martinii var. martinii

Palmarosa

FAMILY: GRAMINACEAE SYNONYMS: *ANDROPOGON MARTINII, A. MARTINII VAR. MOTIA,* EAST INDIAN GERANIUM, TURKISH GERANIUM, INDIAN ROSHA, MOTIA

Herbal/Folk Tradition

'The oil term "Indian" or "Turkish" geranium oil, which formerly was applied to palmarosa oil, dates back to the time when the oil was shipped from Bombay to ports of the Red Sea and transported partly by land, to Constantinople and Bulgaria, where the oil was often used for the adulteration of rose oil.'[32]

A wild-growing herbaceous plant with long slender stems and terminal flowering tops; the grassy leaves are very fragrant.

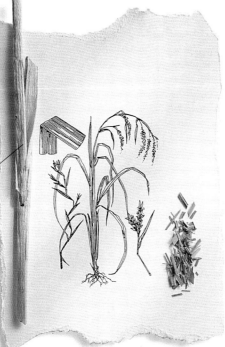

dried palmarosa stem

EXTRACTION
Essential oil by steam or water distillation of the fresh or dried grass.

CHARACTERISTICS
A pale yellow or olive liquid with a sweet, floral, rosy, geranium-like scent. It blends well with cananga, geranium, oakmoss, rosewood, amyris, sandalwood, guaiacwood, cedarwood and floral oils.

ACTIONS
Antiseptic, bactericidal, cicatrizant, digestive, febrifuge, hydrating, stimulant (digestive, circulatory), tonic.

PRINCIPAL CONSTITUENTS
Mainly geraniol; also farnesol, geranyl acetate, methylheptenone, citronellol, citral, dipentene and limonene, among others. Several chemotypes depending upon source – the cultivated varieties are considered of superior quality.

AROMATHERAPY/ HOME USE

Skin Care: *Acne, dermatitis and minor skin infections, scars, sores, wrinkles; valuable for all types of treatment for the face, hands, feet, neck and lips (moisturizes the skin, stimulates cellular regeneration, regulates sebum production).*
Digestive System: *Anorexia, digestive atonia, intestinal infections – 'This is an essence which acts on the pathogenic intestinal flora, in particular on the colibacillus, the Eberth bacillus and the bacillus of dysentery . . . this essence favours the* transmutation of the pathogenic agent into normal cells of intestinal mucous membranes. Thus it arrests the degeneracy of the cells for the latter, swiftly impels groups of normal cells towards an inferior form in their hierarchy. The essence does not appear to contain any acid.'[33]
Nervous System: *Nervous exhaustion, stress-related conditions.*

OTHER USES

Used extensively as a fragrance component in cosmetics, perfumes and especially soaps due to excellent tenacity. Limited use as a flavouring agent, e.g., tobacco. Used for the isolation of natural geraniol.

DISTRIBUTION

Native to India and Pakistan; now grown in Africa, Indonesia, Brazil and the Comoro Islands.

OTHER SPECIES

Of the same family as lemongrass and citronella; also closely related to gingergrass, which is a different chemotype known as C. martinii var. sofia. *Gingergrass is considered an inferior oil, but in some parts of India the two types of grass are distilled together.*

Cymbopogon nardus

Citronella

FAMILY: POACEAE (GRAMINEAE)   SYNONYMS: *ANDROPOGON NARDUS,*
SRI LANKA CITRONELLA, LENABATU CITRONELLA

Herbal/Folk Tradition

The leaves of citronella are used for their aromatic and
medicinal value in many cultures, for fever, intestinal
parasites, digestive and menstrual problems, as a stimulant
and an insect repellent. It is used in Chinese traditional
medicine for rheumatic pain.

EXTRACTION
**Essential oil by steam
distillation of the fresh, part-
dried or dried grass. (The Java
citronella yields twice as much
oil as the Sri Lanka type.)**

CHARACTERISTICS
**A yellow-brown, mobile liquid
with a fresh, powerful, lemony
scent. The Java oil is colourless
to pale yellow with a fresh,
woody-sweet fragrance; it is
considered of superior quality
in perfumery work. It blends
well with geranium, lemon,
bergamot, orange, cedarwood
and pine.**

ACTIONS
**Antiseptic, antispasmodic,
bactericidal, deodorant,
diaphoretic, diuretic,
emmenagogue, febrifuge,
fungicidal, insecticide,
stomachic, tonic, vermifuge.**

PRINCIPAL CONSTITUENTS
**Mainly geraniol (up to 45 per
cent in the Java oil), citronellol
(up to 50 per cent in the Java
oil) with geranyl acetate,
limonene and camphene,
among others. The Sri Lanka
variety contains more
monoterpene hydrocarbons.**

AROMATHERAPY/
HOME USE

Skin Care: *Excessive
perspiration, oily skin, insect
repellent. 'Mixed with cedarwood
oil Virginia, it has been a popular
remedy against mosquito attacks
for many years prior to the
appearance of DDT and other
modern insecticides.'[34]*
Immune System: *Cold, flu,
minor infections.*
Nervous System: *Fatigue,
headaches, migraine, neuralgia.*

OTHER USES

*Extensively used in soaps,
detergents, household goods
and industrial perfumes.
Employed in insect repellent
formulations against moths,
ants, fleas, etc., for use in
the home and in the garden.
The Sri Lanka oil is used in most
major food categories, including
alcoholic and soft drinks. The
Java oil is used as the starting
material for the isolation of
natural geraniol and citronellol.*

DISTRIBUTION

*Native to Sri Lanka, now
extensively cultivated on the
southernmost tip of the country.*

OTHER SPECIES

*An important essential oil
is also produced on a large
scale from the Java or
Maha Pengiri citronella
(C. winterianus). This
variety is cultivated in the
tropics worldwide, especially
in Java, Vietnam, Africa,
Argentina and Central
America. There are many
other related species of
scented grasses.*

Cymbopogon nardus

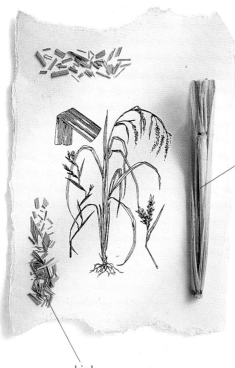

*A tall, aromatic, perennial
grass, which has derived from
the wild-growing 'managrass'
found in Sri Lanka.*

fresh
citronella
grass

dried
citronella

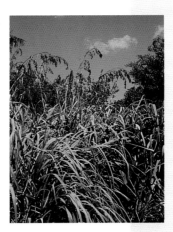

Daucus carota

Carrot seed

FAMILY: APIACEAE (UMBELLIFERAE)   SYNONYMS: WILD CARROT, QUEEN ANNE'S LACE, BIRD'S NEST

Herbal/Folk Tradition

A highly nutritious plant, containing substantial amounts of Vitamins A, C, B_1 and B_2. The roots have a strong tonic action on the liver and gall bladder, good for the treatment of jaundice and other complaints. The seeds are used for the retention of urine, colic, kidney and digestive disorders, and to promote menstruation. In the Chinese tradition it is used to treat dysentery and to expel worms.

The dried leaves are current in the British Herbal Pharmacopoeia for calculus, gout, cystitis and lithuria.

Annual or biennial herb, with a small, inedible, tough whitish root. It has a much-branched stem up to 1.5m (5ft) high with hairy leaves and umbels of white lacy flowers.

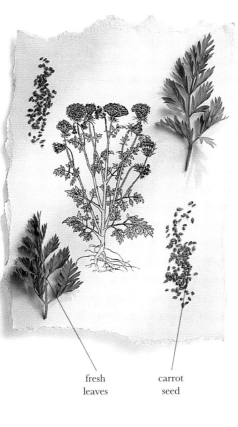

fresh leaves   carrot seed

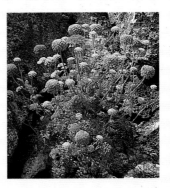

Daucus carota

AROMATHERAPY/ HOME USE

Skin Care: *Dermatitis, eczema, psoriasis, rashes, revitalizing and toning, mature complexions, wrinkles.*
Circulation, Muscles and Joints: *Accumulation of toxins, arthritis, gout, edema, rheumatism.*
Digestive System: *Anemia, anorexia, colic, indigestion, liver congestion.*
Genito-urinary and Endocrine Systems: *Amenorrhea, dysmenorrhea, glandular problems, PMT.*

OTHER USES

Fragrance component in soaps, detergents, cosmetics and perfumes. Flavour ingredient in most major food categories, especially seasonings.

DISTRIBUTION

Native to Europe, Asia and North Africa; naturalized in North America. The essential oil is produced mainly in France.

OTHER SPECIES

An oil is also produced by solvent extraction from the red fleshy root of the common edible carrot (D. carota *subspecies* sativus) *mainly for use as a food colouring.*

EXTRACTION
Essential oil by steam distillation from the dried fruit (seeds).

CHARACTERISTICS
A yellow or amber-coloured liquid with a warm, dry, woody-earthy odour. It blends well with costus, cassie, mimosa, cedarwood, geranium, citrus and spice oils.

ACTIONS
Anthelmintic, antiseptic, carminative, depurative, diuretic, emmenagogue, hepatic, stimulant, tonic, vasodilatory and smooth muscle relaxant.

PRINCIPAL CONSTITUENTS
Pinene, carotol, daucol, limonene, bisabolene, elemene, geraniol, geranyl acetate, caryophyllene, among others.

Dipteryx odorata

Tonka

FAMILY: LEGUMINOSAE **SYNONYMS:** *COUMAROUNA ODORATA*, TONQUIN BEAN, DUTCH TONKA BEAN

Herbal/Folk Tradition

In the Netherlands the fatty substance from the beans is sold as 'taquin butter', which used to be used as an insecticide against moths in linen cupboards. 'The fluid extract has been used with advantage in whooping cough, but it paralyses the heart if used in large doses.'[35]

A very large tropical tree with big elliptical leaves and violet flowers, bearing fruit that contain a single black seed or 'tonka bean', about the size of a butter bean. The beans, known as 'rumara' by the locals, are collected and dried, then soaked in alcohol or rum for twelve to fifteen hours to make them swell. When they are removed from the bath they become dried and shrunken, covered with a whitish powder of crystallized coumarin. The 'curing' of the beans is partly a conventional 'sales promotion' technique rather than an indication of quality, since the frosted appearance has come to be expected of the product.

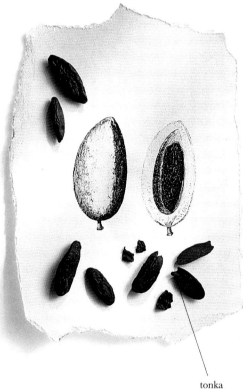

tonka
beans

AROMATHERAPY/
HOME USE
None.

OTHER USES
Used to a limited extent as a pharmaceutical masking agent. The absolute is employed as a fixative and fragrance component in oriental, new-mown hay and chyprès-type perfumes. It is no longer used as a flavouring (due to the coumarin ban in many countries), though it is still used to flavour tobacco.

DISTRIBUTION
Native to South America, especially Venezuela, Guyana and Brazil; cultivated in Nigeria and elsewhere in West Africa. Most beans come from South America after 'curing', to be processed in Europe and the USA.

OTHER SPECIES
There are many other species of Dipteryx that produce beans suitable for extraction.

EXTRACTION
A concrete and absolute by solvent extraction from the 'cured' beans.

CHARACTERISTICS
The absolute is a semi-solid yellow or amber mass with a very rich, warm and sweet herbaceous-nutty odour. It blends well with lavender, lavandin, clary sage, styrax, bergamot, oakmoss, helichrysum and citronella.

ACTIONS
Insecticidal, narcotic, tonic (cardiac).

PRINCIPAL CONSTITUENTS
Mainly coumarin (20–40 per cent) in the absolute.

Dryobalanops aromatica

Borneol

SAFETY DATA *Non-toxic, non-sensitizing, dermal irritant in concentration*

FAMILY: DIPTEROCARPACEAE SYNONYMS: *D. CAMPHORA*, BORNEO CAMPHOR, EAST INDIAN CAMPHOR, BAROS CAMPHOR, SUMATRA CAMPHOR, MALAYAN CAMPHOR

Herbal/Folk Tradition

Borneol has long been regarded as a panacea by many Eastern civilizations, especially in ancient Persia, India and China. It was used as a powerful remedy against plague and other infectious diseases, stomach and bowel complaints. In China it was also used for embalming purposes. 'It is mentioned by Marco Polo in the thirteenth century and Camoens in 1571 who called it the "balsam of disease".'[36] It is valued for ceremonial purposes in the East generally, and in China particularly for funeral rites. Its odour repels insects and ants, and it is therefore highly regarded as timber for the construction of buildings.

The camphora tree grows to a great height, a majestic tree often over 25m (82ft) high, with a thick trunk up to 2m (6ft) in diameter. Borneol is a natural exudation found beneath the bark in crevices and fissures of some mature trees (about 1 per cent); young trees produce only a clear yellow liquid known as 'liquid camphor'.

crystallized borneol

EXTRACTION
The borneol is collected from the tree trunk in its crude crystalline form (the locals test each tree first by making incisions in the trunk to detect its presence). The so-called oil of borneol is extracted by steam distillation of the wood.

CHARACTERISTICS
Watery white to viscous black oil depending upon the amount of camphor it contains, with a distinctive, sassafras-like, camphoraceous odour.

ACTIONS
Mildly analgesic, antidepressant, antiseptic, antispasmodic, antiviral, carminative, rubefacient, stimulant of the adrenal cortex, tonic (cardiac and general).

PRINCIPAL CONSTITUENTS
The crude is made up of mainly d-borneol, which is an alcohol, not a ketone (like Japanese camphor). The oil contains approx. 35 per cent terpenes: pinene, camphene, dipentene; 10 per cent alcohols: d-borneol, terpineol; 20 per cent sesquiterpenes, and 35 per cent resin.

AROMATHERAPY/ HOME USE
Skin Care: *Cuts, bruises, insect repellent.*
Circulation, Muscles and Joints: *Debility, poor circulation, rheumatism, sprains.*
Respiratory System: *Bronchitis, coughs.*
Immune System: *Colds, fever, flu and other infectious diseases.*
Nervous System: *Nervous exhaustion, stress-related conditions, neuralgia.*

OTHER USES
It is used to scent soap in the East but is still relatively unknown in the West in pharmaceutical and perfumery work. In China and Japan it is used for making varnish and ink; also as a diluent for artists' colours. Mainly used for ritual purposes in the East.

DISTRIBUTION
Native to Borneo and Sumatra.

OTHER SPECIES
To be distinguished from the Japanese or Formosa type of camphor, more commonly used in Europe, which is relatively toxic. See also Botanical Classification section.

Elettaria cardamomum

Cardomon

FAMILY: ZINGIBERACEAE **SYNONYMS:** *ELETTARIA CARDOMOMUM VAR. CARDOMOMUM,* CARDOMOM, CARDAMOMI, CARDOMUM, MUSORE CARDOMOM

Herbal/Folk Tradition

Used extensively as a domestic spice, especially in India, Europe, Latin America and Middle Eastern countries. It has been used in traditional Chinese and Indian medicine for over 3,000 years, especially for pulmonary disease, fever, digestive and urinary complaints. Hippocrates recommended it for sciatica, coughs, abdominal pains, spasms, nervous disorders, retention of urine and also for bites of venomous creatures.

Current in the British Herbal Pharmacopoeia as a specific for flatulent dyspepsia.

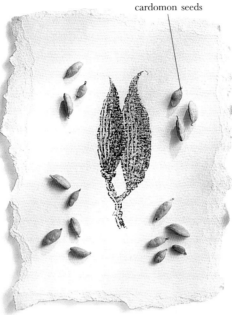

cardomon seeds

A perennial, reed-like herb up to 4m (13ft) high, with long, silk blade-shaped leaves. Its long sheathing stems bear small yellowish flowers with purple tips, followed by oblong red-brown seeds.

EXTRACTION
Essential oil by steam distillation from the dried ripe fruit (seeds). An oleoresin is also produced in small quantities.

CHARACTERISTICS
A colourless to pale yellow liquid with a sweet-spicy, warming fragrance and a woody-balsamic undertone. It blends well with rose, olibanum, orange, bergamot, cinnamon, cloves, caraway, ylang ylang, labdanum, cedarwood, orange blossom, and oriental bases in general.

ACTIONS
Antiseptic, antispasmodic, aphrodisiac, carminative, cephalic, digestive, diuretic, sialagogue, stimulant, stomachic, tonic (nerve).

PRINCIPAL CONSTITUENTS
Terpinyl acetate and cineol (each may be present at up to 50 per cent), limonene, sabiene, linalol, linalyl acetate, pinene, zingiberene, among others.

AROMATHERAPY/ HOME USE

Digestive System: *Anorexia, colic, cramp, dyspepsia, flatulence, griping pains, halitosis, heartburn, indigestion, vomiting.*
Nervous System: *Mental fatigue, nervous strain.*

OTHER USES

Employed in some carminative, stomachic and laxative preparations; also in the form of compound cardomon spirit to flavour pharmaceuticals.

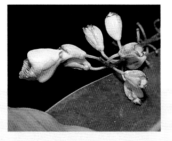

Elettaria cardamomum

Extensively used as a fragrance component in soaps, cosmetics and perfumes, especially oriental types. Important flavour ingredient, particularly in curry and spice products.

DISTRIBUTION

Native to tropical Asia, especially southern India; cultivated extensively in India, Sri Lanka,

Laos, Guatemala and El Salvador. The oil is produced principally in India, Europe, Sri Lanka and Guatemala.

OTHER SPECIES

There are numerous related species found in the East, used as local spices and for medicinal purposes, such as round or Siam cardomon (Amomum cardomomum) found in India and China. An oil is also produced from wild cardomon (E. cardamomum var. major).

Eucalyptus citriodora

Lemon-scented eucalyptus

FAMILY: MYRTACEAE **SYNONYMS:** LEMON-SCENTED GUM, CITRON-SCENTED GUM, SCENTED GUM TREE, SPOTTED GUM, 'BOABO'

Herbal/Folk Tradition

Used traditionally for perfuming the linen cupboard by enclosing the dried leaves in a small cloth sachet. During the last century it was regarded as a good insect repellent, especially for cockroaches and silverfish.

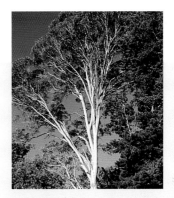

Eucalyptus citriodora

EXTRACTION
Essential oil by steam distillation from the leaves and twigs.

CHARACTERISTICS
A colourless or pale yellow mobile liquid with a strong, fresh, citronella-like odour and sweet balsamic undertone.

ACTIONS
Antiseptic, antiviral, bactericidal, deodorant, expectorant, fungicidal, insecticide.

PRINCIPAL CONSTITUENTS
Citronellal (80–95 per cent), citronellol, geraniol and pinene, among others. (The gum or 'kino' contains the antibiotic substance 'citriodorol'.)

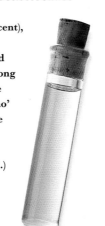

AROMATHERAPY/HOME USE

Not compatible with homeopathic treatment.
Skin Care: *Athlete's foot and other fungal infections (e.g. candida), cuts, dandruff, herpes, insect repellent, scabs, sores, wounds.*
Respiratory System: *Asthma, laryngitis, sore throat.*
Immune System: *Colds, fevers, infectious skin conditions such as chickenpox, infectious disease. 'The essential oil contained in the leaves appears to have bacteriostatic activity towards Staphylococcus aureus; this is due to synergism between the citronellol and citronellal present in the oil.'*[37]

OTHER USES

Used as a fragrance component (in place of E. globulus) in soaps, detergents and perfumes; also used in room sprays and insect repellents. Employed for the isolation of natural citronellal.

DISTRIBUTION

Native to Australia; cultivated mainly in Brazil and China.

OTHER SPECIES

There are numerous other species of eucalyptus – see entry on blue gum eucalyptus. See also Botanical Classification section.

An attractive, tall evergreen tree with a smooth dimpled bark, blotched in grey, cream and pink, cultivated as an ornamental. The trunk grows fast, straight and to considerable height, and is used for timber. The young leaves are oval, the mature leaves narrow and tapering.

dried leaves

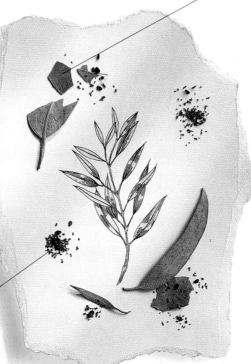

lemon-scented eucalyptus seeds

Eucalyptus dives var. Type

Broad-leaved peppermint eucalyptus

FAMILY: MYRTACEAE **SYNONYMS:** BROAD-LEAF PEPPERMINT, BLUE PEPPERMINT, MENTHOL-SCENTED GUM

> **SAFETY DATA** *Non-toxic, non-irritant (in dilution), non-sensitizing. Eucalyptus oil is toxic if taken internally (see entry on blue gum eucalyptus p.141).*

Herbal/Folk Tradition

The aborigines used the burning leaves in the form of a fumigation for the relief of fever: 'heat went out of sick man and into fire'.

A robust, medium-sized eucalyptus tree, with a short trunk, spreading branches and fibrous grey bark. The young leaves are blue and heart-shaped, the mature leaves are very aromatic, thick and tapering at both ends.

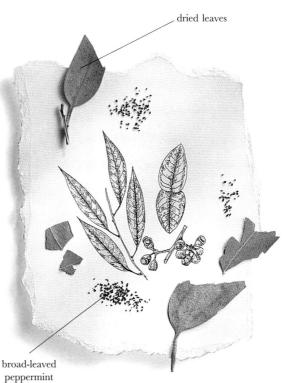

dried leaves

broad-leaved peppermint eucalyptus seeds

EXTRACTION

Essential oil by steam distillation from the leaves and twigs.

CHARACTERISTICS

A colourless or pale yellow mobile liquid with a fresh, camphoraceous, spicy-minty odour.

ACTIONS

Analgesic, antineuralgic, antirheumatic, antiseptic, antispasmodic, antiviral, balsamic, cicatrizant, decongestant, deodorant, depurative, diuretic, expectorant, febrifuge, hypoglycemic, parasiticide, prophylactic, rubefacient, stimulant, vermifuge, vulnerary.

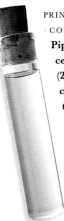

PRINCIPAL CONSTITUENTS

Piperitone (40–50 per cent), phellandrene (20–30 per cent), camphene, cymene, terpinene and thujene, among others. It is sold as Grades A, B or C according to the extract balance of constituents.

AROMATHERAPY/ HOME USE

Not compatible with homeopathic treatment.
Skin Care: *Cuts, sores, ulcers, etc.*
Circulation, Muscles and Joints: *Arthritis, muscular aches and pains, rheumatism, sports injuries, sprains, etc.*
Respiratory System: *Asthma, bronchitis, catarrh, coughs, throat and mouth infections, etc.*
Immune System: *Colds, fevers, flu, infectious illnesses, e.g. measles.*
Nervous System: *Headaches, nervous exhaustion, neuralgia, sciatica.*

OTHER USES

Little used medicinally these days except in deodorants, disinfectants, mouthwashes, gargles and in veterinary practice. 'Piperitone' rich oils are used in solvents. Employed for the manufacture of thymol and menthol (for piperitone).

DISTRIBUTION

Native to Australia, especially New South Wales, Tasmania and Victoria. Oil is also produced in South Africa.

OTHER SPECIES

There are two types of broad-leaved peppermint although they look identical – one is rich in cineol (E. dives var. C.) and one is rich in 'piperitone' (E. dives var. Type). It is also similar to the peppermint eucalyptus (E. piperita) and the grey or narrow-leaved peppermint (E. radiata var. phellandra). See also entry on blue gum eucalyptus and Botanical Classification section.

Eucalyptus globulus var. globulus

Blue gum eucalyptus

FAMILY: MYRTACEAE **SYNONYMS:** GUM TREE, SOUTHERN BLUE GUM, TASMANIAN BLUE GUM, FEVER TREE, STRINGY BARK

Herbal/Folk Tradition

A traditional household remedy in Australia, the leaves and oil are used especially for respiratory ailments such as bronchitis and croup, and the dried leaves are smoked like tobacco for asthma. It is also used for feverish conditions (malaria, typhoid, cholera, etc.) and skin problems such as burns, ulcers and wounds. Aqueous extracts are used for aching joints, bacterial dysentery, ringworms, tuberculosis, etc. and employed for similar reasons in Western and Eastern medicine. The wood is also used for timber production in Spain.

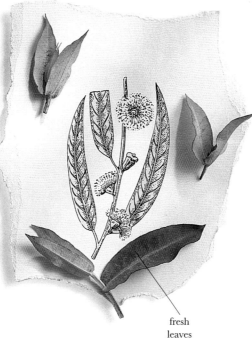

fresh leaves

A beautiful, tall, evergreen tree, up to 90m (295ft) high. The young trees have bluish-green oval leaves while the mature trees develop long, narrow, yellowish leaves, creamy-white flowers and a smooth, pale grey bark often covered with a white powder.

EXTRACTION
Essential oil by steam distillation from the fresh or partially dried leaves and young twigs.

CHARACTERISTICS
A colourless mobile liquid (yellow on aging), with a somewhat harsh camphoraceous odour and woody-scent undertone. It blends well with thyme, rosemary, lavender, marjoram, pine, cedarwood and lemon. (The narrow-leaved eucalyptus (E. radiata var. australiana) is often used in preference to the blue gum in aromatherapy work, being rich in cineol but with a sweeter and less harsh odour.)

ACTIONS
See broad-leaved peppermint eucalyptus.

PRINCIPAL CONSTITUENTS
Cineol (70–85 per cent), pinene, limonene, cymene, phellandrene, terpinene, aromadendrene, among others.

AROMATHERAPY/ HOME USE

Not compatible with homeopathic treatment.

Skin Care: *Burns, blisters, cuts, herpes, insect bites, insect repellent, lice, skin infections, wounds.*

Circulation, Muscles and Joints: *Muscular aches and pains, poor circulation, rheumatoid arthritis, sprains, etc.*

Respiratory System: *Asthma, bronchitis, catarrh, coughs, sinusitis, throat infections.*

Genito-urinary System: *Cystitis, leucorrhea.*

Immune System: *Chickenpox, colds, epidemics, flu, measles.*

Nervous System: *Debility, headaches, neuralgia.*

OTHER USES

The oil and coneol are largely employed in the preparation of liniments, inhalants, cough syrups, ointments, toothpaste and as pharmaceutical flavouring, also used in veterinary practice and dentistry. Used as a fragrance component in soaps, detergents and toiletries – little used in perfumes. Used for the isolation of cineol and employed as a flavour ingredient in most major food categories.

DISTRIBUTION

Native to Australia. Cultivated mainly in Spain and Portugal, also Brazil, California, Russia and China. Very little of this oil now comes from its native country.

OTHER SPECIES

There are over 700 different species of eucalyptus, of which at least 500 produce a type of essential oil. In general, they can be divided into three categories. 1. The medicinal oils. 2. The industrial oils. 3. The perfumery oils. See also Botanical Classification section.

Evernia prunastri

Oakmoss

SAFETY DATA *Extensively compounded or bouquetted by cutting or adulteration with other lichen or synthetic perfume materials*

FAMILY: USNEACEAE **SYNONYMS:** *MOUSSE DE CHÊNE*, TREEMOSS

Herbal/Folk Tradition

Sticta pulmonaceae, a greeny-brown lichen frequently harvested along with *E. prunastri*, is also called oak lungs, lung moss, lungwort or 'lungs of oak' by the Native Americans who use it for respiratory complaints and for treating wounds. It is called lobaria in the British Herbal Pharmacopoeia and is used for asthma, bronchitis and coughs in children. Many types of lichen, especially the *Parmelia* group, are used as vegetable dyes.

A light green lichen found growing primarily on oak trees, sometimes on other species.

oakmoss
lichen

AROMATHERAPY/ HOME USE

As a fixative.

OTHER USES

The concrete is used primarily in soaps; the absolute is the most versatile and is used in all perfume types (oriental, moss, fougère, new-mown hay, floral, colognes, aftershaves, etc.). The absolute oil is used in high-class perfumes. The resins and resinoids, which have a poor solubility, are used in soaps, hair preparations, industrial perfumes and low-cost products.

DISTRIBUTION

The oak (Quercus robur) is indigenous to Europe and North America; the lichen is collected all over central and southern Europe, especially France, former

Yugoslavia, Hungary, Greece, and also Morocco and Algeria. The aromatic materials are prepared mainly in France, but also in the USA, Bulgaria and former Yugoslavia.

OTHER SPECIES

There are many varieties of lichen used for their aromatic qualities, the most common being E. furfuracea and Usnea barbata, which are frequently gathered from spruce and pine trees, and are known as fir moss or tree moss in Europe, but in the USA are also called oakmoss. However, they are less refined than the 'true' oakmoss. Other species include Sticta pulmonaceae or Lobaria pulmonaria, Usnea ceratina, and some members of the Ramalina, Alectoria and Parmelia groups.

EXTRACTION

A range of products is produced: a concrete and an absolute by solvent extraction from the lichen that has often been soaked in lukewarm water prior to extraction; an absolute oil by vacuum distillation of the concrete; resins and resinoids by alcohol extraction of the raw material. Most important of these products is the absolute.

CHARACTERISTICS

**1. The absolute is a dark green or brown, very viscous liquid with an extremely tenacious, earthy-mossy odour and a leather-like undertone.
2. The absolute oil is a pale yellow or olive viscous liquid with a dry-earthy, bark-like odour, quite true to nature.
3. The concrete, resin and resinoids are very dark-coloured semi-solid or solid masses with a heavy, rich-earthy, extremely tenacious odour. They have a high fixative value and blend with virtually all other oils: they are extensively used in perfumery to lend body and rich natural undertones to all perfume types.**

ACTIONS

Antiseptic, demulcent, expectorant, fixative.

PRINCIPAL CONSTITUENTS

Crystalline matter of so-called lichen acids': mainly evernic acid, d-usnic acid, some atranorine and chloratronorine.

Ferula assa-foetida

Asafetida

SAFETY DATA *Available information indicates the oil to be relatively non-toxic and non-irritant. However, it has the reputation for being the most adulterated 'drug' on the market. Before being sold, the oleoresin is often mixed with red clay or similar substitutes*

FAMILY: APIACEAE (UMBELLIFERAE)   **SYNONYMS:** ASAFOETIDA, GUM ASAFETIDA, DEVIL'S DUNG, FOOD OF THE GODS, GIANT FENNEL

Herbal/Folk Tradition

In Chinese medicine it has been used since the seventh century as a nerve stimulant in treating neurasthenia. It is also widely used in traditional Indian medicine, where it is believed to stimulate the brain. In general, it has the reputation of treating various ailments including asthma, bronchitis, convulsions, coughs, constipation, flatulence and hysteria. The foliage of the plant is used as a local vegetable. It is current in the British Herbal Pharmacopoeia as a specific for intestinal flatulent colic.

A large branching perennial herb up to 3m (10ft) high, with a thick fleshy root system and pale yellow-green flowers.

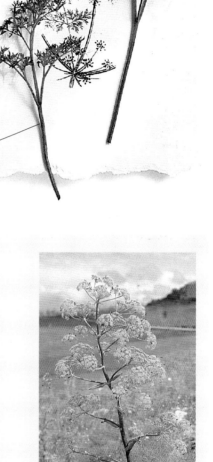

fresh
asafetida

EXTRACTION
The oleoresin is obtained by making incisions into the root and above-ground parts of the plant. The milky juice is left to leak out and harden into dark reddish lumps, before being scraped off and collected. The essential oil is then obtained from the resin by steam distillation. An absolute, resinoid and tincture are also produced.

CHARACTERISTICS
A yellowy-orange oil with a bitter acrid taste and a strong, tenacious odour resembling garlic. However, beneath this odour there is a sweet, balsamic note.

ACTIONS
Antispasmodic, carminative, expectorant, hypotensive, stimulant. Animals are repelled by its odour.

PRINCIPAL CONSTITUENTS
Disulphides, notably 2-butyl propenyl disulphide with momeoterpenes, free ferulic acid, valeric, traces of vanillin, among others.

AROMATHERAPY/ HOME USE

Respiratory System: *'There is evidence that the volatile oil is expelled through the lungs, therefore it is excellent for asthma, bronchitis, whooping cough, etc.'*[39]
Nervous System: *Fatigue, nervous exhaustion and stress-related conditions.*

OTHER USES

Now rarely used in pharmaceutical preparations; formerly used as a local stimulant for the mucous membranes. Occasionally used as a fixative and fragrance component in perfumes, especially rose bases and heavy oriental types. Employed in a wide variety of food categories, mainly condiments and sauces.

DISTRIBUTION
Native to Afghanistan, Iran and other regions of south-west Asia.

Ferula assa-foetida

OTHER SPECIES

There are several other species of Ferula *that yield the oleoresin known as 'asafetida', e.g. Tibetan asafetida, which is also used to a lesser extent in commerce.*

Ferula galbaniflua

Galbanum

FAMILY: APIACEAE (UMBELLIFERAE) **SYNONYMS:** *F. GUMOSA*, GALBANUM GUM, GALBANUM RESIN, 'BUBONION'

Herbal/Folk Tradition

It was used by the ancient civilizations as an incense, and in Egypt for cosmetics and in the embalming process. It is generally used in the East in a similar way to asafetida: for treating wounds, inflammations and skin disorders and also for respiratory, digestive and nervous complaints. Zalou root *(F. hermonic)* is used in Beirut as an aphrodisiac.

EXTRACTION
Essential oil by water or steam distillation from the oleoresin or gum – only the Levant or soft type is used for oil production. A partially deterpenized oil is produced, known as 'galbanol'. (A resinoid is also produced, mainly for use as a fixative.)

CHARACTERISTICS
Crude – A dark amber or brown viscous liquid with a green-woody scent and a soft balsamic undertone. Oil – A colourless, or pale yellow or olive liquid with a fresh green top note and woody-dry balsamic undertone. It blends well with hyacinth, violet, narcissus, lavender, geranium, oakmoss, opopanax, pine, fir, styrax and oriental bases.

ACTIONS
Analgesic, anti-inflammatory, antimicrobial, antiseptic, antispasmodic, aphrodisiac, balsamic, carminative, cicatrizant, digestive, diuretic, emmenagogue, expectorant, hypotensive, restorative, tonic.

PRINCIPAL CONSTITUENTS
Pinene, cadinol, cadinene and myrcene, among others.

AROMATHERAPY/HOME USE

Skin Care: *Abscesses, acne, boils, cuts, heals scar tissue, inflammations, tones the skin, mature skin, wrinkles, wounds - 'signifies drying and preservation'.*[40]

Circulation, Muscles and Joints: *Poor circulation, muscular aches and pains, rheumatism.*

Respiratory System: *Asthma, bronchitis, catarrh, chronic coughs.*

Digestive System: *Cramp, flatulence, indigestion.*

Nervous System: *Nervous tension and stress-related complaints.*

OTHER USES

The Persian gum used to be employed in pharmaceutical products. Both oil and resinoid are used as fixative and fragrance components in soaps, detergents, creams, lotions and perfumes. Also used as a flavour ingredient in most major food categories, alcoholic and soft drinks.

DISTRIBUTION

Native to the Middle East and western Asia; cultivated in Iran, Turkey, Afghanistan and Lebanon. Distillation usually takes place in Europe or the USA.

OTHER SPECIES

There are two distinct types: Levant galbanum, which is liquid or soft, and Persian galbanum, which is solid or hard. Other Ferula species also yield galbanum gum, such as the muskroot; see also Botanical Classification section.

A large perennial herb with a smooth stem, shiny leaflets and small flowers. It contains resin ducts that exude a milky juice, a natural oleoresin. The dried resinous exudation is collected by making incisions at the base of the stem.

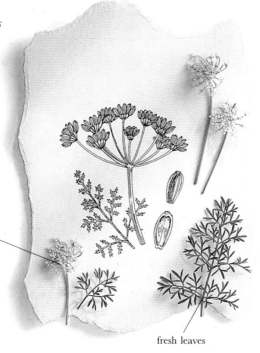

galbanum flowers

fresh leaves

Foeniculum vulgare

Fennel

FAMILY: APIACEAE (UMBELLIFERAE) **SYNONYMS:** *F. OFFICINALE, F. CAPILLACEUM, ANETHUM FOENICULUM,* FENKEL

Herbal/Folk Tradition

A herb of ancient medical repute, believed to convey longevity, courage and strength. It was also used to ward off evil spirits, strengthen the eyesight and neutralize poisons. It is considered good for obstructions of the liver, spleen and gall bladder and for digestive complaints. It has traditionally been used for obesity, which may be due to a type of estrogenic action, which also increases the milk of nursing mothers. Still current in the British Herbal Pharmacopoeia, used locally for conjunctivitis, blepharitis and pharyngitis.

fennel seeds

fresh fennel leaves

Biennial or perennial herb up to 2m (6ft) high, with feathery leaves and golden yellow flowers. There are two main varieties of fennel: bitter or common fennel, slightly taller with less divided leaves occurring in a cultivated or wild form; and sweet fennel (also known as Roman, garden or French fennel), which is always cultivated.

EXTRACTION
Essential oil by steam distillation. 1. Sweet fennel oil from crushed seeds, and 2. bitter fennel oil from crushed seeds or the whole herb (the wild 'weed').

CHARACTERISTICS
1. A colourless to pale yellow liquid with a very sweet, anise-like, slightly earthy-peppery scent. It blends well with geranium, lavender, rose and sandalwood. 2. The seed oil is a pale yellow liquid with a sharp, warm camphoraceous odour; the 'weed' oil is a pale orange-brown with a sharp, peppery-camphoraceous odour.

ACTIONS
Aperitif, anti-inflammatory, antimicrobial, antiseptic, antispasmodic, carminative, depurative, diuretic, emmenagogue, expectorant, galactagogue, laxative, orexigenic, stimulant (circulatory), splenic, stomachic, tonic, vermifuge.

PRINCIPAL CONSTITUENTS
Anethole (50–60 per cent), limonene, phellandrene, pinene, anisic acid, anisic aldehyde, camphene, limonene, among others. Bitter fennel oil contains 18–22 per cent fenchone; sweet fennel oil contains little or none.

AROMATHERAPY/ HOME USE

Bitter fennel: none.
Sweet fennel:
Skin Care: *Bruises, dull, oily, mature complexions, pyorrhea.*
Circulation, Muscles and Joints: *Cellulitis, obesity, edema, rheumatism.*
Respiratory System: *Asthma, bronchitis.*
Digestive System: *Anorexia, colic, constipation, dyspepsia, flatulence, hiccough, nausea.*
Genito-Urinary System: *Amenorrhea, insufficient milk (in nursing mothers), menopausal problems.*

OTHER USES

In pharmaceutical products it is known as 'codex' fennel oil, used in cough drops, lozenges, etc.; also used in carminative and laxative preparations. Used as a flavour ingredient in all major food categories, in soft and alcoholic drinks. Fennel oil is used in soaps, toiletries and perfumes, is a good masking agent for industrial products, room sprays, etc.

DISTRIBUTION

Bitter fennel is native to the Mediterranean region. It is cultivated extensively worldwide, the main oil producers being Hungary, Bulgaria, Germany, France, Italy and India. Sweet fennel is grown principally in France, Italy and Greece.

OTHER SPECIES

Bitter fennel (F. vulgare var. amarga) and sweet fennel (F. vulgare var. dulce) are both closely related to the Florence fennel (F. axoricum). There are also many other cultivated varieties.

Gardenia jasminoides

Gardenia

FAMILY: RUBIACEAE **SYNONYMS:** *G. GRANDIFLORA, G. RADICANS, G. FLORIDA,* GARDINIA, CAPE JASMINE, COMMON GARDENIA

Herbal/Folk Tradition

The flowers are used locally to flavour tea, much like jasmine.

A decorative bush, often grown for ornamental purposes, bearing fragrant white flowers.

AROMATHERAPY/ HOME USE

Perfume.

OTHER USES

Employed in high-class perfumery, especially oriental fragrances.

DISTRIBUTION

Native to the Far East, India and China. Efforts to produce the oil commercially have been largely unsuccessful.

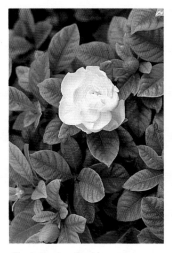

Gardenia jasminoides

OTHER SPECIES

There are several varieties of gardenia depending on location, such as G. citriodora *or G.* calyculata *found in Japan and Indonesia.*

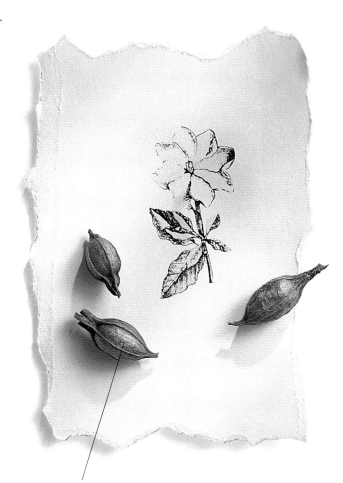

dried gardenia buds

EXTRACTION

An absolute (and concrete) by solvent extraction from the fresh flowers.

CHARACTERISTICS

A dark yellow, oily liquid with a sweet, rich, floral, jasmine-like scent. It blends well with ylang ylang, jasmine, tuberose, orange blossom, rose, spice and citrus oils.

ACTIONS

Antiseptic, aphrodisiac.

PRINCIPAL CONSTITUENTS

Mainly benzyl acetate, with phenyl acetate, linalol, linalyl acetate, terpineol and methyl anthranilate, among others – composition varies according to source.

Gaultheria procumbens

Wintergreen

SAFETY DATA *Toxic, irritant and sensitizing – an environmental hazard or marine pollutant. The true oil is almost obsolete, having been replaced by synthetic methyl salicylate. See also sweet birch oil*

FAMILY: ERICACEAE **SYNONYMS:** AROMATIC WINTERGREEN, CHECKERBERRY, TEABERRY, GAULTHERIA (OIL)

Herbal/Folk Tradition

The plant has been used for respiratory conditions such as chronic mucous discharge, but is employed mainly for joint and muscular problems such as lumbago, sciatica, neuralgia, myalgia, etc. The dried leaf and stem are current in the British Herbal Pharmacopoeia as a specific for rheumatoid arthritis.

The essential oil has been used interchangeably with sweet birch oil, both being made up almost exclusively of methyl salicylate.

A small evergreen herb up to 15cm (6in) high with slender creeping stems shooting forth erect twigs with leathery serrated leaves and drooping white flowers, which are followed by fleshy scarlet berries.

fresh wintergreen

EXTRACTION

Essential oil by steam (or water) distillation from the leaf, previously macerated in warm water. The essential oil does not occur crudely in the plant but is produced only during the process of decomposition in warm water.

CHARACTERISTICS

A pale yellow or pinkish liquid with an intense sweet-woody, almost fruity odour. It blends well with oregano, mints, thyme, ylang ylang, narcissus and vanilla.

ACTIONS

Analgestic (mild), anti-inflammatory, antirheumatic, antitussive, astringent, carminative, diuretic, emmenagogue, galactagogue, stimulant.

PRINCIPAL CONSTITUENTS

Almost exclusively methyl salicylate (up to 98 per cent), with formaldehyde and gaultheriline.

AROMATHERAPY/ HOME USE

None. 'Avoid both internally and externally.'[41]

OTHER USES

Some pharmaceutical use, such as 'Olbas' oil. Some perfumery applications especially in forest-type fragrances. Extensively used as a flavouring agent in the USA for toothpaste, chewing gum, root beer, Coca-Cola, and other soft drinks.

DISTRIBUTION

Native to North America, especially the north-eastern region and Canada. The oil is produced in the USA.

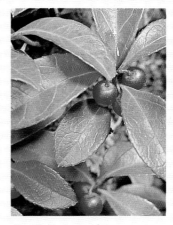

Gaultheria procumbens

OTHER SPECIES

There are several other Gaultheria *species that are also used for oil production, sharing similar properties.*

Helichrysum angustifolium

Helichrysum

FAMILY: ASTERACEAE (COMPOSITAE)   **SYNONYMS:** IMMORTELLE, EVERLASTING, ST JOHN'S HERB

Herbal/Folk Tradition

In Europe it is used for respiratory complaints such as asthma, chronic bronchitis and whooping cough; also for headaches, migraine, liver ailments and skin conditions including burns, allergies and psoriasis. Usually taken in the form of a decoction or infusion.

EXTRACTION

**1. Essential oil by steam distillation from the fresh flowers and flowering tops.
2. An absolute (and concrete) are also produced by solvent extraction.**

CHARACTERISTICS

**1. A pale yellow to red oily liquid with a powerful, rich honey-like scent with a delicate tea-like undertone.
2. A yellowy-brown viscous liquid with a rich, floral, tea-like scent. It blends well with chamomile, boronia, labdanum, lavender, mimosa, oakmoss, geranium, clary sage, rose, Peru balsam, clove and citrus oils.**

ACTIONS

Anti-allergenic, anti-inflammatory, antimicrobial, antitussive, antiseptic, astringent, cholagogue, cicatrizant, diuretic, expectorant, fungicidal, hepatic, nervine.

PRINCIPAL CONSTITUENTS

Nerol and neryl acetate (30–50 per cent), geraniol, pinene, linalol, isovaleric aldehyde, sesquiterpenes, furfurol and eugenol, among others.

AROMATHERAPY/ HOME USE

Skin Care: *Abscess, acne, allergic conditions, boils, burns, cuts, dermatitis, eczema, inflammation, spots, wounds, etc.*
Circulation, Muscles and Joints: *Muscular aches and pains, rheumatism, sprains, strained muscles.*
Respiratory System: *Asthma, bronchitis, chronic coughs, whooping cough.*
Digestive System: *Liver congestion, spleen congestion.*
Immune System: *Bacterial infections, colds, flu, fever.*
Nervous System: *Depression, debility, lethargy, nervous exhaustion, neuralgia, stress-related conditions.*

OTHER USES

Used as fixatives and fragrance components in soaps, cosmetics and perfumes. The absolute is used to flavour certain tobaccos; used for the isolation of natural anethole.

DISTRIBUTION

Native to the Mediterranean region, especially the eastern part and North Africa. It is cultivated mainly in Italy, former Yugoslavia, Spain and France.

OTHER SPECIES

There are several other Helichrysum *species such as* H. arenarium *found in florist shops and* H. stoechas, *which is also used to produce an absolute.* H. orientale *is grown for its oil.*

A strongly aromatic herb, up to 60cm (24in) high with a much-branched stem, woody at the base. The brightly coloured, daisy-like flowers become dry as the plant matures, yet retain their colour.

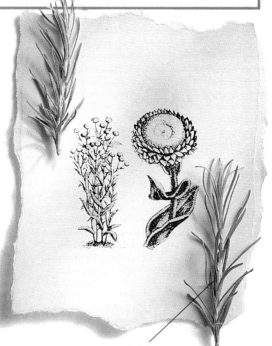

fresh leaves

Humulus lupulus

Hops

FAMILY: MORACEAE **SYNONYMS:** COMMON HOP, EUROPEAN HOP, LUPULUS

Herbal/Folk Tradition

Best known as a nerve remedy, for insomnia, nervous tension, neuralgia, and also for sexual neurosis in both sexes. It supports the female estrogens and is useful for amenorrhea (absence of periods). 'A mild sedative, well known in the form of the hop pillow where the heavy aromatic odour has been shown to relax by direct action at the olfactory centres . . . it is the volatile aromatic component that appears to be the most active.'[42] It has also been used for heart disease, stomach and liver complaints, including bacterial dysentery.

In China it is used for pulmonary tuberculosis and cystitis. It is used to make beer. Current in the British Herbal Pharmacopoeia as a specific for restlessness with nervous headaches and/or indigestion.

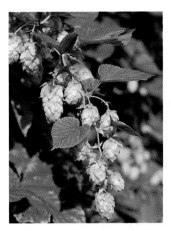

Humulus lupulus

dried
hops

Perennial creeping, twining herb up to 8m (26ft) high, which bears male and female flowers on separate plants. It has dark green, heart-shaped leaves and greeny-yellow flowers. A volatile oil, called lupulin, is formed in the glandular hairs of the cones or 'strobiles'.

AROMATHERAPY/ HOME USE

Skin Care: *Dermatitis, rashes, rough skin, ulcers.*
Respiratory System: *Asthma, spasmodic cough.*
Digestive System: *Indigestion, nervous dyspepsia.*
Genito-urinary and Endocrine Systems: *Amenorrhea, menstrual cramp, supports female estrogens, promotes feminine characteristics, reduces sexual overactivity.*
Nervous system: *Headaches, insomnia, nervous tension, neuralgia, stress-related conditions.*

OTHER USES

Employed as a fragrance ingredient in perfumes, especially spicy or oriental types. Used in flavour work in tobacco, sauces and spice products, but mainly in alcoholic drinks, especially beer.

DISTRIBUTION

Native to Europe and North America; cultivated worldwide, especially in the USA (California and Washington), former Yugoslavia and Germany. The oil is produced mainly in France, Britain and Germany.

EXTRACTION
Essential oil by steam distillation from the dried cones or catkins, known as 'strobiles'. (An absolute is also produced by solvent extraction for perfumery use.

CHARACTERISTICS
A pale yellow to reddish-amber liquid with a rich, spicy-sweet odour. It blends well with pine, hyacinth, nutmeg, copaiba balsam, citrus and spice oils.

ACTIONS
Anodyne, an aphrodisiac, antimicrobial, antiseptic, antispasmodic, astringent, bactericidal, carminative, diuretic, emollient, estrogenic properties, hypnotic, nervine, sedative, soporific.

PRINCIPAL CONSTITUENTS
Mainly humulene, myrcene, caryophyllene and farnesene, with over 100 other trace components.

Hyacinthus orientalis

Hyacinth

FAMILY: LILIACEAE **SYNONYMS:** *SCILLA NUTANS*, BLUEBELL

Herbal/Folk Tradition

The wild bluebell bulbs are poisonous; however, the white juice used to be employed as a substitute for starch or glue. 'The roots, dried and powdered, are balsamic, having some styptic properties that have not fully been investigated.'[43]

A much-loved cultivated plant with fragrant, bell-shaped flowers of many colours, bright lance-shaped leaves and a round bulb.

sliced
hyacinth
bulb

dried
leaf

EXTRACTION
Concrete and absolute by solvent extraction from the flowers. (An essential oil is also obtained by steam distillation from the absolute.)

CHARACTERISTICS
A reddish or greeny-brown viscous liquid with a sweet-green, floral fragrance and soft floral undertone. It blends well with narcissus, violet, ylang ylang, styrax, galbanum, jasmine, orange blossom and with oriental-type bases.

ACTIONS
Antiseptic, balsamic, hypnotic, sedative, styptic.

PRINCIPAL CONSTITUENTS
Phenylethyl alcohol, benzaldehyde, cinnamaldehyde, benzyl alcohol, benzoic acid, benzyl acetate, benzyl benzoate, eugenol, methyl eugenol and hydroquinone, among others.

AROMATHERAPY/ HOME USE

Nervous System: *The Greeks described the fragrance of hyacinth as being refreshing and invigorating to a tired mind. It may also be used for stress-related conditions, 'in self-hypnosis techniques . . . and developing the creative right-hand side of the brain'.*[44]

OTHER USES
Used in high-class perfumery, especially oriental/floral types.

DISTRIBUTION
Native to Asia Minor, said to be of Syrian origin. Cultivated mainly in the Netherlands and southern France.

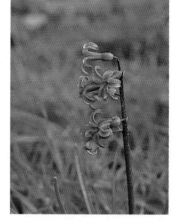

Hyacinthus orientalis

OTHER SPECIES
Closely related to garlic (Allium sativum), onion (A. cepa) and the wild bluebell (H. non-scriptus). At one time bluebell essential oil was produced at Grasse, in the south of France, and had a fresher and more flowery fragrance.

Hyssopus officinalis

Hyssop

FAMILY: LAMIACEAE (LABIATAE) SYNONYM: AZOB

Herbal/Folk Tradition

Although hyssop is mentioned in the Bible, it probably does not refer to this herb but to a form of wild marjoram or oregano, possibly *Oreganum syriacum*. Nevertheless *H. officinalis* has an ancient medical reputation and was used for purifying sacred places and employed as a strewing herb. It is used principally for respiratory and digestive complaints, and externally for rheumatism, bruises, sores, earache and toothache. It is also used to regulate the blood pressure, as a general nerve tonic, and for states of anxiety or hysteria. It is current in the British Herbal Pharmacopoeia as a specific for bronchitis and the common cold.

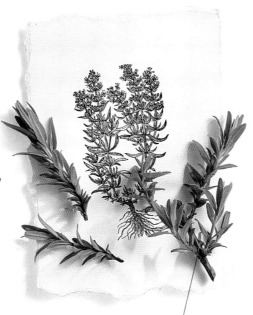

fresh hyssop

An attractive perennial, almost evergreen subshrub up to 60cm (24in) high with a woody stem, small, lance-shaped leaves and purplish-blue flowers.

EXTRACTION
Essential oil by steam distillation from the leaves and flowering tops.

CHARACTERISTICS
A colourless to pale yellowy-green liquid with a sweet, camphoraceous top note and warm spicy-herbaceous undertone. It blends well with lavender, rosemary, myrtle, bay leaf, sage, clary sage, geranium and citrus oils.

ACTIONS
Astringent, antiseptic, antispasmodic, antiviral, bactericidal, carminative, cephalic, cicatrizant, digestive, diuretic, emmenagogue, expectorant, febrifuge, hypertensive, nervine, sedative, sudorific, tonic (heart and circulation), vermifuge, vulnerary.

PRINCIPAL CONSTITUENTS
Pinocamphone, isopinocamphone, estragole, borneol, geraniol, limonene, thujone, myrcene, caryophyllene, among others.

AROMATHERAPY/ HOME USE

Skin Care: *Bruises, cuts, dermatitis, eczema, inflammation, wounds.*
Circulation, Muscles and Joints: *Low or high blood pressure, rheumatism.*
Respiratory System: *Asthma, bronchitis, catarrh, cough, sore throat, tonsillitis, whooping cough.*
Digestive System: *Colic, indigestion.*
Genito-urinary System: *Amenorrhea, leucorrhea.*
Immune System: *Colds, flu.*
Nervous System: *Anxiety, fatigue, nervous tension and stress-related conditions.*

OTHER USES
Employed as a fragrance component in soaps, cosmetics and perfumes, especially eau-de-cologne and oriental bases. Used as a flavour ingredient in many food products, mainly sauces and seasonings; also in alcoholic drinks, especially liqueurs such as chartreuse.

DISTRIBUTION
Native to the Mediterranean region and temperate Asia; now grows wild throughout America, Russia and Europe. It is cultivated mainly in Hungary and France, and to a lesser degree in Albania and former Yugoslavia.

OTHER SPECIES
There are four main subspecies of hyssop, but H. officinalis *is the main oil-producing variety. The species* H. officinalis var. decumbens *is less toxic than many other types, and well suited to aromatherapy use. To be distinguished from hedge hyssop (Gratiola officinalis), which is still used in herbal medicine but belongs to a different family.*

Illicium verum

Star anise

FAMILY: ILLICIACEAE **SYNONYMS:** CHINESE ANISE, ILLICIUM, CHINESE STAR ANISE

Herbal/Folk Tradition

Used in Chinese medicine for over 1,300 years for its stimulating effect on the digestive system and for respiratory disorders such as bronchitis and unproductive coughs. In the East, it is used as a remedy for colic and rheumatism, and often chewed after meals to sweeten the breath and promote digestion. A common oriental domestic spice.

EXTRACTION

Essential oil by steam distillation from the fruits, fresh or partially dried. An oil is also produced from the leaves in small quantities.

CHARACTERISTICS

A pale yellow liquid with a warm, spicy, extremely sweet, liquorice-like scent. It blends well with rose, lavender, orange, pine and other spice oils, and has excellent masking properties.

ACTIONS

Antiseptic, carminative, expectorant, insect repellent, stimulant.

PRINCIPAL CONSTITUENT

Trans-anethole (80–90 per cent).

AROMATHERAPY/ HOME USE

Circulation, Muscles and Joints: *Muscular aches and pains, rheumatism.*
Respiratory System: *Bronchitis, coughs.*
Digestive System: *Colic, cramp, flatulence, indigestion.*
Immune System: *Colds.*

OTHER USES

By the pharmaceutical industry in cough mixtures, lozenges, etc. and to mask undesirable odours and flavours in drugs. As a fragrance component in soaps, toothpaste and detergents as well as cosmetics and perfumes. Widely used for flavouring food, especially confectionery, alcoholic and soft drinks.

DISTRIBUTION

Native to south east China, also Vietnam, India and Japan. Produced mainly in China.

OTHER SPECIES

Several other related species, e.g. Japanese star anise, which is highly poisonous!

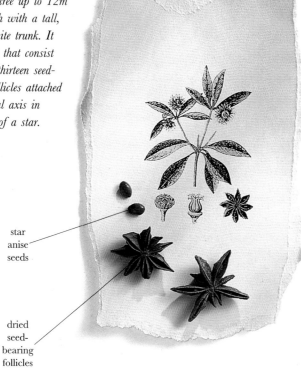

Evergreen tree up to 12m (39ft) high with a tall, slender white trunk. It bears fruit that consist of five to thirteen seed-bearing follicles attached to a central axis in the shape of a star.

star anise seeds

dried seed-bearing follicles

Elecampane

Inula helenium

FAMILY: ASTERACEAE (COMPOSITAE) **SYNONYMS:** *HELENIUM GRANDIFLORUM, ASTER OFFICINALIS, A. HELENIUM,* INULA, SCABWORT, ALANT, HORSEHEAL, YELLOW STARWORT, ELF DOCK, WILD SUNFLOWER, VELVET DOCK, 'ESSENCE D'AUNEE'

Herbal/Folk Tradition

A herb of ancient medical repute, which used to be candied and sold as a sweetmeat. It is used as an important spice, incense and medicine in the East. It is used in both Western and Eastern herbalism, mainly in the form of a tea for respiratory conditions such as asthma, bronchitis and whooping cough, disorders of the digestion, intestines and gall bladder and for skin disorders.

Current in the British Herbal Pharmacopoeia as a specific for irritating coughs or bronchitis. Elecampane root is the richest source of inulin.

A handsome perennial herb up to 1.5m (5ft) high, with a stout stem covered with soft hairs. It has oval pointed leaves that are velvety underneath, large, yellow, daisy-like flowers and large, fleshy rhizome roots.

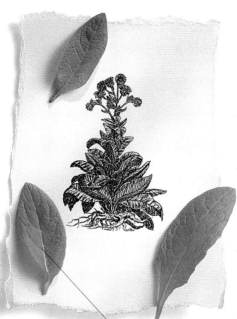

fresh
elecampane

EXTRACTION

Essential oil by steam distillation from the dried roots and rhizomes. (An absolute and concrete are also produced in small quantities.)

CHARACTERISTICS

A semi-solid or viscous dark yellow or brownish liquid with a dry, soft, woody, honey-like odour, often containing crystals. It blends well with cananga, cinnamon, labdanum, lavender, mimosa, frankincense, orris, tuberose, violet, cedarwood, patchouli, sandalwood, cypress, bergamot and oriental fragrances.

ACTIONS

Alterative, anthelminthic, anti-inflammatory, antiseptic, antispasmodic, antitussive, astringent, bactericidal, diaphoretic, diuretic, expectorant, fungicidal, hyperglycemic, hypotensive, stomachic, tonic.

PRINCIPAL CONSTITUENTS

Mainly sesquiterpene lactones, including alantolactone (or helenin), isolactone, dihydroisalantolactone, dihydralantolactone, alantic acid and azulene.

AROMATHERAPY/ HOME USE

None. NB: In Phytoguide I, *sweet inula* (I. odora *or* I. graveolens), *a deep green oil, is described as 'queen of mucolytic essential oils', having properties as diverse as: 'anti-flammatory, hyperthermic, sedative, cardio-regulative, diuretic and depurative'.[46] It is described as being an excellent oil for the cardiopulmonary zone including asthma, chronic bronchitis and unproductive coughs. This variety of* Inula *seems to avoid the sensitization problems of elecampane, at least when it is used as an inhalation or by aerosol treatment.*

OTHER USES

Alantolactone is used as an anthelminthic in Europe (it is also an excellent bactericide). The oil and absolute are used as fixatives and fragrance components in soaps, detergents, cosmetics and perfumes. Used as a flavour ingredient in alcoholic beverages, soft drinks and foodstuffs.

DISTRIBUTION

Native to Europe and Asia, naturalized in North America. Cultivated in Europe (Belgium, France, Germany) and Asia (China, India). The oil is produced mainly from imported roots in southern France.

OTHER SPECIES

There are several varieties of Inula; *the European and Asian species are slightly different having a harsher scent. Other varieties include golden samphire* (I. crithmoides) *and sweet inula* (I. graveolens *or* I. odora).

Iris pallida

Orris

FAMILY: IRIDACEAE **SYNONYMS:** ORRIS ROOT, IRIS, FLAG IRIS, PALE IRIS, ORRIS BUTTER (OIL)

Herbal/Folk Tradition

In ancient Greece and Rome orris root was used extensively in perfumery, and its medicinal qualities were held in high esteem by Dioscorides. In Russia the root was used to make a tonic drink with honey and ginger.

Iris is little used medicinally these days, but it still appears in the British Herbal Pharmacopoeia as being formerly used in upper respiratory tract catarrh, coughs, and for diarrhea in infants.

orris root

A decorative perennial plant up to 1.5m (5ft) high, with sword-shaped leaves, a creeping fleshy rootstock and delicate, highly scented, pale blue flowers.

AROMATHERAPY/ HOME USE

None. However, the powdered orris, which is a common article, may be used as a dry shampoo, a body powder, a fixative for pot pourris, and to scent linen.

OTHER USES

The powder is used to scent dentifrices, toothpowders, etc. The resin is used in soaps, colognes and perfumes; the absolute and 'concrete' oil are reserved for high-class perfumery work. Occasionally used in Europe for confectionery and fruit flavours.

DISTRIBUTION

Native to the eastern Mediterranean region; also found in northern India and North Africa. Most commercial orris is produced in Italy where it grows wild. The oil is produced mainly in France and Morocco and to a lesser extent in Italy and the USA.

OTHER SPECIES

There are many species of iris; cultivation has also produced further types. In Italy the pale iris (I. pallida) is collected indiscriminately with the Florentine orris (I. florentina), which has white flowers tinged with pale blue, and the common or German iris (I. germanica), which has deep purple flowers with a yellow beard. Other species that have been used medicinally include the American blue flag (I. versicolor), and the yellow flag iris (I. pseudacorus).

EXTRACTION

1. An essential oil (often called a 'concrete') by steam distillation from the rhizomes that have been peeled, washed, dried and pulverized. The rhizomes must be stored for a minimum of three years prior to extraction otherwise they have virtually no scent! 2. An absolute produced by alkali washing in ethyl ether solution to remove the myristic acid from the 'concrete' oil. 3. A resin or resinoid by alcohol extraction from the peeled rhizomes.

CHARACTERISTICS

1. The oil solidifies at room temperature to a cream-coloured mass with a woody, violet-like scent and a soft, floral-fruity undertone. 2. The absolute is a water-white or pale yellow oily liquid with a delicate, sweet, floral-woody odour. 3. The resin is a brown or dark orange viscous mass with a deep, woody-sweet, tobacco-like scent – very tenacious. Orris blends well with cedarwood, sandalwood, vetiver, cypress, mimosa, labdanum, bergamot, clary sage, rose, violet and other florals.

ACTIONS

Dried root – antidiarrheal, demulcent, expectorant. Fresh root – diuretic, cathartic, emetic.

PRINCIPAL CONSTITUENTS

Myristic acid, an odourless substance that makes the 'oil' solid (85–90 per cent), alpha-irone and oleic acid.

Jasminum officinale

Jasmine

SAFETY DATA *Non-toxic, non-irritant, generally non-sensitizing (an allergic reaction has been known to occur in some individuals)*

FAMILY: OLEACEAE **SYNONYMS:** JASMIN, JESSAMINE, COMMON JASMINE, POET'S JESSAMINE

Herbal/Folk Tradition

In China the flowers of *J. officinale var. grandiflorum* are used to treat hepatitis, liver cirrhosis and dysentery; the flowers of *J. sambac* are used for conjunctivitis, dysentery, skin ulcers and tumours. The root is used to treat headaches, insomnia, pain due to dislocated joints and rheumatism.

In the West, the common jasmine was said to 'warm the womb . . . and facilitate the birth; it is useful for cough, difficulty of breathing, etc. It disperses crude humours, and is good for cold and catarrhous constitutions, but not for the hot.'[47] It was also used for hard, contracted limbs and problems with the nervous and reproductive systems.

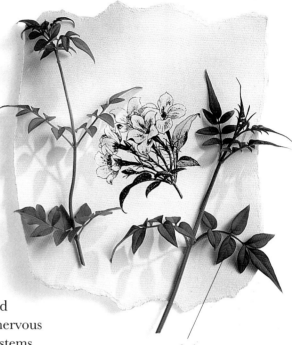

fresh jasmine

An evergreen shrub or vine up to 10m (33ft) high with delicate, bright green leaves and star-shaped very fragrant white flowers.

EXTRACTION

A concrete is produced by solvent extraction; the absolute is obtained from the concrete by separation with alcohol. An essential oil is produced by steam distillation of the absolute.

CHARACTERISTICS

The absolute is a dark orange-brown, viscous liquid with an intensely rich, warm, floral scent and a tea-like undertone. It blends well with rose, sandalwood, clary sage, and all citrus oils. It has the ability to round off any rough notes and blend with virtually everything.

ACTIONS

Analgesic (mild), antidepressant, anti-inflammatory, antiseptic, antispasmodic, aphrodisiac, carminative, cicatrizant, expectorant, galactagogue, parturient, sedative, tonic (uterine).

PRINCIPAL CONSTITUENTS

There are over one hundred constituents in the oil including benzyl acetate, linalol, phenylacetic acid, benzyl alcohol, farnesol, methyl anthranilate, cis-jasmone, methyl jasmonate, among others.

AROMATHERAPY/ HOME USE

Skin Care: *Dry, greasy, irritated, sensitive skin.*
Circulation, Muscles and Joints: *Muscular spasm, sprains.*
Respiratory System: *Catarrh, coughs, hoarseness, laryngitis.*
Genito-urinary System: *Dysmenorrhea, frigidity, labour pains, uterine disorders.*
Nervous System: *Depression, nervous exhaustion and stress-related conditions. 'It . . . produces a feeling of optimism, confidence and euphoria. It is most useful in cases where there is apathy, indifference or listlessness.'[48]*

OTHER USES

Extensively used in soaps, toiletries, cosmetics and perfumes, especially high-class floral and oriental fragrances. The oil and absolute are used in a wide range of food products, alcoholic and soft drinks. The dried flowers of J. sambac are used in jasmine tea.

DISTRIBUTION

Native to China, northern India and west Asia; cultivated in the Mediterranean region, China and India (depending on the exact species). The concrete is produced in Italy, France, Morocco, Egypt, China, Japan, Algeria and Turkey; the absolute is produced mainly in France.

Juniperus ashei

Texas cedarwood

FAMILY: CUPRESSACEAE **SYNONYMS:** *J. MEXICANA*,
MOUNTAIN CEDAR, MEXICAN CEDAR, ROCK CEDAR,
MEXICAN JUNIPER

Herbal/Folk Tradition

In New Mexico the Native Americans use cedarwood oil for
skin rashes. It is also used for arthritis and rheumatism.

EXTRACTION

**Essential oil by steam
distillation from the heartwood
and wood shavings, etc. (Unlike
the Virginian cedar, the tree is
felled especially for its
essential oil.)**

CHARACTERISTICS

**Crude – a dark orange to
brownish viscous liquid with a
smoky-woody, sweet tar-like
odour.
Rectified – a colourless or pale
yellow liquid with a sweet,
balsamic, 'pencil-wood' scent,
similar to Virginian cedarwood
but harsher. It blends well with
patchouli, spruce, vetiver, pine
and leather-type scents.**

ACTIONS

**Antiseptic,
antispasmodic,
astringent,
diuretic,
expectorant,
sedative (nervous),
stimulant
(circulatory).**

PRINCIPAL CONSTITUENTS

**Cedrene, cedrol
(higher than the
Virginian oil),
thujopsene and sabinene,
among others. Otherwise
similar to Virginian cedarwood.**

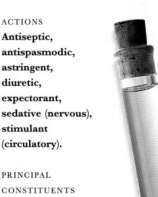

AROMATHERAPY/ HOME USE

Skin Care: *Acne, dandruff,
eczema, greasy hair, insect
repellent, oily skin, psoriasis.*
**Circulation, Muscles and
Joints:** *Arthritis, rheumatism.*
Respiratory System:
*Bronchitis, catarrh, congestion,
coughs, sinusitis.*
Genito-urinary System:
Cystitis, leucorrhea.
Nervous System: *Nervous
tension and stress-related disorders.*

OTHER USES

*Extensively used in room sprays
and household insect repellents.
Employed as a fragrance
component in soaps, cosmetics
and perfumes. Used as the
starting material for the
isolation of cedrene.*

DISTRIBUTION

*Native to south-western USA,
Mexico and Central America; the
oil is produced mainly in Texas.*

OTHER SPECIES

The name **J.** mexicana *has
erroneously been applied to many
species; botanically related to the
so-called Virginian cedarwood
(*J. virginiana*) and the East
African cedarwood (*J. procera*).*

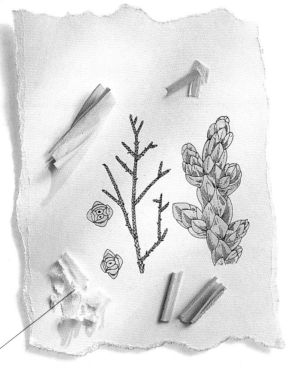

*A small, alpine
evergreen tree up
to 7m (23ft)
high with stiff
green needles and
an irregular
shaped trunk and
branches, which
tend to be crooked
or twisted. The
wood also tends to
crack easily, so it
is not used for
timber.*

Texas
cedarwood
chippings

Juniperus communis

Juniper

FAMILY: CUPRESSACEAE **SYNONYM:** COMMON JUNIPER

Herbal/Folk Tradition

Used medicinally for urinary infections, for respiratory problems as well as gastro-intestinal infections and worms. It helps expel the build-up of uric acid in the joints and is employed in gout, rheumatism and arthritis. Current in the British Herbal Pharmacopoeia for rheumatic pain and cystitis.

An evergreen shrub or tree up to 6m (20ft) high, with bluish-green stiff needles. It has small flowers and berries that are green in the first year, black in the second and third.

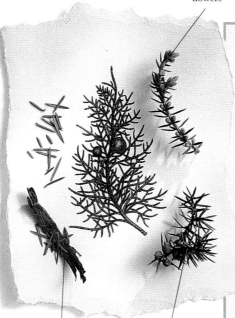

flowers

bark and needles

juniper berries

EXTRACTION

Essential oil by steam distillation from 1. the berries (sometimes fermented first as a by-product of juniper-brandy manufacture – the oil is considered an inferior product), and 2. the needles and wood. A resinoid, concrete and absolute are also produced on a small scale.

CHARACTERISTICS

1. A water-white or pale yellow mobile liquid with a sweet, fresh, woody-balsamic odour. It blends well with vetiver, sandalwood, cedarwood, mastic, oakmoss, galbanum, elemi, cypress, clary sage, pine, lavender, lavandin, labdanum, fir needle, rosemary, benzoin, balsam tolu, geranium and citrus oils. 2. A water-white or pale yellow mobile liquid with a sweet-balsamic, fresh, turpentine-like odour.

ACTIONS

Antirheumatic, antiseptic, antispasmodic, antitoxic, aphrodisiac, astringent, carminative, cicatrizant, depurative, diuretic, emmenagogue, nervine, parasiticide, rubefacient, sedative, stomachic, sudorific, tonic, vulnerary.

PRINCIPAL CONSTITUENTS

Mainly monoterpenes: pinene, myrcene, sabinene with limonene, cymene, terpinene, thujene and camphene, among others.

AROMATHERAPY/ HOME USE

The wood oil is usually adulterated with turpentine oil. It is best to use only juniper berry oil, in moderation.
Skin Care: *Acne, dermatitis, eczema, hair loss, hemorrhoids, oily complexions, as a skin toner, wounds.*
Circulation, Muscles and Joints: *Accumulation of toxins, arteriosclerosis, cellulitis, gout, obesity, rheumatism.*
Immune System: *Colds, flu, infections.*
Genito-urinary System: *Amenorrhea, cystitis, dysmenorrhea, leucorrhea.*
Nervous System: *Anxiety, nervous tension and stress-related conditions.*

OTHER USES

Berries and extracts are used in diuretic and laxative preparations; also veterinary preventatives of ticks and fleas. Employed as a fragrance component in soaps, detergents, cosmetics and perfumes, especially spicy fragrances and aftershaves. Extensively used in many food products but especially alcoholic and soft drinks: the berries are used to flavour gin.

DISTRIBUTION

Native to the northern hemisphere: Scandinavia, Siberia, Canada, northern Europe and northern Asia. The oil is produced mainly in Italy, France, former Yugoslavia, Austria, former Czechoslovakia, Spain, Germany and Canada.

OTHER SPECIES

There are various other species of juniper such as J. oxycedrus, *which produces cade oil,* J. virginiana, *which produces the so-called Virginian cedarwood oil, and* J. sabina, *which produces savin oil. See also Botanical Classification section.*

Juniperus oxycedrus

Cade

FAMILY: CUPRESSACEAE   **SYNONYMS:** JUNIPER TAR, PRICKLY CEDAR, MEDLAR TREE, PRICKLY JUNIPER

Herbal/Folk Tradition

Used in the treatment of cutaneous diseases, such as chronic eczema, parasites, scalp disease, hair loss, etc. especially in France and other European countries. It is also used as an antiseptic wound dressing and for toothache.

A large evergreen shrub up to 4m (13ft) high, with long dark needles and brownish-black berries about the size of hazelnuts.

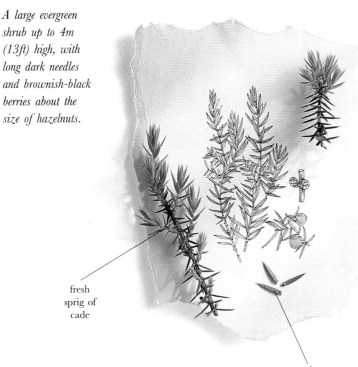

fresh sprig of cade

cade needles

EXTRACTION
The crude oil or tar is obtained by destructive distillation from the branches and heartwood (usually in the form of shavings or chips). A rectified oil is produced from the crude by steam or vacuum distillation. In addition, an oil is occasionally produced from the berries by steam distillation.

CHARACTERISTICS
The rectified oil is an orange-brown, oily liquid with a woody, smoky, leather-like odour. It blends well with thyme, origanum, clove, cassia, tea tree, pine and medicinal-type bases.

ACTIONS
Analgesic, antimicrobial, antipruritic, antiseptic, disinfectant, parasiticide, vermifuge.

PRINCIPAL CONSTITUENTS
Cadinene, cadinol, p-cresol, guaiacol, among others.

AROMATHERAPY/ HOME USE

Skin Care: *Cuts, dandruff, dermatitis, eczema, spots, etc.*

OTHER USES

Extensively used in pharmaceutical work as a solvent for chemical drugs, in dermatological creams and ointments, as well as in veterinary medicine. Rectified cade is used in fragrance work, in soaps, lotions, creams and perfumes (especially leather and spice).

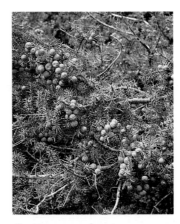

Juniperus oxycedrus

DISTRIBUTION

Native to southern France; now common throughout Europe and North Africa. The tar is produced mainly in Spain and former Yugoslavia.

OTHER SPECIES

There are many varieties of juniper used commercially apart from the prickly juniper: J. communis *produces juniper oil,* J. virginiana *produces Virginian cedarwood oil, and in former Yugoslavia an oil is produced from the fruits and twigs of* J. smerka.

Juniperus sabina

Savine

FAMILY: CUPRESSACEAE   **SYNONYMS:** *SABINA CACUMINA*, SAVIN (OIL)

Herbal/Folk Tradition

It was used at one time as an ointment or dressing for blisters, in order to promote discharge, and for syphilitic warts and other skin problems. In Britain the fresh, dried shoots of *Juniperus sabina* were once collected in spring for topical use. The powdered leaves mixed with an equal part of verdigris were also used to destroy warts. It is a powerful emmenagogue and should never be used in pregnancy. It is rarely administered nowadays because of its possible toxic effects. NB: red cedar, *Juniperus virginiana*, is sometimes referred to as savin and is occasionally substituted commercially.

A compact evergreen shrub about 1m (3ft) high (though much taller in the Mediterranean countries), which tends to spread horizontally. It has a pale green bark becoming rough with age, small, dark green leaves and purplish-black berries containing three seeds. An essential oil gland is clearly visible on the dorsal side of each leaf.

fresh sprig
of savine

EXTRACTION
Essential oil by steam distillation from the twigs and leaves.

CHARACTERISTICS
A pale yellow or olive oily liquid with a disagreeable, bitter, turpentine-like odour.

ACTIONS
Powerful anthelmintic, diuretic, emmenagogue, rubefacient, stimulant, vermifuge.

PRINCIPAL CONSTITUENTS
Sabinol, sabinyl acetate, terpinene, pinene, sabinene, decyl aldehyde, citronellol, geraniol, cadinene and dihydro-cuminyl alcohol.

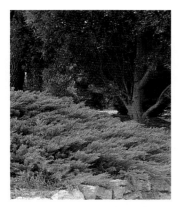

Juniperus sabina

AROMATHERAPY/ HOME USE

None. 'Should not be used in therapy, whether internally or externally.' [50]

OTHER USES

Occasional perfumery use. Little employed nowadays.

DISTRIBUTION

Native to North America, middle and southern Europe. The oil is produced mainly in Austria (the Tirol), a little in France and former Yugoslavia.

OTHER SPECIES

*Closely related to the common juniper (*J. communis*) and other members of the family — see juniper.*

Juniperus virginiana

Virginian cedarwood

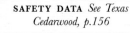

SAFETY DATA *See Texas Cedarwood, p.156*

FAMILY: CUPRESSACEAE **SYNONYMS:** RED CEDAR, EASTERN RED CEDAR, SOUTHERN RED CEDAR, BEDFORD CEDARWOOD (OIL)

Herbal/Folk Tradition

The Native Americans used it for respiratory infections, especially those involving an excess of catarrh. Decoctions of leaves, bark, twigs and fruit were used to treat a variety of ailments: menstrual delay, rheumatism, arthritis, skin rashes, venereal warts, gonorrhea, pyelitis and kidney infections.

It is an excellent insect and vermin repellent (mosquitoes, moths, woodworm, rats, etc.) and was once used with citronella as a commercial insecticide.

EXTRACTION
Essential oil by steam distillation from the timber waste, sawdust, shavings, etc. (At one time a superior oil was distilled from the red heartwood, from trees over twenty-five years old.)

CHARACTERISTICS
A pale yellow or orange oily liquid with a mild, sweet-balsamic, 'pencil-wood' scent. It blends well with sandalwood, rose, juniper, cypress, vetiver, patchouli and benzoin.

ACTIONS
Abortifacient, antiseborrheic, antiseptic (pulmonary, genito-urinary), antispasmodic, astringent, balsamic, diuretic, emmenagogue, expectorant, insecticide, sedative (nervous), stimulant (circulatory).

PRINCIPAL CONSTITUENTS
Mainly cedrene (up to 80 per cent), cedrol (3–14 per cent), and cedrenol, among others.

AROMATHERAPY/ HOME USE

Skin Care: *Acne, dandruff, eczema, greasy hair, insect repellent, oily skin, psoriasis.*
Circulation, Muscles and Joints: *Arthritis, rheumatism.*
Respiratory System: *Bronchitis, catarrh, congestion, coughs, sinusitis.*
Genito-urinary System: *Cystitis, leucorrhea.*
Nervous System: *Nervous tension and stress-related disorders.*

OTHER USES

Extensively used in room sprays and household insect repellents. Employed as a fragrance component in soaps, cosmetics and perfumes. Used as the starting material for the isolation of cedrene.

DISTRIBUTION

Native to North America, especially mountainous regions east of the Rocky Mountains.

OTHER SPECIES

There are many cultivars of the red cedar; its European relative is the shrubby red cedar (J. sabina) also known as savine – see entry. It is also closely related to the East African cedarwood (J. procera).

A coniferous, slow-growing, evergreen tree up to 33m (108ft) high with a narrow, dense and pyramidal crown, a reddish heartwood and brown cones. The tree can attain a majestic stature with a trunk diameter of over 1.5m (5ft).

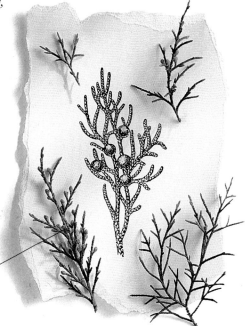

fresh Virginian cedarwood

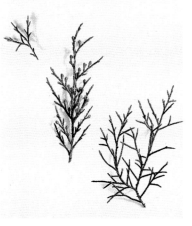

Laurus nobilis

Bay laurel

FAMILY: LAURACEAE **SYNONYMS:** SWEET BAY, LAUREL, GRECIAN LAUREL, TRUE BAY, MEDITERRANEAN BAY, ROMAN LAUREL, NOBLE LAUREL LEAF (OIL)

Herbal/Folk Tradition

A popular culinary herb throughout Europe. The leaves were used by the ancient Greeks and Romans to crown their victors. Both leaf and berry were formerly used for a variety of afflictions including hysteria, colic, indigestion, loss of appetite, to promote menstruation and for fever. It is little used internally these days, due to its narcotic properties. A 'fixed' oil of bay, expressed from the berries, is still used for sprains, bruises, earache, etc.

An evergreen tree up to 20m (65ft) high with dark green, glossy leaves and black berries; often cultivated as an ornamental shrub.

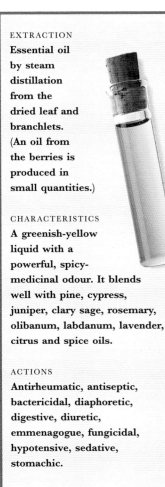

fresh bay
leaves

EXTRACTION

Essential oil by steam distillation from the dried leaf and branchlets. (An oil from the berries is produced in small quantities.)

CHARACTERISTICS

A greenish-yellow liquid with a powerful, spicy-medicinal odour. It blends well with pine, cypress, juniper, clary sage, rosemary, olibanum, labdanum, lavender, citrus and spice oils.

ACTIONS

Antirheumatic, antiseptic, bactericidal, diaphoretic, digestive, diuretic, emmenagogue, fungicidal, hypotensive, sedative, stomachic.

PRINCIPAL CONSTITUENTS

Cineol (30–50 per cent), pinene, linalol, terpineol acetate, and traces of methyl eugenol.

AROMATHERAPY/ HOME USE

Digestive System: *Dyspepsia, flatulence, loss of appetite.*
Genito-urinary System: *Scanty periods.*
Immune System: *Colds, flu, tonsillitis and viral infections.*

OTHER USES

Used as a fragrance component in detergents, cosmetics, toiletries and perfumes, especially aftershaves. Extensively used in processed food of all types, as well as alcoholic and soft drinks.

DISTRIBUTION

Native to the Mediterranean region; extensively cultivated, especially for its berries, in France, Spain, Italy, Morocco, former Yugoslavia, China, Israel, Turkey and Russia. The oil is produced mainly in former Yugoslavia.

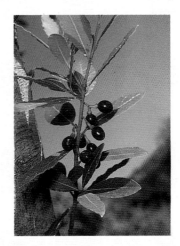

Laurus nobilis

OTHER SPECIES

There are several related species, all of which are commonly called bay: Californian bay (Umbellularia california), West Indian bay (Pimenta racemosa) and the cherry laurel (Prunus laurocerasus), which is poisonous.

Lavandula angustifolia

True lavender

FAMILY: LAMIACEAE (LABIATAE) **SYNONYMS:** *L. VERA, L. OFFICINALIS,* GARDEN LAVENDER, COMMON LAVENDER

Herbal/Folk Tradition

Lavender has a well-established tradition as a folk remedy, and its scent is still familiar to almost everyone. It was used to 'comfort the stomach' but above all as a cosmetic water, an insect repellent, to scent linen, and as a reviving yet soothing oil. Generally regarded as the most versatile essence therapeutically.

fresh lavender

An evergreen woody shrub, up to 1m (3ft) tall, with pale green, narrow, linear leaves and flowers on blunt spikes of a beautiful violet-blue colour. The whole plant is highly aromatic.

EXTRACTION

1. Essential oil by steam distillation from the fresh flowering tops. 2. An absolute and concrete are also produced by solvent extraction in smaller quantities.

CHARACTERISTICS

1. The oil is a colourless to pale yellow liquid with a sweet, floral-herbaceous scent and balsamic-woody undertone; it has a more fragrant floral scent than spike lavender. It blends well with most oils, especially citrus and florals; also cedarwood, clove, clary sage, pine, geranium, labdanum, oakmoss, vetiver, patchouli, etc. 2. The absolute is a dark green viscous liquid with a very sweet herbaceous, somewhat floral odour.

ACTIONS

Analgesic, anticonvulsive, antidepressant, antimicrobial, antirheumatic, antiseptic, antispasmodic, antitoxic, carminative, cholagogue, choleretic, cicatrizant, cordial, cytophylactic, deodorant, diuretic, emmenagogue, hypotensive, insecticide, nervine, parasiticide, rubefacient, sedative, stimulant, sudorific, tonic, vermifuge, vulnerary.

PRINCIPAL CONSTITUENTS

Over 100 constituents including linalyl acetate (up to 40 per cent), linalol, lavandulol, lavandulyl acetate, terpineol, cineol, limonene, ocimene, caryophyllene, among others. Constituents vary according to source: high altitudes generally produce more esters.

AROMATHERAPY/ HOME USE

Skin Care: *Abscesses, acne, allergies, athlete's foot, boils, bruises, burns, dandruff, dermatitis, earache, eczema, inflammations, insect bites and stings, insect repellent, lice, psoriasis, ringworm, scabies, sores, spots, all skin types, sunburn, wounds.*

Circulation, Muscles and Joints: *Lumbago, muscular aches and pains, rheumatism, sprains.*

Respiratory System: *Asthma, bronchitis, catarrh, halitosis, laryngitis, throat infections, whooping cough.*

Digestive System: *Abdominal cramps, colic, dyspepsia, flatulence, nausea.*

Genito-urinary System: *Cystitis, dysmenorrhea, leucorrhea.*

Immune System: *flu.*

Nervous System: *Depression, headache, hypertension, insomnia, migraine, nervous tension and stress-related conditions, PMT, sciatica, shock, vertigo.*

OTHER USES

Used in pharmaceutical antiseptic ointments and as a fragrance. Extensively employed in all types of soaps, lotions, perfumes, etc. Employed as a flavouring agent in most categories of food as well as alcoholic and soft drinks.

DISTRIBUTION

Indigenous to the Mediterranean, now grown all over the world. The oil mainly comes from France.

OTHER SPECIES

L. angustifolia *is divided into two subspecies –* L. delphinensis *and* L. fragrans. *See also spike lavender, lavandin and the Botanical Classification section.*

Lavandula latifolia

Spike lavender

FAMILY: LAMIACEAE (LABIATAE) **SYNONYMS:** *L. SPICA*, ASPIC, BROAD-LEAVED LAVENDER, LESSER LAVENDER, SPIKE

Herbal/Folk Tradition

Culpeper recommends spike lavender for a variety of ailments including 'pains of the head and brain which proceed from cold, apoplexy, falling sickness, the dropsy, or sluggish malady, cramps, convulsions, palsies, and often faintings.' He also warns that 'the oil of spike is of a fierce and piercing quality, and ought to be carefully used, a very few drops being sufficient for inward or outward maladies.'[51] The preparation 'oleum spicae' was made by mixing ¼ spike oil with ½ turpentine, and used for paralysed limbs, old sprains and stiff joints (it was also said to encourage hair growth). Current in the British Herbal Pharmacopoeia, indicated for flatulent dyspepsia, colic, depressive headaches, and the oil (topically) for rheumatic pain.

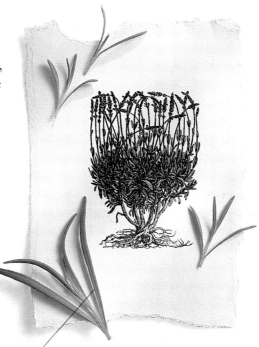

An aromatic evergreen sub-shrub up to 1m (3ft) high with lance-shaped leaves, broader and rougher than those of true lavender. The flower is more compressed and of a dull grey-blue colour.

fresh leaves

EXTRACTION
Essential oil by water or steam distillation from the flowering tops.

CHARACTERISTICS
A water-white or pale yellow liquid with a penetrating, fresh-herbaceous, camphoraceous odour. It blends well with rosemary, sage, lavandin, eucalyptus, rosewood, lavender, petitgrain, pine, cedarwood, oakmoss, patchouli and spice oils, particularly clove.

ACTIONS
See true lavender.

PRINCIPAL CONSTITUENTS
Mainly cineol and camphor (40–60 per cent), with linalol and linalyl acetate, among others.

AROMATHERAPY/
HOME USE
See true lavender.

OTHER USES
It is used in some pharmaceutical preparations and especially in veterinary practice as a prophylactic, in incipient paralysis, for rheumatism and arthritis and to get rid of lice. It is extensively employed as a fragrance component especially in soaps and industrial perfumes such as deodorants, disinfectants and cleansing agents, as well as insecticides and room sprays, etc. It is also used in the food industry and in the production of fine varnishes and lacquers.

DISTRIBUTION
Native to the mountainous regions of France and Spain, also found in North Africa, Italy, former Yugoslavia and the eastern Mediterranean countries. It is cultivated internationally; the oil is produced mainly in France and Spain.

OTHER SPECIES
There are many different chemotypes of lavender in general, and this also applies to spike lavender. The French spike oil is reputed to be a more delicate, aromatic scent than the Spanish variety. For other varieties, see entries on lavandin, true lavender; also the Botanical Classification section.

Lavandula × intermedia

Lavandin

FAMILY: LAMIACEAE (LABIATAE)   **SYNONYMS:** *LAVANDULA HYBRIDA*, *L. HORTENSIS*, BASTARD LAVENDER

Herbal/Folk Tradition

Sixty years ago, when *A Modern Herbal* was written by Mrs Grieve, lavandin was still unknown, so it does not have a long history of therapeutic use. Its properties seem to combine those of the true lavender and aspic.

A hybrid plant developed by crossing true lavender (L. angustifolia) *with spike lavender or aspic* (L. latifolia). *Due to its hybrid nature, lavandin has a variety of forms: in general, it is a larger plant than true lavender, with woody stems. Its flowers may be blue like true lavender, or greyish like aspic.*

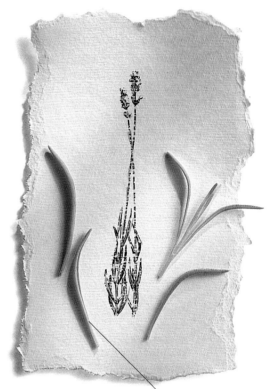

fresh
lavandin
leaf

EXTRACTION
Essential oil by steam distillation from the fresh flowering tops; it has a higher yield of oil than either true lavender or aspic. (A concrete and absolute are also produced by solvent extraction.)

CHARACTERISTICS
A colourless or pale yellow liquid with a fresh camphoraceous top note (which should not be too strong in a good-quality oil), and a woody herbaceous undertone. It blends well with clove, bay leaf, cinnamon, citronella, cypress, pine, clary sage, geranium, thyme, patchouli, rosemary and citrus oils, especially bergamot and lime.

ACTIONS
See true lavender.

PRINCIPAL CONSTITUENTS
Linalyl acetate (30–32 per cent), linalol, cineol, camphene, pinene and other trace constituents.

AROMATHERAPY/ HOME USE
Similar uses to true lavender, but it is more penetrating and rubefacient with a sharper scent – good for respiratory, circulatory or muscular conditions.

OTHER USES
Extensively employed in soaps, detergents, room sprays, hair preparations and industrial perfumes. Used as a flavour ingredient in most major food categories, and also as a natural source of linalol and linalyl acetate.

DISTRIBUTION
A natural lavandin occurs in the mountainous regions of southern France where both parent plants grow wild, though at different altitudes. Still cultivated mainly in France, but also Spain, Hungary, former Yugoslavia and Argentina.

OTHER SPECIES
There are cultivars of lavender, such as 'Dwarf Blue', 'Hidcote Pink' and 'Bowles Early'; there are also many cultivars of lavandin such as 'Grey Hedge', 'Silver Grey' and 'Alba'. For further information see entries on true lavender and spike lavender; also the Botanical Classification section.

Levisticum officinale

Lovage

SAFETY DATA *Non-toxic, non-irritant, possible sensitization/ phototoxic effects. Use with care. Avoid during pregnancy*

FAMILY: APIACEAE (UMBELLIFERAE) **SYNONYMS:** *ANGELICA LEVISTICUM, LIGUSTICUM LEVISTICUM,* SMELLAGE, MAGGI HERB, GARDEN LOVAGE, COMMON LOVAGE, OLD ENGLISH LOVAGE, ITALIAN LOVAGE, CORNISH LOVAGE

Herbal/Folk Tradition

A herb of ancient medical repute, used mainly for digestive complaints, edema, skin problems, menstrual irregularities and fever. It was also believed to be good for the sight. The leaf stalks used to be blanched and used as a vegetable or in salads. The root is current in the British Herbal Pharmacopoeia as a specific for flatulent dyspepsia and anorexia.

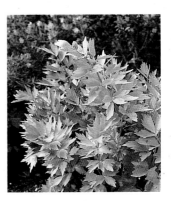

Levisticum officinale

EXTRACTION

Essential oil by steam distillation from 1. the fresh roots, and 2. the herb – fresh leaves and stalks.

CHARACTERISTICS

**1. An amber or olive-brown liquid with a rich, spicy-warm, root-like odour.
2. A very pale yellow mobile liquid with a spicy, warm odour and sweet-floral undertone. It blends well with rose, galbanum, costus, opopanax, oakmoss, bay, lavandin and spice oils.**

ACTIONS

Antimicrobial, antiseptic, antispasmodic, diaphoretic, digestive, diuretic, carminative, depurative, emmenagogue, expectorant, febrifuge, stimulant (digestive), stomachic.

PRINCIPAL CONSTITUENTS

Mainly phthalides (up to 70 per cent) such as butylidene, dihydrobutylidene, butylphthalides and ligostilides, with lesser amounts of terpenoids, volatile acids, coumarins and furocoumarins.

AROMATHERAPY/ HOME USE

Circulation, Muscles and Joints: *Accumulation of toxins, congestion, gout, edema, poor circulation, rheumatism, water retention.*
Digestive System: *Anemia, flatulence, indigestion, spasm.*
Genito-urinary System: *Amenorrhea, dysmenorrhea, cystitis.*

OTHER USES

The root oil is used as a fragrance component in soaps, cosmetics and perfumes. The oils and extracts are used as savoury flavouring agents and in liqueurs and tobacco.

DISTRIBUTION

Native to southern Europe and western Asia; naturalized in North America. It is cultivated in central and southern Europe, especially in France, Belgium, former Czechoslovakia, Hungary, former Yugoslavia and Germany.

OTHER SPECIES

Several related plants are also used to produce essential oils, such as sea lovage (Ligusticum scoticum) and alpine lovage (L. mutellina).

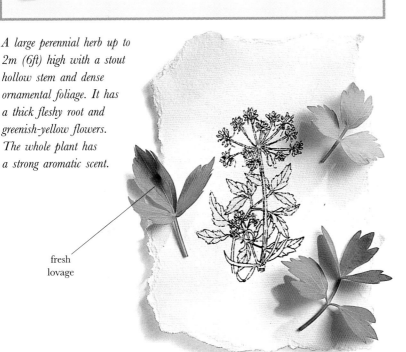

A large perennial herb up to 2m (6ft) high with a stout hollow stem and dense ornamental foliage. It has a thick fleshy root and greenish-yellow flowers. The whole plant has a strong aromatic scent.

fresh lovage

Liquidambar orientalis

Levant styrax

FAMILY: HAMAMELIDACEAE **SYNONYMS:** *BALSAM STYRACIS*, ORIENTAL SWEETGUM, TURKISH SWEETGUM, ASIATIC STYRAX, STYRAX, STORAX, LIQUID STORAX

Herbal/Folk Tradition

In China it is used for coughs, colds, epilepsy and skin problems, including cuts, wounds and scabies. In the West it has been recommended as a remedy for catarrh, diphtheria, gonorrhea, leucorrhea, ringworm, etc. A syrup made from the bark of the American styrax is used for diarrhea and dysentery in the western USA.

A deciduous tree, up to 15m (49ft) high, with a purplish-grey bark, leaves arranged into five three-lobed sections, and white flowers. The styrax is a pathological secretion produced by pounding the bark, which induces the sapwood to produce a liquid from beneath the bark. It hardens to form a semi-solid, greenish-brown mass with a sweet balsamic odour.

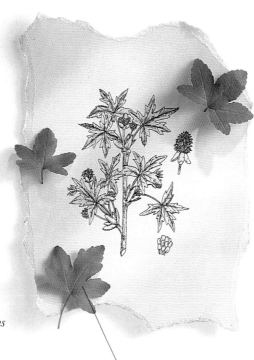

fresh leaves

AROMATHERAPY/ HOME USE

Skin Care: *Cuts, ringworm, scabies, wounds.*
Respiratory System: *Bronchitis, catarrh, coughs.*
Nervous System: *Anxiety, stress-related conditions.*

OTHER USES

Used in compound benzoin tincture, mainly for respiratory conditions. The oil and resinoid are used as fixatives and fragrance components mainly in soaps, floral and oriental perfumes. The resinoid and absolute are used in most major food categories, including alcoholic and soft drinks.

DISTRIBUTION

Native to Asia Minor. It forms forests around Bodrum, Milas, Mugla and Marmaris in Turkey.

OTHER SPECIES

Very similar to the American styrax (L. styraciflua) or red gum, which produces a natural exudation slightly darker and harder than the Levant type. There are also many other types of styrax; Styrax officinale produced the styrax of ancient civilizations.
NB: Styrax benzoin is the botanical name for benzoin, with which it shares similar qualities.

EXTRACTION
Essential oil by steam distillation from the crude. (A resinoid and absolute are also produced by solvent extraction.)

CHARACTERISTICS
A water-white or pale yellow liquid with a sweet-balsamic, rich, tenacious odour. It blends well with ylang ylang, jasmine, mimosa, rose, lavender, carnation, violet, cassie and spice oils.

ACTIONS
Anti-inflammatory, antimicrobial, antiseptic, antitussive, bactericidal, balsamic, expectorant, nervine, stimulant.

PRINCIPAL CONSTITUENTS
Mainly styrene with vanillin, phenylpropyl alcohol, cinnamic alcohol, benzyl alcohol and ethyl alcohol, among others.

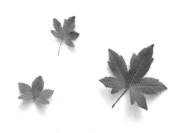

Litsea cubeba

Litsea cubeba

FAMILY: LAURACEAE **SYNONYMS:** *L. CITRATA*, 'MAY CHANG', EXOTIC VERBENA, TROPICAL VERBENA

Herbal/Folk Tradition

The root and stem are used in traditional Chinese medicine to treat dysmenorrhea, indigestion, lower back pain, chills, headaches, muscular aches and pains and travel sickness. Recent research has shown it may be valuable in the treatment of cardiac arrythmia (disordered heart rhythm).

A small tropical tree with fragrant, lemongrass-scented leaves and flowers. The small fruits are shaped like peppers, from which the name 'cubeba' derives.

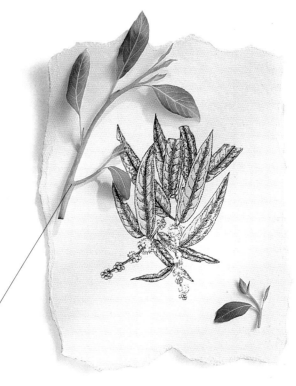

fresh
litsea
cubeba

EXTRACTION
Essential oil by steam distillation from the fruits.

CHARACTERISTICS
A pale yellow mobile liquid with an intense, lemony, fresh-fruity odour (sweeter than lemongrass but less tenacious).

ACTIONS
Antiseptic, deodorant, digestive, disinfectant, insecticidal, sedative, stomachic.

PRINCIPAL CONSTITUENTS
Mainly citral (up to 85 per cent); also limonene, miycrene, methyl hepetone, linalol and linlyl acetate, among others.

AROMATHERAPY/ HOME USE

Skin Care: *Acne, dermatitis, excessive perspiration, greasy skin, insect repellent, spots.*
Digestive System: *Flatulence, indigestion.*
Immune System: *Epidemics, sanitation.*
Nervous System: *Arrhythmia, high blood pressure, nervous tension and stress-related conditions.*

OTHER USES

Extensively used as a fragrance component in air fresheners, soaps, deodorants, colognes, toiletries and perfumes. Employed in flavouring work, especially fruit products. It serves as a source of natural 'citral' all over the world.

DISTRIBUTION

Native to east Asia, especially China; cultivated in Taiwan

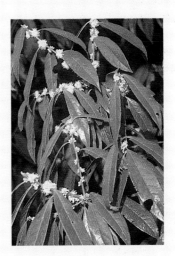

Litsea cubeba

and Japan. China is the main producer of the oil, much of which is used by the Chinese themselves.

OTHER SPECIES

Despite its folk names, this plant is not related to lemon verbena (Aloysia triphylla). It belongs to the same family as the laurel tree, rosewood and cinnamon.

Matricaria recutica

German chamomile

FAMILY: ASTERACEAE (COMPOSITAE) **SYNONYMS:** *M. CHAMOMILLA,* CAMOMILE, BLUE CHAMOMILE, MATRICARIS, HUNGARIAN CHAMOMILE, SWEET FALSE CHAMOMILE, SINGLE CHAMOMILE, CHAMOMILE BLUE (OIL)

Herbal/Folk Tradition

This herb has a long-standing medicinal tradition, especially in Europe, for 'all states of tension and the visceral symptoms that can arise therefrom, such as nervous dyspepsia, and nervous bowel, tension headaches, and sleeplessness; especially useful for all children's conditions, calming without depressing . . . '[52]

An excellent skin care remedy, it has many of the same qualities as Roman chamomile, except that its anti-inflammatory properties are greater because of the higher percentage of azulene.

An annual, strongly aromatic herb, up to 60cm (24in) tall with a hairless, erect, branching stem. It has delicate feathery leaves and simple daisy-like white flowers on single stems. In appearance it is very similar to the corn chamomile (Anthemis arvensis) *but can be distinguished from it because the latter is scentless.*

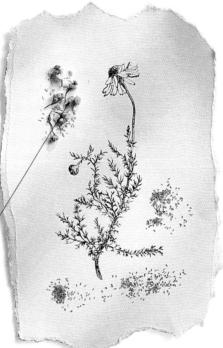

German chamomile seeds

EXTRACTION
Essential oil by steam distillation from the flower heads (up to 1.9 per cent yield). An absolute is also produced in small quantities, which is a deeper blue colour and has greater tenacity and fixative properties.

CHARACTERISTICS
An inky-blue viscous liquid with a strong, sweetish warm-herbaceous odour. It blends well with geranium, lavender, patchouli, rose, benzoin, orange blossom, bergamot, marjoram, lemon, ylang ylang, jasmine, clary sage and labdanum.

ACTIONS
Analgesic, anti-allergenic, anti-inflammatory, antiphlogistic, antispasmodic, bactericidal, carminative, cicatrizant, cholagogue, digestive, emmenagogue, febrifuge, fungicidal, hepatic, nerve sedative, stimulant of leucocyte production, stomachic, sudorific, vermifuge, vulnerary.

PRINCIPAL CONSTITUENTS
Chamazulene, farnesene, bisabolol oxide, en-yndicycloether, among others. (NB: The chamazulene is not present in the fresh flower but is only produced during the process of distillation.)

AROMATHERAPY/ HOME USE

See Roman chamomile.

OTHER USES

See Roman chamomile.

DISTRIBUTION

Native to Europe and north and west Asia; naturalized in North America and Australia. It is cultivated extensively, especially in Hungary and eastern Europe, *where the oil is produced. It is no longer grown in Germany, despite the herbal name.*

OTHER SPECIES

There are many varieties of chamomile, such as the pineapple weed (Chamaemelum suaveolens) *and the Roman chamomile* (C. nobile), *both of which are used to produce an essential oil.*

Melaleuca alternifolia

Tea tree

SAFETY DATA *Non-toxic, non-irritant, possible sensitization in some individuals*

FAMILY: MYRTACEAE **SYNONYMS:** NARROW-LEAVED PAPERBARK TEA TREE, TI-TREE, TI-TROL, MELASOL

Herbal/Folk Tradition

The name derives from its local usage as a type of herbal tea, prepared from the leaves. Our present knowledge of the properties and uses of tea tree is based on a very long history of use by the aboriginal people of Australia. It has been extensively researched recently by scientific methods with the following results:

'1. This oil is unusual in that it is active against all three varieties of infectious organisms: bacteria, fungi and viruses. 2. It is a very powerful immuno-stimulant, so when the body is threatened by any of these organisms ti-tree increases its ability to respond.'[53]

A small tree or shrub (smallest of the tea tree family), with needle-like leaves similar to cypress, with heads of sessile yellow or purplish flowers.

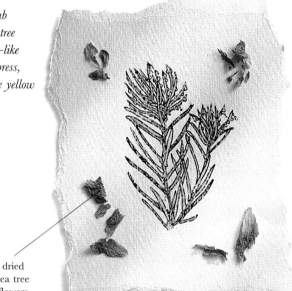

dried
tea tree
flowers

EXTRACTION
Essential oil by steam or water distillation from the leaves and twigs.

CHARACTERISTICS
A pale yellowy-green or water-white liquid with a warm, fresh, spicy-camphoraceous odour. It blends well with lavandin, lavender, clary sage, rosemary, oakmoss, pine, cananga, geranium, marjoram and spice oils, especially clove and nutmeg.

ACTIONS
Anti-infectious, anti-inflammatory, antiseptic, antiviral, bactericidal, balsamic, cicatrizant, diaphoretic, expectorant, fungicidal, immuno-stimulant, parasiticide, vulnerary.

PRINCIPAL
CONSTITUENTS
Terpinene-4-ol (up to 30 per cent), cineol, pinene, terpinenes, cymene, sesquiterpenes, sesquiterpene alcohols, among others.

AROMATHERAPY/ HOME USE

Skin Care: *Abscess, acne, athlete's foot, blisters, burns, cold sores, dandruff, herpes, insect bites, oily skin, rashes (nappy rash), spots, veruccae, warts, wounds (infected).*
Respiratory System: *Asthma, bronchitis, catarrh, coughs, sinusitis, tuberculosis, whooping cough.*
Genito-urinary System: *Thrush, vaginitis, cystitis, pruritis.*
Immune System: *Colds, fever, flu, infectious illnesses such as chicken pox.*

OTHER USES

Employed in soaps, toothpastes, deodorants, disinfectants, gargles, germicides and, increasingly, in aftershaves and spicy colognes.

DISTRIBUTION

Native to Australia, mainly in New South Wales. Other varieties have been cultivated elsewhere, but M. alternifolia *is not produced outside Australia.*

OTHER SPECIES

Tea tree is a general name for members of the Melaleuca *family, which exists in many physiological forms including cajeput (*M. cajeputi*), niaouli (*M. viridiflora*), and many others such as* M. bracteate *and* M. linariifolia *– see Botanical Classification section.*

Melaleuca cajeputi

Cajeput

| SAFETY DATA *Non-toxic, non-sensitizing, may irritate the skin in high concentration* |

FAMILY: MYRTACEAE **SYNONYMS:** *M. MINOR*, CAJUPUT, WHITE TEA TREE, WHITE WOOD, SWAMP TEA TREE, PUNK TREE, PAPERBARK TREE

fresh cajeput

Herbal/Folk Tradition

Held in high regard in the East, it is used locally for colds, headaches, throat infections, toothache, sore and aching muscles, fever (cholera), rheumatism and various skin diseases. Only the oil is used in the Western herbal tradition, and is known for producing a sensation of warmth and quickening the pulse. It is used for chronic laryngitis and bronchitis, cystitis, rheumatism and to expel roundworm.

A tall evergreen tree up to 30m (98ft) high, with thick pointed leaves and white flowers. The flexible trunk has a whitish spongy bark that flakes off easily. In Malaysia it is called 'caju-puti', meaning 'white wood', because of the colour of the timber.

EXTRACTION

Essentials oil by steam distillation from the fresh leaves and twigs.

CHARACTERISTICS

A pale yellowy-green, mobile liquid (the green tinge derives from traces of copper found in the tree), with a penetrating, camphoraceous-medicinal odour. Compared with eucalyptus oil, it has a slightly milder fruity body note.

ACTIONS

Mildly analgesic, antimicrobial, antineuralgic, antispasmodic, antiseptic (pulmonary, urinary, intestinal), anthelminthic, diaphoretic, carminative, expectorant, febrifuge, insecticide, sudorific, tonic.

PRINCIPAL CONSTITUENTS

Cineol (14–65 per cent depending on source), terpineol, terpinyl acetate, pinene, nerolidol and other traces.

AROMATHERAPY/ HOME USE

Skin Care: *Insect bites, oily skin, spots.*
Circulation, Muscles and Joints: *Arthritis, muscular aches and pains, rheumatism.*
Respiratory System: *Asthma, bronchitis, catarrh, coughs, sinusitis, sore throat.*
Genito-urinary System: *Cystitis, urethritis, urinary infection.*
Immune System: *Colds, flu, viral infections.*

OTHER USES

Used in dentistry and pharmaceutical work as an antiseptic; in expectorant and tonic formulations, throat lozenges, gargles, etc. Used as a fragrance and freshening agent in soaps, cosmetics, detergents and perfumes. Occasionally employed as a flavour component in food products and soft drinks.

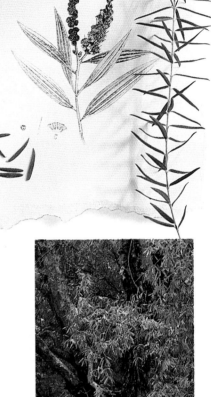

Melaleuca cajeputi

DISTRIBUTION

It grows wild in Malaysia, Indonesia, the Philippines, Vietnam, Java, Australia and south-eastern Asia.

OTHER SPECIES

Several other varieties of Melaleuca *are used to produce cajeput oil, such as* M. quinquenervia. *See Botanical Classification section. Closely related to other members of the* Melaleuca *group, notably eucalyptus, clove, niaouli and tea tree.*

Melaleuca viridiflora

Niaouli

FAMILY: MYRTACEAE **SYNONYMS:** *M. QUINQUENERVIA,* 'GOMENOL'

Herbal/Folk Tradition

It is used locally for a wide variety of ailments, such as aches and pains, respiratory conditions, cuts and infections; it is also used to purify the water. The name 'gomenol' derives from the fact that it used to be shipped from Gomen in the French East Indies.

An evergreen tree with a flexible trunk and spongy bark, pointed linear leaves and bearing spikes of sessile yellowish flowers. The leaves have a strong aromatic scent when they are crushed.

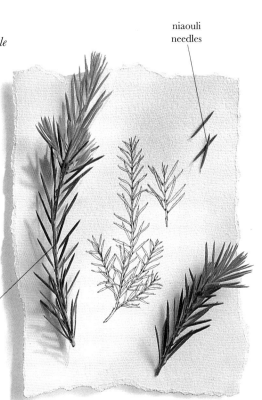

niaouli needles

sprig of fresh niaouli

EXTRACTION
Essential oil by steam distillation from the leaves and young twigs. (Usually rectified to remove irritant aldehydes.)

CHARACTERISTICS
A colourless, pale yellow or greenish liquid with a sweet, fresh, camphoraceous odour.

ACTIONS
Analgesic, anthelminthic, anticatarrhal, antirheumatic, antiseptic, antispasmodic, bactericidal, balsamic, cicatrizant, diaphoretic, expectorant, regulator, stimulant, vermifuge.

PRINCIPAL CONSTITUENTS
Cineol (50–65 per cent), terpineol, pinene, limonene, citrene, terebenthene, valeric ester, acetic ester, butyric ester.

AROMATHERAPY/ HOME USE

Skin Care: *Acne, boils, burns, cuts, insect bites, oily skin, spots, ulcers, wounds.*
Circulation, Muscles and Joints: *Muscular aches and pains, poor circulation, rheumatism.*
Respiratory System: *Asthma, bronchitis, catarrhal conditions, coughs, sinusitis, sore throat, whooping cough.*
Genito-urinary System: *Cystitis, urinary infection.*

Immune System:
Colds, fever, flu.

OTHER USES

Used in pharmaceutical preparations such as gargles, cough drops, toothpastes, mouth sprays, etc.

DISTRIBUTION

Native to Australia, New Caledonia and the French Pacific Islands. The majority of the oil is produced in Australia.

OTHER SPECIES

A typical member of the 'tea tree' group of oils; the oil is similar to cajeput. There is another physiological form of **M.** *viridiflora called 'Variety A', which was originally developed to provide a natural source of nerolidol, the main constituent of its essential oil.*

Melilotus officinalis

Melilotus

FAMILY: FABACEAE (LEGUMINOSAE) **SYNONYMS:** COMMON MELILOT, YELLOW MELILOT, WHITE MELILOT, CORN MELILOT, MELILOT TREFOIL, SWEET CLOVER, PLASTER CLOVER, SWEET LUCERNE, WILD LABURNUM, KING'S CLOVER, MELILOTIN (OLEORESIN)

Herbal/Folk Tradition

The leaves and shoots are used in continental Europe for conditions that include sleeplessness, thrombosis, nervous tension, varicose veins, intestinal disorders, headache, earache and indigestion. In the form of an ointment or plaster, it is used externally for inflamed or swollen joints, abdominal and rheumatic pain, also bruises, cuts and skin eruptions.

A bushy perennial herb up to 1m (3ft) high with smooth erect stems, trifoliate oval leaves and small sweet-scented white or yellow flowers. The scent of the flowers becomes stronger on drying.

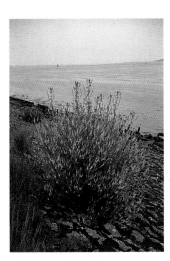

Melilotus officinalis

AROMATHERAPY/ HOME USE

None.

OTHER USES

The oleoresin is used in high-class perfumery work. Extensively used for flavouring tobacco in countries without the coumarin ban.

DISTRIBUTION

Native to Europe and Asia Minor. Other similar species are found in Asia, the USA and Africa. The flowers are mainly cultivated in Britain, France, Germany and Russia.

OTHER SPECIES

There are several similar species such as M. arvensis, *the oil of which is also used in perfumery and flavouring work.*

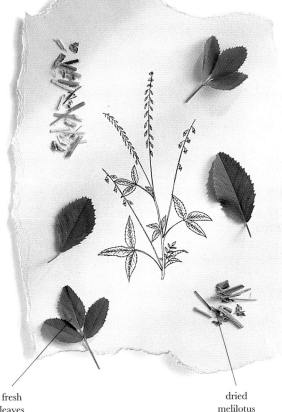

fresh
leaves

dried
melilotus

EXTRACTION
A concrete (usually called a resinoid or oleoresin) by solvent extraction from the dry flowers.

CHARACTERISTICS
A viscous dark green liquid with a rich, sweet-herbaceous 'new-mown hay' scent.

ACTIONS
Anti-inflammatory, antirheumatic, antispasmodic, astringent, emollient, expectorant, digestive, insecticidal (against moth), sedative.

PRINCIPAL CONSTITUENTS
Mainly coumarins – melilotic acid and orthocoumaric acid.

Melissa officinalis

Lemon balm

SAFETY DATA *Non-toxic. Possible sensitization and dermal irritation: use in low dilutions only. One of the most frequently adulterated oils. Most commercial so-called melissa contains some or all of the following: lemon, lemongrass or citronella*

FAMILY: LAMIACEAE (LABIATAE) **SYNONYMS:** MELISSA, COMMON BALM, BEE BALM, SWEET BALM, HEART'S DELIGHT, HONEY PLANT

Herbal/Folk Tradition

One of the earliest known medicinal herbs – Paracelsus called it the 'Elixir of Life'. It was associated particularly with nervous disorders, the heart and the emotions. It was used for anxiety, melancholy, etc., and to strengthen and revive the vital spirit. Generally employed for digestive and respiratory complaints of nervous origin such as asthma, indigestion and flatulence. It also helps to regulate the menstrual cycle and promote fertility. Effective remedy for wasp and bee stings. In France the leaves are still used a great deal in pharmaceutical and herbal products. Current in the British Herbal Pharmacopoeia for flatulent dyspepsia, neurasthenia and depressive illness.

fresh leaves

A sweet-scented herb about 60cm (24in) high, soft and bushy, with bright green serrated leaves, square stems and tiny white or pink flowers.

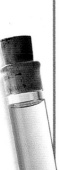

EXTRACTION
Essential oil by steam distillation from the leaves and flowering tops.

CHARACTERISTICS
A pale yellow liquid with a light, fresh lemony fragrance. It blends well with lavender, geranium, floral and citrus oils.

ACTIONS
Antidepressant, antihistaminic, antispasmodic, bactericidal, carminative, cordial, diaphoretic, emmenagogue, febrifuge, hypertensive, insect-repellent, nervine, sedative, stomachic, sudorific, tonic, uterine, vermifuge.

PRINCIPAL CONSTITUENTS
Mainly citronellal and geranial with neral, citronellol caryophyllene, caryophyllene oxide, linalol and limonene, among others.

AROMATHERAPY/ HOME USE

Skin Care: *Allergies, insect bites, insect repellent. 'Melissa in very low concentration is a very valuable oil indeed in treating eczema and other skin problems.'[54]*
Respiratory System: *Asthma, bronchitis, chronic coughs.*
Digestive System: *Colic, indigestion, nausea.*
Genito-urinary System: *Menstrual problems.*
Nervous System: *Anxiety, depression, hypertension, insomnia, migraine, nervous tension, shock and vertigo.*

OTHER USES

Used extensively as a fragrance component in toiletries, cosmetics and perfumes. Employed in most major food categories including alcoholic and soft drinks.

DISTRIBUTION

Native to the Mediterranean region, now common throughout Europe, middle Asia, North America, North Africa and Siberia. Cultivated mainly in Hungary, Egypt and Italy; the major oil-producing country is the Republic of Ireland.

OTHER SPECIES

Several varieties, e.g. a variegated leaf type, common in gardens.

Mentha arvensis

Cornmint

FAMILY: LAMIACEAE (LABIATAE)   **SYNONYMS:** FIELD MINT, JAPANESE MINT

Herbal/Folk Tradition

It is used therapeutically in many of the same ways as peppermint; the bruised leaves are applied to the forehead to relieve nervous headache. In the East it is used to treat rheumatic pain, neuralgia, toothache, laryngitis, indigestion, colds and bronchitis. In Chinese medicine, it is also employed for relieving earache, treating tumours and some skin conditions.

A rather fragile herb with leafy stems up to 60cm (24in) high, lance-shaped leaves and lilac-coloured flowers borne in clustered whorls in the axils of the upper leaves.

fresh
cornmint
leaves

EXTRACTION

Essential oil by steam distillation from the flowering herb. The oil is usually dementholized since it contains so much menthol that it is otherwise solid at room temperature.

CHARACTERISTICS

Dementholized oil – a colourless or pale yellow liquid with a strong, fresh, bitter-sweet minty odour, somewhat like peppermint.

ACTIONS

Anesthetic, antimicrobial, antiseptic, antispasmodic, carminative, cytotoxic, digestive, expectorant, stimulant, stomachic.

PRINCIPAL CONSTITUENTS

Menthol (70–95 per cent), menthone (10–20 per cent), pinene, menthyl acetate, isomenthone, thujone, phellandrene, piperitone and menthofuran, among others. Constituents vary according to source.

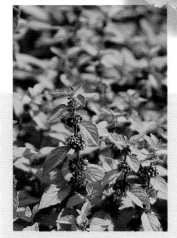

Mentha arvensis

AROMATHERAPY/ HOME USE

Not compatible with homeopathic treatment. Use peppermint in preference, since it is not fractionated like the commercial cornmint oil and has a more refined fragrance.

OTHER USES

Used in some pharmaceutical preparations, such as cough lozenges, herb teas and syrups, mainly in the form of menthol. Extensively employed in soaps, toothpastes, detergents, cosmetics, perfumes and especially industrial fragrances. Used by the food industry especially for flavouring confectionery, liqueurs and chewing gum. However, it is used mainly for the isolation of natural menthol.

DISTRIBUTION

Native to Europe and parts of Asia (Japan and China); naturalized in North America. Major producers of the oil include China, Brazil, Argentina, India and Vietnam.

OTHER SPECIES

There are many varieties and chemotypes of this herb, which is used for large-scale oil production, such as the Chinese type M. arvensis var. glabrata, and the Japanese species M. arvensis var. piperascens.

Mentha piperita

Peppermint

FAMILY: LAMIACEAE (LABIATAE) **SYNONYMS:** BRANDY MINT, BALM MINT

Herbal/Folk Tradition

Mints have been cultivated since ancient times in China and Japan. In Egypt evidence of a type of peppermint has been found in tombs dating from 1000 BC. It has been used extensively in Eastern and Western medicine for a variety of complaints, including indigestion, nausea, sore throat, diarrhea, headaches, toothaches and cramp. It is current in the British Herbal Pharmacopoeia for intestinal colic, flatulence, common cold, vomiting in pregnancy and dysmenorrhea.

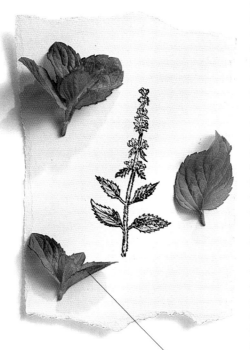

fresh peppermint leaves

A perennial herb up to 1m (3ft) high with underground runners by which it is easily propagated. The 'white' peppermint has green stems and leaves; the 'black' peppermint has dark green serrated leaves, purplish stems and reddish-violet flowers.

EXTRACTION
Essential oil by steam distillation from the flowering herb (approx. 3–4 per cent yield).

CHARACTERISTICS
A pale yellow or greenish liquid with a highly penetrating, grassy-minty camphoraceous odour. It blends well with benzoin, rosemary, lavender, marjoram, lemon, eucalyptus and other mints.

ACTIONS
Analgesic, anti-inflammatory, antimicrobial, antiphlogistic, antipruritic, antiseptic, antispasmodic, antiviral, astringent, carminative, cephalic, cholagogue, cordial, emmenagogue, expectorant, febrifuge, hepatic, nervine, stomachic, sudorific, vasoconstrictor, vermifuge.

PRINCIPAL CONSTITUENTS
Menthol (29–48 per cent), menthone (20–31 per cent), menthyl acetate, menthofuran, limonene, pulegone, cineol, among others.

AROMATHERAPY/ HOME USE
Not compatible with homeopathic treatment.
Skin Care: *Acne, dermatitis, ringworm, scabies, toothache.*
Circulation, Muscles and Joints: *Neuralgia, muscular pain, palpitations.*
Respiratory System: *Asthma, bronchitis, halitosis, sinusitis, spasmodic cough – 'When inhaled (in steam) it checks catarrh temporarily, and will provide relief from head colds and bronchitis: its antispasmodic action combines well with this to make it a most useful inhalation in asthma.'*[55]
Digestive System: *Colic, cramp, dyspepsia, flatulence, nausea.*
Immune System: *Colds, flu, fevers.*
Nervous System: *Fainting, headache, mental fatigue, migraine, nervous stress, vertigo.*

OTHER USES
Flavouring agent in pharmaceuticals, and ingredient in cough, cold and digestive remedies. Flavouring agent in many foods, especially chewing gum and confectionery, alcoholic and soft drinks; also tobacco. Fragrance component in soaps, toothpaste, detergents, cosmetics, perfumes, etc.

DISTRIBUTION
Originally a cultivated hybrid between M. viridis and M. aquatica. It is cultivated worldwide.

OTHER SPECIES
There are several different strains or chemotypes of peppermint and numerous other species of mint. See Botanical Classification section.

Mentha pulegium

Pennyroyal

FAMILY: LAMIACEAE (LABIATAE) **SYNONYMS:** PULEGIUM, EUROPEAN PENNYROYAL, PUDDING GRASS

Herbal/Folk Tradition

A herbal remedy of ancient repute, used for a wide variety of ailments. It was believed to purify the blood and be able to communicate its purifying qualities to water. 'Pennyroyal water was distilled from the leaves and given as an antidote to spasmodic, nervous and hysterical affections. It was also used against cold and "affections of the joints".'[56]

It is still current in the British Herbal Pharmacopoeia, indicated for flatulent dyspepsia, intestinal colic, the common cold, delayed menstruation, cutaneous eruptions and gout.

A perennial herb up to 50cm (20in) tall with smooth roundish stalks, small, pale purple flowers and very aromatic, grey-green, oval leaves. Like other members of the mint family, it has a fibrous creeping root.

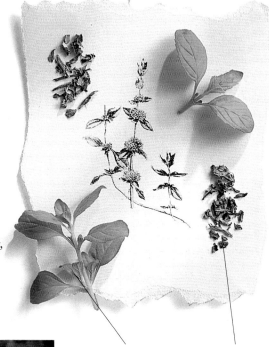

fresh sprig of
pennyroyal

dried
pennyroyal

EXTRACTION
Essential oil by steam distillation from the fresh or slightly dried herb.

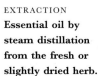

CHARACTERISTICS
A colourless or pale yellow liquid with a very fresh, minty-herbaceous odour. It blends well with geranium, rosemary, lavandin, sage and citronella.

ACTIONS
Antiseptic, antispasmodic, diaphoretic, carminative, digestive, emmenagogue, insect repellent, refrigerant, stimulant.

PRINCIPAL CONSTITUENTS
Mainly pulegone, with menthone, iso-menthone, octanol, piperitenone and trans-iso-pulegone. Constituents vary according to source – the Moroccan oil contains up to 96 per cent pulegone.

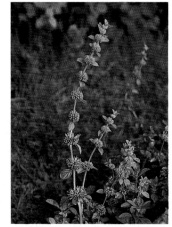

Mentha pulegium

**AROMATHERAPY/
HOME USE**

None. 'Should not be used in aromatherapy whether internally or externally.'[57]

OTHER USES

Used as a fragrance material mainly in detergents or low-cost industrial perfumes. Employed mainly as a source of natural pulegone.

DISTRIBUTION

Native to Europe and parts of Asia; it is cultivated mainly in southern Spain, Morocco, Tunisia, Portugal, Italy, former Yugoslavia and Turkey.

OTHER SPECIES

There are several different varieties of pennyroyal according to location: in Britain the 'erecta' and 'decumbens' types are most common. The North American pennyroyal (Hedeoma pulegoides), which is also used to produce an essential oil, belongs to a slightly different species, though it shares similar properties with the European variety.

Mentha spicata

Spearmint

FAMILY: LAMIACEAE (LABIATAE) **SYNONYMS:** *M. VIRIDIS*, COMMON SPEARMINT, GARDEN SPEARMINT, SPIRE MINT, GREEN MINT, LAMB MINT, PEA MINT, FISH MINT

Herbal/Folk Tradition

Valued all over the world as a culinary herb, as shown by its folk names. It was used by the ancient Greeks as a restorative and to scent their bathwater. The distilled water is used to relieve hiccough, colic, nausea, indigestion and flatulence. 'Applied to the forehead and temples, it eases the pains in the head, and is good to wash the heads of young children with, against all manner of breakings out, sores or scabs . . . being smelled unto, it is comforting to the head.'[58]

EXTRACTION

Essential oil by steam distillation from the flowering tops.

CHARACTERISTICS

A pale yellow or olive mobile liquid with a warm, spicy-herbaceous, minty odour. It blends well with lavender, lavandin, jasmine, eucalyptus, basil and rosemary and is often used in combination with peppermint.

ACTIONS

Anesthetic (local), antiseptic, antispasmodic, astringent, carminative, cephalic, cholagogue, decongestant, digestive, diuretic, expectorant, febrifuge, hepatic, nervine, stimulant, stomachic, tonic.

PRINCIPAL CONSTITUENTS

L-carvone (50–70 per cent), dihydrocarvone, phellandrene, limonene, menthone, menthol, pulegone, cineol, linalol, pinenes, among others.

AROMATHERAPY/ HOME USE

Not compatible with homeopathic treatment. 'The properties of spearmint oil resemble those of peppermint but its effects are less powerful . . . it is better adapted to children's maladies.'[59]
Skin Care: *Acne, dermatitis, congested skin.*
Respiratory System: *Asthma, bronchitis, catarrhal conditions, sinusitis.*
Digestive System: *Colic, dyspepsia, flatulence, hepatobiliary disorders, nausea, vomiting.*
Immune System: *Colds, fevers, flu.*
Nervous System: *Fatigue, headache, migraine, nervous strain, neurasthenia, stress.*

OTHER USES

Used as a fragrance component, mainly in soaps and colognes. Used primarily as a flavour ingredient in a wide range of products, including toothpaste, chewing gum, confectionery, alcoholic and soft drinks.

DISTRIBUTION

Native to the Mediterranean region, now common throughout Europe, western Asia and the Middle East. It was introduced to the USA where it has become a very popular flavouring. The oil is produced in midwest USA, Hungary, Spain, former Yugoslavia, Russia and China.

OTHER SPECIES

*There are several different types of spearmint, especially in the USA, such as the curly mint (**M.** spicata var. crispa). In Russia the oil from **M.** verticellata is also sold as spearmint oil.*

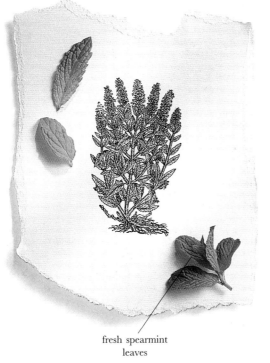

A hardy branched perennial herb with bright green, lance-shaped, sharply serrated leaves, quickly spreading underground runners and pink or lilac-coloured flowers in slender cylindrical spikes.

fresh spearmint leaves

Myristica fragrans

Nutmeg

FAMILY: MYRISTICACEAE **SYNONYMS:** *M. OFFICINALIS, M. AROMATA, NUX MOSCHATA,* MYRISTICA (OIL), MACE (HUSK), MACIS (OIL)

Herbal/Folk Tradition

Nutmeg and mace are widely used as domestic spices and have been used for centuries as a remedy mainly for digestive and kidney problems. Grated nutmeg with lard is used for piles. A fixed oil of nutmeg is also used in soap and candle-making. Current in the British Herbal Pharmacopoeia for flatulent dyspepsia, nausea, diarrhea, dysentery and rheumatism.

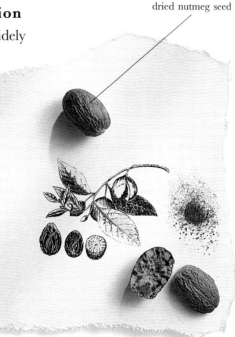

dried nutmeg seed

An evergreen tree up to 20m (65ft) high with a greyish-brown smooth bark, dense foliage and small dull-yellow flowers.

AROMATHERAPY/ HOME USE

'Large quantities are hallucinogenic and excitant to the motor cortex.' [60] *Nutmeg (especially the West Indian type) is probably safer to use than mace. Use in moderation, and with care in pregnancy.*
Circulation, Muscles and Joints: *Arthritis, gout, muscular aches and pains, poor circulation, rheumatism.*
Digestive System: *Flatulence, indigestion, nausea, sluggish digestion.*
Immune System: *Bacterial infection.*
Nervous System: *Frigidity, impotence, neuralgia, nervous fatigue.*

OTHER USES

Used as a flavouring agent in pharmaceuticals, especially analgesic and tonic preparations.

Nutmeg and mace oil are used in soaps, lotions, detergents, cosmetics and perfumes. Mace oleoresin is used in colognes and perfumes, especially men's fragrances. Both oils and oleoresin are used in most major food categories, including alcoholic and soft drinks.

DISTRIBUTION

Native to the Moluccas and nearby islands; cultivated in Indonesia, Sri Lanka and the West Indies, especially Grenada. The essential oil is also distilled in the USA and Europe from imported nutmegs.

OTHER SPECIES

Indonesia and Sri Lanka produce the so-called East Indian nutmeg, which is considered superior, while Grenada produces the 'West Indian' nutmeg. See also Botanical Classification section.

EXTRACTION

Essential oil by steam (or water) distillation from 1. the dried worm-eaten nutmeg seed (the worms eat away all the starch and fat content); 2. the dried orange-brown aril or husk – mace; and 3. an oleoresin is also produced by solvent extraction from mace.

CHARACTERISTICS

1. A water-white or pale yellow mobile liquid with a sweet, warm-spicy odour and a terpeney top note. 2. A water-white or pale yellow mobile liquid with a sweet, warm-spicy scent. 3. An orange-brown viscous liquid with a fresh, spicy-warm, balsamic fragrance. It has good masking power. They blend well with oakmoss, lavandin, bay leaf, Peru balsam, orange, geranium, clary sage, rosemary, lime, petitgrain, mandarin, coriander and other spice oils.

ACTIONS

Analgesic, anti-emetic, anti-oxidant, antirheumatic, antiseptic, antispasmodic, aphrodisiac, carminative, digestive, emmenagogue, gastric secretory stimulant, larvicidal, orexigenic, prostaglandin inhibitor, stimulant, tonic.

PRINCIPAL CONSTITUENTS

Mainly monoterpene hydrocarbons (88 per cent approx.): camphene, pinene, dipentene, sabinene, cymene, with lesser amounts of geraniol, borneol, linalol, terpineol, myristicin (4–8 per cent), safrol and elemincin, among others.

Myrocarpus fastigiatus

Cabreuva

SAFETY DATA *Non-toxic, non-irritant, non-sensitizing*

FAMILY: FABACEAE (LEGUMINOSAE)   SYNONYMS: CABUREICIA, 'BAUME DE PEROU BRUN'

Herbal/Folk Tradition

The wood is highly appreciated for carving and furniture making. It is used by the local people to heal wounds, ulcers, and to obviate scars. It was once listed in old European pharmacopeias for its antiseptic qualities.

A graceful, tall tropical tree, 12–15m (39–49ft) high, with a very hard wood, extremely resistant to moisture and mould growth. It yields a balsam when the trunk is damaged, like many other South American trees.

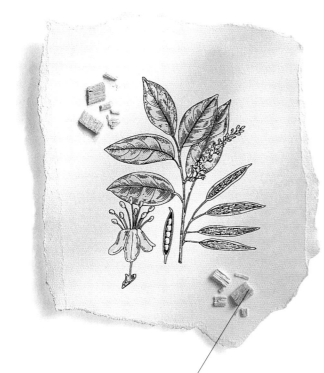

cabreuva
wood
chippings

AROMATHERAPY/ HOME USE

Skin Care: *Cuts, scars, wounds.*
Respiratory System: *Chills, coughs.*
Immune System: *Colds.*

OTHER USES

Fragrance component and fixative in soaps and high-class perfumes, especially floral, woody or oriental types. Previously used for the isolation of nerolidol, now produced synthetically.

DISTRIBUTION

Found in Brazil, Paraguay, Chile and north Argentina.

OTHER SPECIES

Many varieties of Myrocarpus *yield cabreuva oil, such as* M. frondosus. *It is also botanically related to the trees that yield copaiba, Peru and Tolu balsam.*

EXTRACTION
Essential oil by steam distillation from wood chippings (waste from the timber mills).

CHARACTERISTICS
A pale yellow, viscous liquid with a sweet, woody-floral scent, very delicate but having great tenacity. It blends well with rose, cassie, mimosa, cedarwood, rich woody and oriental bases.

ACTIONS
Antiseptic, balsamic, cicatrizant.

PRINCIPAL CONSTITUENTS
Mainly merolidol (80 per cent approx.), farnesol, bisabolol, among others.

Myroxylon balsamum var. balsamum

Tolu balsam

> **SAFETY DATA** *Available information indicates it to be non-toxic, non-irritant, possible sensitization; see Peru Balsam*

FAMILY: FABACEAE (LEGUMINOSAE) **SYNONYMS:** *TOLUIFERA BALSAMUM, BALSAMUM TOLUTANUM, B. AMERICANUM, MYROSPERMUM TOLUIFERUM,* THOMAS BALSAM, RESIN TOLU, OPOBALSAM

Herbal/Folk Tradition

The balsam works primarily on the respiratory mucous membranes and is good for chronic catarrh and non-inflammatory chest complaints, laryngitis and croup. It is still used as a flavour and mild expectorant in cough syrups and lozenges. As an ingredient in compound benzoin tincture and similar formulations, it is helpful in the treatment of cracked nipples, lips, cuts, bedsores, etc.

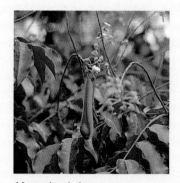

Myroxylon balsamum var. balsamum

A tall, graceful tropical tree, similar in appearance to the Peru balsam tree. The balsam is a pathological product, obtained by making V-shaped incisions into the bark and sap wood, often after the trunk has been beaten and scorched. It is a 'true' balsam.

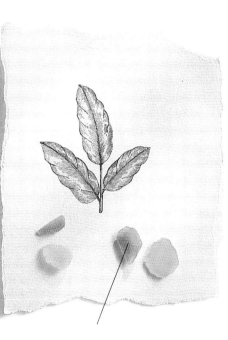

Tolu balsam

AROMATHERAPY/ HOME USE

Skin Care: *Dry, chapped and cracked skin, eczema, rashes, scabies, sores, wounds.*
Respiratory System: *Bronchitis, catarrh, coughs, croup, laryngitis. 'It may be used as an inhalant by putting about a teaspoon into a steam bath.'*[61]

OTHER USES

As a fixative and fragrance component in colognes, cosmetics and perfumes (especially the dry distilled type). Some use in pharmaceutical preparations, e.g. cough syrups. Low levels used in many major food products, especially baked goods.

DISTRIBUTION

Native to South America, mainly Venezuela, Colombia and Cuba; also cultivated in the West Indies.

OTHER SPECIES

There are many types of South American balsam-yielding trees, such as the Peru balsam – see entry.

EXTRACTION
The crude balsam is collected from the trees. It appears first in liquid form, then hardens and solidifies into an orange-brown brittle mass. An 'essential oil' is obtained from the crude by 1. steam distillation, or
2. dry distillation. (A resinoid and absolute are also produced for use primarily as fixatives.)

CHARACTERISTICS
1. A pale yellow-brown liquid with a sweet-floral scent and peppery undertone.

2. An amber-coloured liquid with a rich balsamic-floral scent, which slowly solidifies on cooling into a crystalline mass. Tolu balsam blends well with mimosa, ylang ylang, sandalwood, labdanum, neroli, patchouli, cedarwood, and oriental, spicy and floral bases.

ACTIONS
Antitussive, antiseptic, balsamic, expectorant, stimulant.

PRINCIPAL CONSTITUENTS
The balsam contains approx. 80 per cent resin, 20 per cent oil, with cinnamic and benzoic acids, small amounts of terpenes, and traces of eugenol and vanillin.

Myroxylon balsamum var. pereirae

Peru balsam

FAMILY: FABACEAE (LEGUMINOSAE) **SYNONYMS:** *TOLUIFERA PEREIRA, MYROSPERUM PEREIRA, MYROXYLON PEREIRAE,* PERUVIAN BALSAM, INDIAN BALSAM, BLACK BALSAM

Herbal/Folk Tradition

It stimulates the heart, increases blood pressure, and lessens mucus secretions; useful for respiratory disorders such as asthma, chronic coughs and bronchitis. Traditionally employed for rheumatic pain and skin problems including scabies, nappy rash, bedsores, prurigo, eczema, sore nipples and wounds; it also destroys the itch acarus and its eggs.

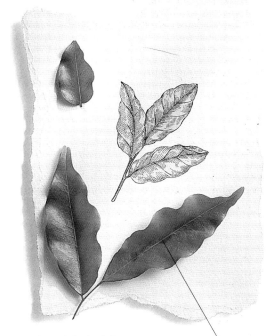

Peru balsam leaves

EXTRACTION

A resin-free essential oil is produced from the crude balsam by high vacuum dry distillation. (A wood oil is also produced by steam distillation from the wood chippings, which is considered of inferior quality. A white balsam called 'myroxocarpin' is made from the fruit, and an extract called 'balsamito' from the young fruit.)

CHARACTERISTICS

The oil is a pale amber or brown viscous liquid with a rich, sweet, balsamic, 'vanilla-like' scent. It blends well with ylang ylang, patchouli, petitgrain, sandalwood, rose, spices, floral and oriental bases.

ACTIONS

Anti-inflammatory, antiseptic, balsamic, expectorant, parasiticide, stimulant; promotes the growth of epithelial cells.

PRINCIPAL CONSTITUENTS

Benzoic and cinnamic acid esters such as benzyl benzoate, benzyl cinnamate, and cinnamyl cinnamate as well as other traces. The crude balsam contains approximately 50–64 per cent oil, referred to as 'cinnamein', and 20–28 per cent resin.

A large tropical tree up to 25m (82ft) high, with a straight smooth trunk, beautiful foliage and very fragrant flowers. Every part of the tree, including the fibrous fruit, contains a resinous juice. The balsam is a pathological product, obtained from the exposed lacerated wood, after strips of the bark have been removed. It is a 'true' balsam, which is collected in the form of a dark brown or amber semi-solid mass.

AROMATHERAPY/ HOME USE

The balsam (not the oil) is a common contact allergen, which may cause dermatitis. Those who have this sensitivity may also react to benzoin resinoid; this is called 'cross-sensitization'. The commercial oil is often a water-white liquid, being diluted with a solvent such as benzyl alcohol.
Skin Care: *Dry and chapped skin, eczema, rashes, sores and wounds.*
Circulation, Muscles and Joints: *Low blood pressure, rheumatism.*
Respiratory System: *Asthma, bronchitis, coughs.*
Immune System: *Colds.*
Nervous System: *Nervous tension, stress; like other balsams it has a warming, opening, comforting quality.*

OTHER USES

The balsam is extensively used in tropical medicinal preparations, and to some extent in pharmaceutical products, for example, cough syrup. Used as a fixative and fragrance component in soaps, detergents, creams, lotions and perfumes; the oil is often used in perfumery since this avoids any resin deposits or discolouration; used in most food categories, including alcoholic and soft drinks.

DISTRIBUTION

Native to Central America; production takes place mainly in El Salvador.

OTHER SPECIES

Myroxylon frutescens and guina-guina are close relations, as is Tolu balsam.

Myrtus communis

Myrtle

SAFETY DATA *Non-toxic, non-irritant, non-sensitizing*

FAMILY: MYRTACEAE SYNONYM: CORSICAN PEPPER

Herbal/Folk Tradition

The leaves and berries have been used for 'drying and binding, good for diarrhea and dysentery, spitting of blood and catarrhous defluctions upon the breast'.[62] Dioscorides prescribed it for lung and bladder infections in the form of an extract made by macerating the leaves in wine. The leaves and flowers were a major ingredient of 'angel's water', a sixteenth-century skin care lotion.

A large bush or small tree with many tough but slender branches, a brownish-red bark and small sharp-pointed leaves. It has white flowers followed by small black berries; both leaves and flowers are very fragrant.

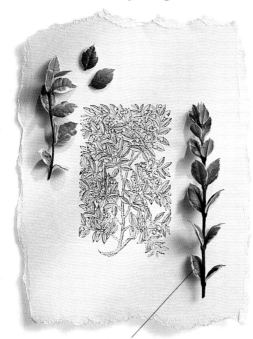

fresh myrtle

EXTRACTION
Essential oil by steam distillation from the leaves and twigs (sometimes the flowers).

CHARACTERISTICS
A pale yellow or orange liquid with a clear, fresh, camphoraceous, sweet-herbaceous scent somewhat similar to eucalyptus. It blends well with bergamot, lavandin, lavender, rosemary, clary sage, hyssop, bay leaf, lime, laurel, ginger, clove and other spice oils.

ACTIONS
Anticatarrhal, antiseptic (urinary, pulmonary), astringent, balsamic, bactericidal, expectorant, regulator, slightly sedative.

PRINCIPAL CONSTITUENTS
Cineol, myrtenol, pinene, geraniol, linalol, camphene, among others.

AROMATHERAPY/ HOME USE

Skin Care: *Acne, hemorrhoids, oily skin, open pores.*
Respiratory System: *Asthma, bronchitis, catarrhal conditions, chronic coughs, tuberculosis – 'Because of its relative mildness, this is a very suitable oil to use for children's coughs and chest complaints.'* [63]
Immune System: *Colds, flu, infectious disease.*

OTHER USES

Used mainly in eau-de-colognes and toilet waters. Employed as a flavouring ingredient in meat sauces and seasonings, generally in combination with other herbs.

DISTRIBUTION

Native to North Africa, it now grows freely all over the Mediterranean region; it is also cultivated as a garden shrub throughout Europe. The oil is produced mainly in Corsica, Spain, Tunisia, Morocco, Italy, former Yugoslavia and France.

OTHER SPECIES

*Part of the same large aromatic family that includes eucalyptus and tea tree; also bayberry or wax myrtle (*Myrica cerifera*) and the Dutch myrtle or English bog myrtle (*Myrica gale*), which are used in herbal medicine (though their essential oils are said to be poisonous). Not to be confused*

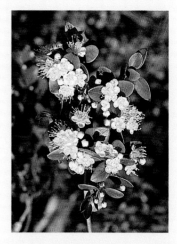

Myrtus communis

with iris, sometimes called 'myrtle flower' or calamus, which is also known as 'myrtle grass' or 'sweet myrtle'.

Narcissus poeticus

Narcissus

SAFETY DATA *All members of the Amaryllidaceae family, especially the bulbs, have a profound effect on the nervous system, causing paralysis and even in some cases death*

FAMILY: AMARYLLIDACEAE **SYNONYMS:** PINKSTER LILY, PHEASANT'S EYE, POET'S NARCISSUS

Herbal/Folk Tradition

The name derives from the Greek *narkao* – to be numb – because of its narcotic properties. The Roman perfumers used 'narcissum', a solid unguent made from narcissus flowers, in the preparation of their elaborate fragrances. In France the flowers were used at one time for their antispasmodic properties, said to be useful in hysteria and epilepsy.

In India the oil is applied to the body before prayer in temples, along with rose, sandalwood and jasmine. The Arabians recommend the oil as a cure for baldness, and as an aphrodisiac.

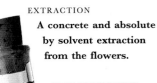

EXTRACTION
A concrete and absolute by solvent extraction from the flowers.

CHARACTERISTICS
The absolute is a dark orange, olive or green viscous liquid with a sweet, green-herbaceous odour and heavy floral undertone. It blends well with clove bud, jasmine, orange blossom, ylang ylang, rose, mimosa, sandalwood, oriental and floral fragrances.

ACTIONS
Antispasmodic, aphrodisiac, emetic, narcotic, sedative.

PRINCIPAL CONSTITUENTS
Quercetin, possibly narcissine (the alkaloid that causes nausea).

A familiar garden flower up to 50cm (20in) high, with long sword-shaped leaves and very fragrant white flowers having a short yellow trumpet and crisped red edge.

narcissus bulb

AROMATHERAPY/ HOME USE

Perfume.
'The bulbs of N. poeticus *are more dangerous than those of the daffodil, being powerfully emetic and irritant. The scent of the flowers is deleterious, if they are present in any quantity in a closed room, producing in some persons headache and even vomiting.'[64]*

OTHER USES

The absolute and concrete are used almost exclusively in high-class perfumes of the narcotic/ floral type.

DISTRIBUTION

Native to the Middle East or the eastern Mediterranean region; naturalized in southern France. It is cultivated extensively for its flowers. Only the Netherlands and the Grasse region of France produce the concrete and absolute.

OTHER SPECIES

There are two main types produced in France: the cultivated or des plaines *variety and the wild or* des montagnes *type. Narcissus is also closely related to the jonquil (*N. jonquilla*) and campernella (*N. odorus*), which are also occasionally used to produce an absolute, as well as to the daffodil (*N. pseudo-narcissus*).*

Nardostachys jatamansi

Spikenard

FAMILY: VALERIANANCEAE   **SYNONYMS:** NARD, 'FALSE' INDIAN VALERIAN ROOT (OIL)

Herbal/Folk Tradition

Spikenard is one of the early aromatics used by the ancient Egyptians and is mentioned in the Song of Solomon in the Bible. It is also the herb that Mary used to anoint Jesus before the Last Supper: 'Then took Mary a pound of ointment of spikenard, very costly, and anointed the feet of Jesus, and wiped his feet with her hair; and the house was filled with the odour of the ointment.'[65]

The oil was also used by the Roman perfumers, or *unguentarii*, in the preparation of *nardinum*, one of their most celebrated scented oils, and by the Mughal empress Nur Jehan in her rejuvenating cosmetic preparations.

It was also a herb known to Dioscorides as 'warming and drying', good for nausea, flatulent indigestion, menstrual problems, inflammations and conjunctivitis.

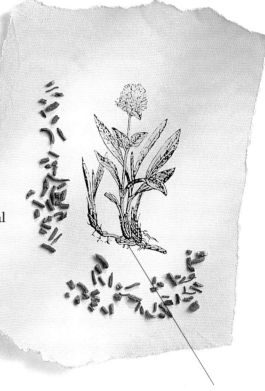

A tender aromatic herb with a pungent rhizome root.

dried
spikenard
root

EXTRACTION
Essential oil by steam distillation from the dried and crushed rhizome and roots.

CHARACTERISTICS
A pale yellow or amber-coloured liquid with a heavy, sweet-woody, spicy-animal odour, somewhat similar to valerian oil. It blends well with labdanum, lavender, oakmoss, patchouli, pine needle, vetiver and spice oils.

ACTIONS
Anti-inflammatory, antipyretic, bactericidal, deodorant, fungicidal, laxative, sedative, tonic.

PRINCIPAL CONSTITUENTS
Bornyl acetate, isobornyl valerianate, borneol, patchouli alcohol, terpinyl valerianate, terpineol, eugenol and pinenes, among others.

AROMATHERAPY/
HOME USE
Skin Care: *Allergies, inflammation, mature skin (rejuvenating), rashes, etc.*
Nervous System: *Insomnia, nervous indigestion, migraine, stress and tension.*

OTHER USES
Little used these days, usually as a substitute for valerian oil.

DISTRIBUTION
Native to the mountainous regions of northern India; also China and Japan (see other species). The oil is distilled mainly in Europe or the USA.

OTHER SPECIES
Closely related to the common valerian (Valeriana officinalis) and the Indian valerian (V. wallichii) with which it shares many qualities. There are also several other similar species, notably the Chinese spikenard (N. chinensis), which is also used to produce an essential oil. Not to be confused with aspic or spike lavender (Lavandula latifolia) or with essential oils from the musk root (Ferula sumbul), which is collected from the same area. The roots of several other plants are also commonly sold as 'Indian valerian root'.

Ocimum basilicum

Exotic basil

FAMILY: LAMIACEAE (LABIATAE)   **SYNONYMS:** SWEET BASIL, COMORAN BASIL (OIL), REUNION BASIL (OIL)

Herbal/Folk Tradition

Widely used in Far Eastern medicine especially in the Ayurvedic tradition, where it is called tulsi. It is used for respiratory problems such as bronchitis, coughs, colds, asthma, flu and emphysema but is also used as an antidote to poisonous insect or snake bites. It has also been used against epidemics and fever, such as malaria. It improves blood circulation and the digestive system, and in China it is used for stomach and kidney ailments.

In the West it is considered a 'cooling' herb and is used for rheumatic pain, irritable skin conditions and for those of a nervous disposition. It is a popular culinary herb, especially in Italy and France.

Botanically classified as identical with French basil, though it is a larger plant with a harsher odour and different constituents.

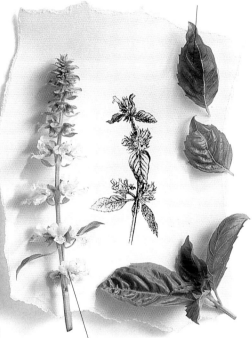

fresh leaves

fresh basil flowers

AROMATHERAPY/ HOME USE

None.
'The methyl chavicol content of Comoran basil is sufficient reason to discard it for therapeutic usage in favour of the French type.'[66]

OTHER USES

The oil is employed in high-class fragrances, soaps and dental products; used extensively in major food categories especially meat products and savouries.

DISTRIBUTION

Mainly produced in the Comoro Islands, but it is also processed in Madagascar.

OTHER SPECIES

The exotic basil is a dramatically different chemotype to the French basil and probably a separate sub-species (possibly a form of O. canum), although this has not been specified. Essential oils are also produced in Morocco, Egypt, South Africa, Brazil and Indonesia from various chemotypes of the East Indian or shrubby basil (O. gratissimum), which contain a high percentage of either thymol or eugenol. The hairy or hoary basil (O. canum), originating in East Africa and found in India and South America, is also used to extract oils rich in either methyl cinnamate or camphor, which are produced in West and East Africa, India, the West Indies and Indonesia. See also entry on French basil.

EXTRACTION
Essential oil by steam distillation from the leaves and flowering tops.

CHARACTERISTICS
The Exotic-type oil is yellow or pale green, with a slightly coarse sweet-herbaceous odour with a camphoraceous tinge. Its scent does not compare with the 'true' sweet basil oil.

ACTIONS
Antidepressant, antiseptic, antispasmodic, carminative, cephalic, digestive, emmenagogue, expectorant, febrifuge, galactagogue, nervine, prophlyactic, restorative, stimulant of adrenal cortex, stomachic, tonic.

PRINCIPAL CONSTITUENTS
Mainly methyl chavicol (70–88 per cent), with small amounts of linalol, cineol, camphor, eugenol, limonene and citronellol.

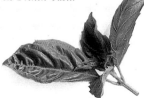

Ocimum basilicum

French basil

FAMILY: LAMIACEAE (LABIATAE) **SYNONYMS:** COMMON BASIL, JOY-OF-THE-MOUNTAIN, 'TRUE' SWEET BASIL, EUROPEAN BASIL

Herbal/Folk Tradition
See Exotic basil.

A tender annual herb, with very dark green, ovate leaves, greyish-green beneath, an erect square stem up to 60cm (24in) high, bearing whorls of two-lipped greenish or pinky-white flowers. The whole plant has a powerful aromatic scent.

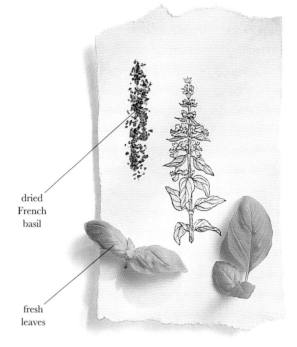

dried French basil

fresh leaves

EXTRACTION
Essential oil by steam distillation from the flowering herb.

CHARACTERISTICS
'True' sweet basil oil is a colourless or pale yellow liquid with a light fresh sweet-spicy scent and balsamic undertone. It blends well with bergamot, clary sage, lime, opopanax, oakmoss, citronella, geranium, hyssop and other 'green' notes.

ACTIONS
See Exotic basil.

PRINCIPAL CONSTITUENTS
Linalol (40–45 per cent), methyl chavicol (23.8 per cent) and small amounts of eugenol, limonene and citronellol, among others.

AROMATHERAPY/ HOME USE

Skin Care: *Insect bites (mosquito, wasp), insect repellent.*
Circulation, Muscles and Joints: *Gout, muscular aches and pains, rheumatism.*
Respiratory System: *Bronchitis, coughs, earache, sinusitis.*
Digestive System: *Dyspepsia, flatulence, nausea.*
Genito-urinary System: *Cramps, scanty periods.*
Immune System: *Colds, fever, flu, infectious disease.*
Nervous System: *Anxiety, depression, fatigue, insomnia, migraine, nervous tension: 'Oil of Basil is an excellent, indeed perhaps the best, aromatic nerve tonic. It clears the head, relieves intellectual fatigue, and gives the mind strength and clarity.'* [67]

OTHER USES
The oil is used in soaps, cosmetics and perfumery; it is also used extensively in major food categories, especially savouries.

DISTRIBUTION
Native to tropical Asia and Africa, it is now widely cultivated throughout Europe, the Mediterranean region, the Pacific Islands, North and South America. The European, French or 'true' sweet basil oil is produced in France, Italy, Egypt, Bulgaria, Hungary and the USA.

OTHER SPECIES
There are many varieties of basil occurring all over the world, used both for their culinary and medicinal applications, such as bush basil (O. minimum), holy basil (O. sanctum), both from India, camphor basil (O. kilimanjaricum) from East Africa (also grown in India), and the fever plant (O. viride) from West Africa. However, there are two principal chemotypes most commonly used for the extraction of essential oil: the so-called French basil and the Exotic basil — see separate entry.

Origanum marjorana

Sweet marjoram

FAMILY: LAMIACEAE (LABIATAE) **SYNONYMS:** *MARJORANA HORTENSIS*, KNOTTED MARJORAM

Herbal/Folk Tradition

A traditional culinary herb and folk remedy. It was used by the ancient Greeks in their fragrances, cosmetics and medicines; the name oregano derives from a Greek word meaning 'joy of the mountains'. It is a versatile herb that has a soothing, fortifying and warming effect; it aids digestive and menstrual problems, as well as nervous and respiratory complaints.

It is 'comforting in cold diseases of the head, stomach, sinews and other parts, taken inwardly or outwardly applied . . . helps diseases of the chest, obstructions of the liver and spleen.'[68] It is also very helpful for muscular and rheumatic pain, sprains, strains, stiff joints, bruises, etc.

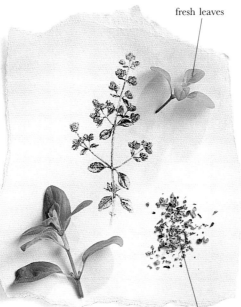

fresh leaves

dried sweet marjoram

A tender bushy perennial plant (cultivated as an annual in colder climates), up to 60cm (24in) high with a hairy stem, dark green oval leaves and small greyish-white flowers in clusters or 'knots'. The whole plant is strongly aromatic.

EXTRACTION
Essential oil by steam distillation of the dried flowering herb. An oleoresin is also produced in smaller quantities.

CHARACTERISTICS
A pale yellow or amber-coloured mobile liquid with a warm, woody, spicy-camphoraceous odour. It blends well with lavender, rosemary, bergamot, chamomile, cypress, cedarwood, tea tree and eucalyptus.

ACTIONS
Analgesic, anaphrodisiac, anti-oxidant, antiseptic, antispasmodic, antiviral, bactericidal, carminative, cephalic, cordial, diaphoretic, digestive, diuretic, emmenagogue, expectorant, fungicidal, hypotensive, laxative, nervine, sedative, stomachic, tonic, vasodilator, vulnerary.

PRINCIPAL CONSTITUENTS
Terpinenes, terpineol, sabinenes, linalol, carvocrol, linalyl acetate, ocimene, cadinene, geranyl acetate, citral, eugenol, among others.

AROMATHERAPY/ HOME USE

Skin Care: *Chilblains, bruises, ticks.*
Circulation, Muscles and Joints: *Arthritis, lumbago, muscular aches and stiffness, rheumatism, sprains, strains.*
Respiratory System: *Asthma, bronchitis, coughs.*
Digestive System: *Colic, constipation, dyspepsia, flatulence.*
Genito-urinary System: *Amenorrhea, dysmenorrhea, leucorrhea, PMT.*
Immune System: *Colds.*
Nervous System: *Headache, hypertension, insomnia, migraine, nervous tension and stress-related conditions.*

OTHER USES
The oil and oleoresin are used as fragrance components in soaps, detergents, cosmetics and perfumes. Employed in most major food categories, especially meats, seasonings and sauces, as well as soft drinks and alcoholic beverages.

DISTRIBUTION
Native to the Mediterranean region, Egypt and North Africa.

OTHER SPECIES
The most common types are the pot or French marjoram (Origanum onites *or* Marjorana onites), *which is a hardier plant than the sweet marjoram; the Spanish marjoram or oregano* (Thymus mastichina) *and the wild or common marjoram or oregano* (Origanum vulgare), *which is used to produce the so-called oregano oil. See common oregano, Spanish oregano and the Botanical Classification section.*

Origanum vulgare

Common oregano

FAMILY: LAMIACEAE (LABIATAE) **SYNONYMS:** EUROPEAN OREGANO, WILD MARJORAM, COMMON MARJORAM, GROVE MARJORAM, JOY-OF-THE-MOUNTAIN, ORIGANUM (OIL)

Herbal/Folk Tradition

This is the 'true' oregano of the herb garden, which also has a very ancient medical reputation. It has been used as a traditional remedy for digestive upsets, respiratory problems (asthma, bronchitis, coughs, etc.), colds and flu as well as for inflammations of the mouth and throat.

In China it is also used to treat fever, vomiting, diarrhea, jaundice and itchy skin conditions. The (diluted) oil has been used externally in herbal medicine for headaches, rheumatism, general aches and pains, and applied to stings and bites.

A hardy, bushy, perennial herb up to 90cm (35in) high with an erect hairy stem, dark green ovate leaves and pinky-purple flowers. A common garden plant with a strong aroma when the leaves are bruised.

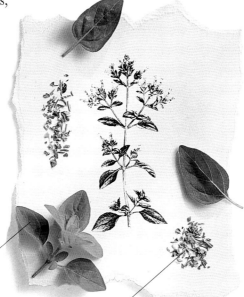

fresh leaves

dried herb

AROMATHERAPY/ HOME USE

None. 'Should not be used on the skin at all.' [69]

OTHER USES

Used as a fragrance component in soaps, colognes and perfumes, especially men's fragrances. Employed to some extent as a flavouring agent, mainly in meat products and pizzas.

DISTRIBUTION

Native to Europe, now cultivated all over the world, including the USA, India and South America; the oil is produced mainly in Russia, Bulgaria and Italy.

OTHER SPECIES

There is much confusion concerning the exact botanical classification of the marjoram and oregano species. There are over thirty varieties, some of which are used to produce essential oils, such as the winter or Greek marjoram O. heracleoticum, *the African species* O. glandulosum, *the Moroccan species* O. virens, *as well as the Mexican oregano* Lippia graveolens *or* L. palmeri *and the Syrian oregano* O. maru. *However, most commercial 'oregano oil' is derived from the Spanish oregano* (Thymus capitatus) *and to a lesser degree from the common oregano or wild marjoram. See entries on Spanish oregano and sweet marjoram.*

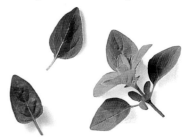

EXTRACTION
Essential oil by steam distillation from the dried flowering herb.

CHARACTERISTICS
A pale yellow liquid (browning with age), with a warm, spicy-herbaceous, camphoraceous odour. It blends well with lavandin, oakmoss, pine, spike lavender, citronella, rosemary, camphor and cedarwood.

ACTIONS
Analgesic, anthelminthic, antirheumatic, **antiseptic, antispasmodic, antitoxic, antiviral, bactericidal, carminative, choleretic, cytopylactic, diaphoretic, diuretic, emmenagogue, expectorant, febrifuge, fungicidal, parasiticide, rubefacient, stimulant, tonic.**

PRINCIPAL CONSTITUENTS
Carvacrol, thymol, cymene, caryophyllene, pinene, bisabolene, linalol, borneol, geranyl acetate, linalyl acetate, terpinene. NB: Constituents are highly variable according to source, but oils classified as 'oregano' or 'origanum' have thymol and/or carvacrol as their major components.

Ormenis multicaulis

Maroc chamomile

FAMILY: ASTERACEAE (COMPOSITAE) **SYNONYMS:** *O. MIXTA, ANTHEMIS MIXTA,* MOROCCAN CHAMOMILE

Herbal/Folk Tradition

This is one of the more recent oils to appear on the market, and as such it does not have a long history of usage. The oil is often mistaken for a 'true' chamomile, though it should more correctly be called 'Ormenis oil' since, 'Chemically and olfactorily, the oil is distinctly different from the German or the Roman chamomile oils, and cannot be considered as a replacement for them.'[70]

EXTRACTION
Essential oil by steam distillation from the flowering tops.

CHARACTERISTICS
Pale yellow to brownish-yellow mobile liquid with a fresh-herbaceous top note and a sweet rich-balsamic undertone. It blends well with cypress, lavender, lavandin, vetiver, cedarwood, oakmoss, labdanum, olibanum and artemisia oils.

ACTIONS
Antispasmodic, cholagogue, emmenagogue, hepatic, sedative.

PRINCIPAL CONSTITUENTS
Trans pinocarueol, borneol, bornyl acetate, bisabolene, b. caryophellene, a. pinene, 1-8 cineole, yomogi alcohol, santelena alcohol and artemisia, among others.

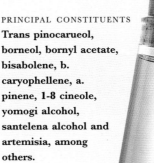

AROMATHERAPY/ HOME USE

'Sensitive skin, colic, colitis, headache, insomnia, irritability, migraine, amenorrhoea, menopause, liver and spleen congestion.'[71] Little is known about its therapeutic history and usage.

OTHER USES

Employed extensively in perfumery work, especially in colognes, chyprès and fougère fragrance.

DISTRIBUTION

Native to north-west Africa and southern Spain, having probably evolved from the very common Ormenis *species that grows all around the Mediterranean. Also found growing on the plains in Israel. The oil is distilled in Morocco.*

OTHER SPECIES

It is distantly related to the German and Roman chamomile botanically, although it does not resemble them physically.

A handsome plant, 90–125cm (35–49in) high with very hairy leaves and tubular yellow flowers, surrounded by white ligulets.

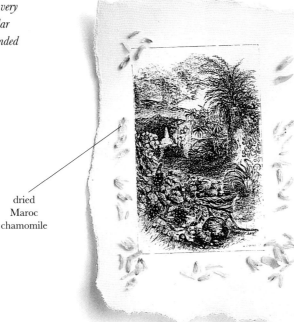

dried Maroc chamomile

Pelargonium graveolens

Geranium

FAMILY: GERANIACEAE **SYNONYMS:** ROSE GERANIUM, PELARGONIUM

Herbal/Folk Tradition

The British plant herb robert *(Geranium robertanium)* and the American cranesbill *(G. maculatum)* are the most widely used types in herbal medicine today, having been used since antiquity. They have many properties in common with the rose geranium, being used for conditions such as dysentery, hemorrhoids, inflammations, metrorrhagia and menorrhagia (excessive blood loss during menstruation). The root and herb of cranesbill is specifically indicated in the British Herbal Pharmacopoeia for diarrhea and peptic ulcer.

A perennial hairy shrub up to 1m (3ft) high with pointed leaves, serrated at the edges and small pink flowers. The whole plant is aromatic.

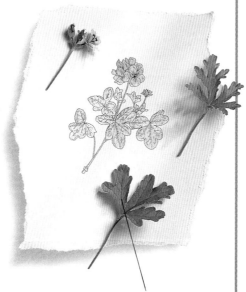

fresh leaves

EXTRACTION

Essential oil by steam distillation from the leaves, stalks and flowers. An absolute and concrete are also produced in Morocco.

CHARACTERISTICS

The Bourbon oil is a greenish-olive liquid with a rosy-sweet, minty scent, preferred in perfumery work; it blends well with lavender, patchouli, clove, rose, orange blossom, sandalwood, jasmine, juniper, bergamot and other citrus oils.

ACTIONS

Antidepressant, anti-hemorrhagic, antiflammatory, antiseptic, astringent, cica-trizant, deodorant, diuretic, fungicidal, hemostatic, stimulant (adrenal cortex), styptic, tonic, vermifuge, vulnerary.

PRINCIPAL CONSTITUENTS

Citronellol, geraniol, linalol, isomenthone, menthone, phellandrene, sabinene, limonene, among others.

AROMATHERAPY/ HOME USE

Skin Care: *Acne, bruises, broken capillaries, burns, congested skin, cuts, dermatitis, eczema, hemorrhoids, lice, mature skin, mosquito repellent, oily complexion, ringworm, ulcers, wounds.*
Circulation, Muscles and Joints: *Cellulitis, engorgement of breasts, edema, poor circulation.*
Respiratory System: *Sore throat, tonsillitis.*
Genito-urinary and Endocrine Systems: *Adrenocortical glands and menopausal problems, PMS.*

Nervous System: *Nervous tension, neuralgia and stress-related conditions.*

OTHER USES

Used as a fragrance component in all kinds of cosmetic products: soaps, creams, perfumes, etc. Employed as a flavouring agent in most major food categories, alcoholic and soft drinks.

DISTRIBUTION

Native to South Africa; widely cultivated in Russia, Egypt, Congo, Japan, Central America and Europe. With regard to essential oil production, there are three main regions: Reunion (Bourbon), Egypt and Russia (also China).

OTHER SPECIES

There are over 700 varieties of cultivated geranium and pelargonium, many of which are grown for ornamental purposes. There are several oil-producing species such as P. odorantis-simum and P. radens, but P. graveolens is the main one commercially cultivated for its oil. See also Botanical Classification.

Petroselinum sativum

Parsley

SAFETY DATA *Both oils are moderately toxic and irritant, otherwise non-sensitizing. Use in moderation. Avoid during pregnancy*

FAMILY: APIACEAE (UMBELLIFERAE) **SYNONYMS:** *P. HORTENSE, APIUM PETROSELINUM, CARUM PETROSELINUM*, COMMON PARSLEY, GARDEN PARSLEY

Herbal/Folk Tradition

It is used extensively as a culinary herb, both fresh and dried. It is a very nutritious plant, high in vitamins A and C; also used to freshen the breath. The herb and seed are used medicinally, principally for kidney and bladder problems, but it has also been employed for menstrual difficulties, digestive complaints and for arthritis, rheumatism, rickets and sciatica. It is said to stimulate hair growth and help eliminate head lice.

The root is current in the British Herbal Pharmacopoeia as a specific for flatulent dyspepsia with intestinal colic.

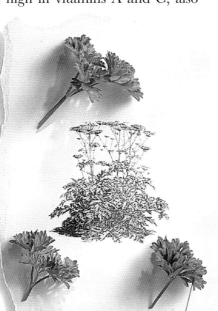

fresh parsley

A biennial or short-lived perennial herb up to 70cm (28in) high with crinkly bright green foliage, small greenish-yellow flowers and producing small brown seeds.

EXTRACTION
Essential oil by steam distillation from 1. the seed, and 2. the herb. (An essential oil is occasionally extracted from the roots; an oleoresin is also produced by solvent extraction from the seeds.)

CHARACTERISTICS
1. A yellow, amber or brownish liquid with a warm woody-spicy herbaceous odour. 2. A pale yellow or greenish liquid with a heavy, warm, spicy-sweet odour, reminiscent of the herb. It blends well with rose, orange blossom, cananga, tea tree, oakmoss, clary sage and spice oils.

ACTIONS
Antimicrobial, antirheumatic, antiseptic, astringent, carminative, diuretic, depurative, emmenagogue, febrifuge, hypotensive, laxative, stimulant (mild), stomachic, tonic (uterine).

PRINCIPAL CONSTITUENTS
1. Mainly apiol, with myristicin, tetramethoxyally-benzene, pinene and volatile fatty acids. 2. Mainly myristicin (up to 85 per cent), with phellandrene, myrcene, apiol, terpenolene, menthatriene, pinene and carotel, among others.

AROMATHERAPY/HOME USE

Circulation, Muscles and Joints: *Accumulation of toxins, arthritis, broken blood vessels, cellulites, rheumatism, sciatica.*
Digestive System: *Colic, flatulence, indigestion, hemorrhoids.*
Genito-urinary System: *Amenorrhea, dysmenorrhea, to aid labour, cystitis, urinary infection.*

OTHER USES

Used in some carminative and digestive remedies, such as 'gripe waters'. The seed oil is used in soaps, detergents, colognes, cosmetics and perfumes, especially men's fragrances. The herb and seed oil as well as the oleoresin are used extensively in many types of food flavourings, especially meats, pickles and sauces, as well as alcoholic and soft drinks.

DISTRIBUTION

Native to the Mediterranean region, especially Greece. It is cultivated extensively, mainly in California, Germany, France, Belgium, Hungary and parts of Asia. The principal oil-producing countries are France, Germany, the Netherlands and Hungary.

OTHER SPECIES

There are over thirty-seven different varieties of parsley, such as the curly-leaved type (P. crispum), which is used in herbal medicine.

Peumus boldus

Boldo leaf

FAMILY: MONIMIACEAE   **SYNONYMS:** *BOLDUS BOLDUS*, *BOLDOA FRAGRANS*, BOLDUS, BOLDU

Herbal/Folk Tradition

The bark is used for tanning, the wood utilized in charcoal making and the fruit eaten by locals. In South America it has long been recognized as a valuable cure for gonorrhea. In Western herbalism, the dried leaves are used for genito-urinary inflammation, gallstones, liver or gall bladder pain, cystitis and rheumatism. The dried leaves are current in the British Herbal Pharmacopoeia as a specific for cholelithiasis with pain.

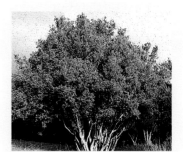

Peumus boldus

An evergreen shrub or small tree up to 6m (20ft) high, with slender branches, sessile coarse leaves and bearing yellowish-green fruit; dried the leaves turn a deep reddish-brown colour. The whole plant is aromatic.

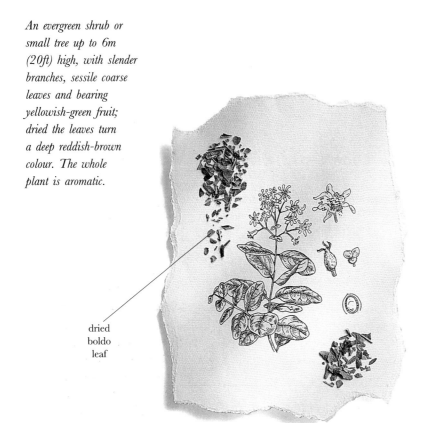

dried
boldo
leaf

AROMATHERAPY/ HOME USE

None.
'*The oil has powerful therapeutic effects, and it can be considered harmful to the human organism even when used in very small doses . . . should not be used in therapy, either internally or externally.*'[72]

OTHER USES

Used in pharmaceuticals in minute amounts for its therapeutic properties.

DISTRIBUTION

Native to Chile; naturalized in the Mediterranean region. Some essential oil is produced in Nepal and Vietnam.

OTHER SPECIES

The Australian tree Monimia rotundifolia *contains a similar oil, which has been used as a substitute. The oil of chenopodium or wormseed is also chemically related.*

EXTRACTION
Essential oil by steam distillation of the leaves.

CHARACTERISTICS
A yellow liquid with a powerful spicy-camphoraceous, disagreeable odour.

ACTIONS
Antiseptic, cholagogue, diaphoretic, diuretic, hepatic, sedative, tonic, urinary demulcent.

PRINCIPAL CONSTITUENTS
Cymene, ascaridole, cineol, linalol.

Pilocarpus jaborandi

Jaborandi

SAFETY DATA *Oral toxin, skin irritant, abortifacient*

FAMILY: RUTACEAE **SYNONYMS:** *PERNAMBUCO JABORANDI, P. PENNATIFOLIUS,* IABORANDI, JAMBORANDI, ARRUDO DO MATO, ARRUDA BRAVA, JAMGUARADDI, JUARANDI

Herbal/Folk Tradition

Jaborandi induces salivation and most gland secretions; it was also used at one time to promote hair growth. 'Useful in psoriasis, prurigo, deafness . . . chronic catarrh, tonsillitis and particularly dropsy.'[73]

A woody shrub up to 2m (6ft) high with a smooth, greyish bark, large brownish-green leathery leaves containing big oil glands and reddish-purple flowers.

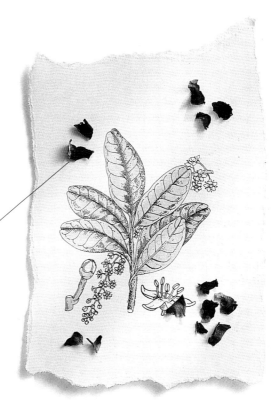

dried jaborandi flowers

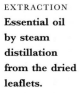

EXTRACTION
Essential oil by steam distillation from the dried leaflets.

CHARACTERISTICS
An orange or yellow liquid with a sweet-herbaceous fruity odour.

ACTIONS
Antiseptic, diaphoretic, emmenagogue, galactagogue, stimulant (nerve).

PRINCIPAL CONSTITUENTS
Pilocarpine is the main active constituent; also isopilocarpine, pilocarpidine, methyl nonyl ketone, dipentene and other hydrocarbons.

AROMATHERAPY/ HOME USE
None.

OTHER USES
Various hypodermic solutions are prepared from pilocarpine: the crude oil is rarely used. Little used in perfumery or flavour work due to toxicity.

DISTRIBUTION
Native to Brazil; other species are found in Paraguay, Cuba, the West Indies and Central America.

OTHER SPECIES
There are many members of the Rutaceae *and* Piperaceae *family known simply as jaborandi, such as* Piper jaborandi. *Others include maranham jaborandi (P.* microphyllus)*, ceara jaborandi (P.* trachylophus) *and aracti jaborandi (P.* spicatus)*. There is consequently some confusion about the exact botanical source of this oil.*

Pimenta dioica

Allspice

FAMILY: MYRTACEAE   **SYNONYMS:** *P. OFFICINALIS*, PIMENTO, PIMENTA, JAMAICA PEPPER

Herbal/Folk Tradition

Used for flatulent indigestion and externally for neuralgic or rheumatic pain. Pimento water is used as a vehicle for medicines that ease dyspepsia and constipation since it helps prevent griping pains. It is used extensively as a domestic spice – allspice is so called because it tastes like a combination of cloves, juniper berries, cinnamon and pepper.

An evergreen tree that reaches about 10m (33ft) high and begins to produce fruit in its third year. Each fruit contains two kidney-shaped green seeds, which turn glossy black upon ripening.

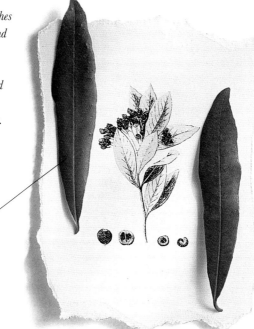

fresh
allspice
leaf

AROMATHERAPY/ HOME USE

Circulation, Muscles and Joints: *Arthritis, fatigue, muscle cramp, rheumatism, stiffness, etc. 'Used in tiny amounts . . . in a massage oil for chest infections, for severe muscle spasm to restore mobility quickly, or where extreme cold is experienced.'* [74]
Respiratory System: *Chills, congested coughs, bronchitis.*
Digestive System: *Cramp, flatulence, indigestion, nausea.*
Nervous System: *Depression, nervous exhaustion, neuralgia, tension and stress.*

OTHER USES

Used in aromatic carminative medicines; as a fragrance component in cosmetics and perfumes, especially soaps, aftershaves, spicy and oriental fragrances. Both leaf and berry oil are used extensively for flavouring foods, especially savoury and frozen foods, as well as alcoholic and soft drinks.

DISTRIBUTION

Indigenous to the West Indies and South America, it is cultivated in Jamaica, Cuba and, to a lesser extent, in Central America. Imported berries are distilled in Europe and America.

OTHER SPECIES

Four other varieties of pimento are found in Venezuela, Guyana and the West Indies and used locally as spices.

EXTRACTION

Essential oil by steam distillation from 1. the leaves, and 2. the fruit. The green unripe berries contain more oil than the ripe berries, but the largest percentage of oil is contained in the shell of the fruit. An oleoresin from the berries is also produced in small quantities.

CHARACTERISTICS

**1. Pimenta leaf oil is a yellowish-red or brownish liquid with a powerful sweet-spicy scent, similar to cloves.
2. Pimenta berry oil is a pale yellow liquid with a sweet warm balsamic-spicy bodynote (middle note) and fresh, clean**

top note. It blends well with ginger, geranium, lavender, opopanax, labdanum, ylang ylang, patchouli, orange blossom, oriental and spicy bases.

ACTIONS

Anesthetic, analgesic, antioxidant, antiseptic, carminative, muscle relaxant, rubefacient, stimulant, tonic.

PRINCIPAL CONSTITUENTS

Mainly eugenol, less in the fruit (60–80 per cent) than in the leaves (up to 96 per cent), also methyl eugenol, cineol, phellandrene and caryophyllene, among others.

Pimenta racemosa

West Indian bay

FAMILY: MYRTACEAE **SYNONYMS:** *MYRCIA ACRIS,*
PIMENTA ACRIS, MYRCIA, BAY, BAY RUM TREE, WILD CINNAMON, BAYBERRY, BAY LEAF (OIL)

Herbal/Folk Tradition

The West Indian bay tree is often grown in groves together with the allspice or pimento bush, then the fruits of both are dried and powdered for the preparation of the household allspice. The so-called bay rum tree also provides the basic ingredient for the famous old hair tonic, which is made from the leaves by being distilled in rum. 'A hair application with both fragrant and tonic virtues . . . useful for those who suffer from greasy hair and need a spirit-based, scalp-stimulating lotion to help them to control their locks!'[75]

A wild-growing tropical evergreen tree up to 8m (26ft) high, with large leathery leaves and aromatic fruits.

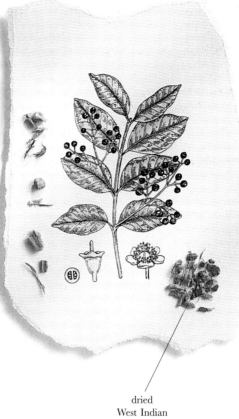

dried
West Indian
bay bark

EXTRACTION
Essential oil by water or steam distillation from the leaves. An oleoresin is also produced in small quantities.

CHARACTERISTICS
A dark yellow mobile liquid with a fresh-spicy top note and a sweet-balsamic undertone. It blends well with lavender, lavandin, rosemary, geranium, ylang ylang, citrus and spice oils.

ACTIONS
Analgesic, anticonvulsant, antineuralgic, expectorant, antirheumatic, antiseptic, astringent, stimulant, tonic (for hair).

PRINCIPAL CONSTITUENTS
Eugenol (up to 56 per cent), myrcene, chavicol and, in lesser amounts, methyl eugenol, linalol, limonene, among others.

**AROMATHERAPY/
HOME USE**

Skin Care: *Scalp stimulant, hair rinse for dandruff, greasy, lifeless hair, and promoting growth.*
Circulation, Muscles and Joints: *Muscular and articular aches and pains, neuralgia, poor circulation, rheumatism, sprains, strains.*
Immune System: *Colds, flu, infectious diseases.*

OTHER USES
Extensively used in fragrance work, in soaps, detergents, perfumes, aftershaves and hair lotions, including bay rum. Employed as a flavour ingredient in many major food categories,
especially condiments, as well as alcoholic and soft drinks.

DISTRIBUTION
Native to the West Indies, particularly Dominica where the essential oil is produced.

OTHER SPECIES
There are several other varieties, for example, the anise-scented and lemon-scented bay, the oils of which have a totally different chemical composition. Not to be confused with bay laurel, the common household spice, nor with the North American bayberry or wax myrtle (Myrica cerifera), well known for its wax yielding berries.

Pimpinella anisum

Aniseed

FAMILY: APIACEAE (UMBELLIFERAE)   **SYNONYMS:** *ANISUM OFFICINALIS, A. VULGARE,* ANISE, SWEET CUMIN

Herbal/Folk Tradition

Widely used as a domestic spice. The volatile oil content provides the basis for its medicinal applications: dry irritable coughs, bronchitis and whooping cough. The seed can be used in smoking mixtures. Aniseed tea is used for infant catarrh, also flatulence, colic and griping pains, and for painful periods and to promote breast milk. In Turkey a popular alcoholic drink, raki, is make from the seed.

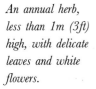

Pimpinella anisum

An annual herb, less than 1m (3ft) high, with delicate leaves and white flowers.

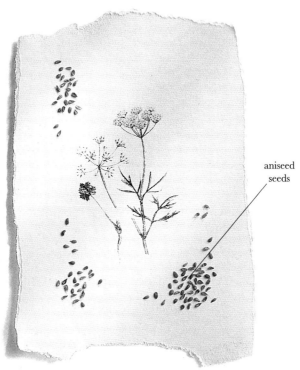

aniseed seeds

AROMATHERAPY/ HOME USE

See star anise.

OTHER USES

Used by the pharmaceutical industry in cough mixtures and lozenges and to mask undesirable flavours in drugs. Also used in dentifrices and as a fragrance component in soaps, toothpaste, detergents, cosmetics and perfumes, mostly of the industrial type. Employed in all major food categories.

DISTRIBUTION

Native to Greece and Egypt, now widely cultivated mainly in India and China and to a lesser extent in Mexico and Spain.

OTHER SPECIES

There are several different chemotypes of aniseed according to the country of origin. Not to be confused with star anise, which belongs to a different family altogether.

EXTRACTION
Essential oil by steam distillation from the seeds.

CHARACTERISTICS
Colourless to pale yellow liquid with a warm, spicy-sweet characteristic scent. Like star anise, it is a good masking agent.

ACTIONS
Antiseptic, antispasmodic, carminative, diuretic, expectorant, galactagogue, stimulant, stomachic.

PRINCIPAL CONSTITUENTS
Trans-anethole (75–90 per cent).

Pinus mugo var. pumilio

Dwarf pine

SAFETY DATA *Dermal irritant, common sensitizing agent; otherwise non-toxic*

FAMILY: PINACEAE **SYNONYMS:** *P. MUGO, P. MONTANA, P. PUMILIO,* MOUNTAIN PINE, SWISS MOUNTAIN PINE, PINE NEEDLE (OIL)

Herbal/Folk Tradition

A preparation made from the needles has been used internally for bladder, kidney and rheumatic complaints, as a liniment for rheumatism and muscular pain, and as an inhalant for bronchitis, catarrh, colds, etc.

EXTRACTION
Essential oil by steam distillation from the needles and twigs.

CHARACTERISTICS
A water-white liquid with a very pleasant, balsamic-sweet, spicy-woody scent of good tenacity. This is the favoured pine fragrance for perfumery use because of its unique delicate odour, which blends well with cedarwood, lavandin, rosemary, sage, cananga, labdanum, juniper and other coniferous oils.

ACTIONS
Analgesic, antimicrobial, antiseptic, antitussive, antiviral, balsamic, diuretic, expectorant, rubefacient.

PRINCIPAL CONSTITUENTS
Mainly monoterpene hydrocarbons; limonene, pinene, phellandrene, dipentene, camphene, myrcene and bornyl acetate among others. The unusual scent is believed to be due to its aldehyde content.

AROMATHERAPY/ HOME USE

None. It is best avoided therapeutically due to irritant hazards.

OTHER USES

Used as a fragrance and flavour component in pharmaceutical preparations for coughs and colds, nasal congestion and externally in analgesic ointments and liniments. Employed extensively in soaps, bath preparations, toiletries, cosmetics and perfumes, especially 'leather' and 'woody' type fragrances. It is also used in most major food categories, alcoholic and soft drinks.

DISTRIBUTION

Native to the mountainous regions of central and southern Europe. The oil is produced mainly in Austria (Tirol), former Yugoslavia, Denmark and Italy.

OTHER SPECIES

There are very many species of pine used to produce essential oil from their needles and wood or employed in the production of turpentine. NB: The so-called huon pine (Dacrydium franklinii), the essential oil of which is also a skin irritant, belongs to a different family, the Podcarpaceae. For further details see Scotch pine and the Botanical Classification section.

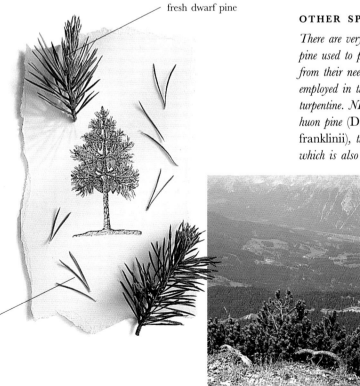

A pyramidal shrub or small tree up to 12m (39ft) high with a black bark, stiff and twisted needles borne in clusters, and brown cones, initially of a bluish hue.

fresh dwarf pine

dwarf pine needles

Pinus mugo var. pumilio

Pinus palustris

Longleaf pine

FAMILY: PINACEAE   **SYNONYMS:** LONGLEAF YELLOW PINE, SOUTHERN YELLOW PINE, PITCH PINE, PINE (OIL)

Herbal/Folk Tradition

Pine sawdust has been used for centuries as a highly esteemed household remedy for a variety of ailments. 'It is a grand, gentle, although powerful external antiseptic remedy, applied as a poultice in rheumatism when localised, hard cancerous tumours, tuberculosis in the knee or ankle joints, disease of the bone, in short, all sluggish morbid deposits . . . I have used it behind the head for failing sight, down the spine for general debility, on the loins for lumbago, etc. all with the best results.'[76]

EXTRACTION

The crude oil is obtained by steam distillation from the sawdust and wood chips from the heartwood and roots of the tree (wastage from the timber mills), and then submitted to fractional distillation under atmospheric pressure to produce pine essential oil.

A tall evergreen tree with long needles and a straight trunk, grown extensively for its timber. It exudes a natural oleoresin from the trunk, which provides the largest source for the production of turpentine in the USA. See also entry on turpentine.

stem with bark

fresh pine needles

CHARACTERISTICS

A water-white or pale yellow liquid with a sweet-balsamic, pinewood scent. It blends well with rosemary, pine needle, cedarwood, citronella, rosewood, ho leaf and oakmoss.

ACTIONS

Analgesic (mild), antirheumatic, antiseptic, bactericidal, expectorant, insecticidal, stimulant.

PRINCIPAL CONSTITUENTS

Terpineol, estragole, fenchone, fenchyl alcohol and borneol, among others.

AROMATHERAPY/
HOME USE

Circulation, Muscles and Joints: *Arthritis, debility, lumbago, muscular aches and pains, poor circulation, rheumatism, stiffness, etc.*
Respiratory System: *Asthma, bronchitis, catarrh, sinusitis.*

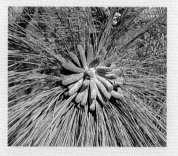

Pinus palustris

OTHER USES

Used extensively in medicine, particularly in veterinary antiseptic sprays, disinfectants, detergents and insecticides (as a solvent carrier). Employed as a fragrance component in soaps, toiletries, bath products and perfumes. Also used in paint manufacture although it is increasingly being replaced by synthetic 'pine oil'.

DISTRIBUTION

Native to south-eastern USA, where the oil is largely produced.

OTHER SPECIES

There are numerous other species of pine all over the world that are used to produce pine oil, as well as pine needle and turpentine oil. See Botanical Classification section.

Pinus palustris and other *Pinus* species

Turpentine

FAMILY: PINACEAE SYNONYMS: TEREBINTH,
THEREBENTINE, GUM THUS, GUM TURPENTINE, TURPENTINE BALSAM, SPIRIT OF TURPENTINE (OIL)

SAFETY DATA *Enviromental hazard – marine pollutant. Relatively non-toxic and non-irritant; possible sensitization in some individuals. Avoid therapeutic use or employ in moderation only*

Herbal/Folk Tradition

Known to Galen and Hippocrates for its many applications, especially with regard to pulmonary and genito-urinary infections, digestive complaints and externally as a treatment for rheumatic or neuralgic pain and skin conditions. In China the oleoresin has been used (both internally and externally) for centuries for excess phlegm, bronchitis, rheumatism, stiff joints, toothache, boils, sores, ringworm and dermatitis.

The turpentine essence or spirit of turpentine is said to be four times more active than the crude turpentine.

fresh turpentine

'Gum turpentine' is a term loosely applied to the natural oleoresin formed as a physiological product in the trunks of various Pinus, Picea and Abies species. Turpentine refers both to the crude oleoresin (a mixture of oil and resin) and to the distilled and rectified essential oils.

AROMATHERAPY/ HOME USE

See Mastic.

OTHER USES

Used in many ointments and lotions for aches and pains; and in cough and cold remedies. Neither oil nor oleoresin is used in perfumery work, although resin derivatives are used as fixative agents and in pine and industrial perfumes. Mainly known as a paint and stain remover, solvent and insecticide. Also used as a starting material for the production of terpineol, etc.

DISTRIBUTION

· *All over the world. The largest producer is the USA.*

OTHER SPECIES

Apart from the longleaf pine (Pinus palustris), which is the leading source of American gum turpentine, other sources in the USA include the slash pine (P. elliottii) and the Mexican white pine (P. ayacahuite). In India the chir pine (P. roxburghii); in Tasmania the lodgepole pine (contorta var. atifolia); in China the masson or southern red pine (P. massoniana); in Europe and Scandinavia the Scotch pine (P. sylvestris) and the sea pine (P. pinaster), as well as many others. See Botanical Classification section.

EXTRACTION
Essential oil by steam (or water) distillation from the crude oleoresin, then rectified. 'It has to be purified because it is viscous, coloured and acidic.' [77]

CHARACTERISTICS
A colourless, water-white mobile liquid with a fresh, warm-balsamic, familiar odour.

ACTIONS
Analgesic, antimicrobial, antirheumatic, antiseptic, antispasmodic, balsamic, diuretic, cicatrizant, counter-irritant, expectorant, hemostatic, parasiticide, rubefacient, stimulant, tonic, vermifuge.

PRINCIPAL CONSTITUENTS
Mainly alphapinene (approx. 50 per cent), betapinene (25–35 per cent) and carene (20–60 per cent) in the American oils. In European oils the alphapinene can constitute up to 95 per cent – constituents vary accordingly to source.

Pinus sylvestris

Scotch pine

FAMILY: PINACEAE   **SYNONYMS:** FOREST PINE, SCOTS PINE, NORWAY PINE, PINE NEEDLE (OIL)

Herbal/Folk Tradition

It was used by the Native Americans to prevent scurvy, and to stuff mattresses to repel lice and fleas.

As an inhalation it helps relieve bronchial catarrh, asthma, blocked sinuses, etc. The pine kernels are said to be excellent restoratives for consumptives, and after long illness.

A tall evergreen tree, up to 40m (131ft) high with a flat crown. It has a reddish-brown, deeply fissured bark, long stiff needles that grow in pairs, and pointed brown cones.

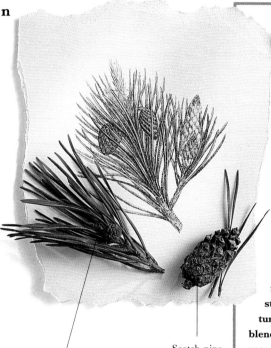

fresh needles

Scotch pine cone

AROMATHERAPY/ HOME USE

Skin Care: *Cuts, lice, excessive perspiration, scabies, sores.*
Circulation, Muscles and Joints: *Arthritis, gout, muscular aches and pains, poor circulation, rheumatism.*
Respiratory System: *Asthma, bronchitis, catarrh, coughs, sinusitis, sore throat.*
Genito-urinary System: *Cystitis, urinary infection.*
Immune System: *Colds, flu.*
Nervous System: *Fatigue, nervous exhaustion and stress-related conditions, neuralgia.*

OTHER USES

Used as a fragrance component in soaps, detergents, cosmetics, toiletries (especially bath products) and, to a limited extent, perfumes. Employed as a flavour ingredient in major food products, alcoholic and soft drinks.

DISTRIBUTION

Native to Eurasia; cultivated in the eastern USA, Europe, Russia, the Baltic States and Scandinavia, especially Finland.

OTHER SPECIES

Numerous species of pine yield an essential oil from their heartwood as well as from their twigs and needles and are also used to produce turpentine. The oil from the needles of the Scotch pine is one of the most useful and safest therapeutically. Other species that produce pine needle oil include eastern white pine (P. strobus), dwarf pine (P. mugo var. pumilio), and black pine (P. nigra). Many varieties, such as the longleaf pine (Pinus palustris), are used to produce turpentine. Siberian pine needle oil is actually from the Siberian fir (Abies sibirica). See also dwarf pine and the Botanical Classification section.

EXTRACTION

1. Essential oil by dry distillation of the needles.
2. Gum turpentine is produced by steam distillation from the oleoresin: see entry on turpentine. (An inferior essential oil is also produced by dry distillation from the wood chippings, etc.)

CHARACTERISTICS

1. Pine needle oil is a colourless or pale yellow mobile liquid with a strong, dry-balsamic, turpentine-like aroma. It blends well with cedarwood, rosemary, tea tree, sage, lavender, juniper, lemon, niaouli, eucalyptus and marjoram. **2.** See entry on turpentine.

ACTIONS

Antimicrobial, antineuralgic, antirheumatic, antiscorbutic, antiseptic (pulmonary, urinary, hepatic), antiviral, bactericidal, balsamic, cholagogue, choleretic, deodorant, diuretic, expectorant, hypertensive, insecticidal, restorative, rubefacient, stimulant (adrenal cortex, circulatory, nervous), vermifuge.

PRINCIPAL CONSTITUENTS

50–90 per cent monoterpene hydrocarbons: pinene, carene, dipentene, limonene, terpinenes, myrcene, ocimene, camphene, sabinene; also bornyl acetate, cineol, citral, chamazulene, among others.

Piper cubeba

Cubeb

FAMILY: PIPERACEAE **SYNONYMS:** *CUBEBA OFFICINALIS*, CUBEBA, TAILED PEPPER, CUBEB BERRY, FALSE PEPPER

Herbal/Folk Tradition

The seeds are used locally as a domestic spice. It has been traditionally used for treating genito-urinary infections, such as gonorrhea, cystitis, urethritis, abscess of the prostate gland and leucorrhea. It is also used for digestive upsets and respiratory problems such as chronic bronchitis. The seeds have a local stimulating effect on the mucous membrane of the urinary and respiratory tracts, and the powder was found '90 per cent clinically effective in treating amoebic dysentery'.[78]

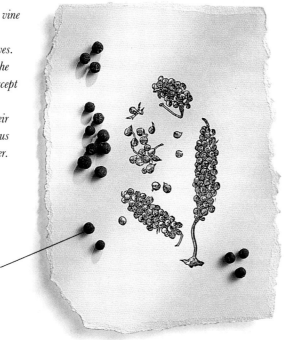

An evergreen climbing vine up to 6m (20ft) high with heart-shaped leaves. Altogether similar to the black pepper plant, except that the fruit or seeds of the cubeb retain their peduncle or stem — thus the name, tailed pepper.

dried
cubeb
seed

EXTRACTION
Essential oil by steam distillation from the unripe but fully grown fruits or berries. (An oleoresin is also produced in small quantities.)

CHARACTERISTICS
A pale greenish or bluish-yellow viscous liquid with a warm woody-spicy, slightly camphoraceous odour. It blends well with cananga, galbanum, lavender, rosemary, black pepper, allspice and other spices.

ACTIONS
Antiseptic (pulmonary, genito-urinary), antispasmodic, antiviral, bactericidal, carminative, diuretic, expectorant, stimulant.

PRINCIPAL
CONSTITUENTS
Mainly sesquiterpenes and monoterpenes, which include caryophyllene, cadinene, cubebene, sabinene, among others.

AROMATHERAPY/ HOME USE

Respiratory System: *Bronchitis, catarrh, congestion, chronic coughs, sinusitis, throat infections.*
Digestive System: *Flatulence, indigestion, piles, sluggish digestion.*
Genito-urinary System: *Cystitis, leucorrhea, urethritis.*

OTHER USES
Employed in diuretic and urinary antiseptic preparations and as a fragrance component in soaps, detergents, toiletries, cosmetics and perfumes. Used as a flavouring agent in most major food categories; also used for flavouring tobacco.

DISTRIBUTION
Native to Indonesia, cultivated throughout south-east Africa,

usually together with coffee crops. The oil is produced mainly at source in Indonesia.

OTHER SPECIES
Closely related to the black pepper plant (P. nigrum) and to the South American matico (P. angustifolium). There are also many other related species grown in Indonesia that are often used for adulteration, such as false cubeb (P. crassipes).

Piper nigrum

Black pepper

FAMILY: PIPERACEAE **SYNONYMS:** PIPER, PEPPER

Herbal/Folk Tradition

Both black and white pepper have been used in the East for over 4,000 years for medicinal and culinary purposes. In Chinese medicine, white pepper is used to treat malaria, cholera, dysentery, diarrhea, stomach ache and other digestive problems. In Greece it is used for intermittent fever and to fortify the stomach. 'The mendicant monks of India who cover daily considerable distances on foot, swallow 7–9 grains of pepper a day. This gives them remarkable endurance.'[79]

A perennial woody vine up to 5m (16ft) high with heart-shaped leaves and small white flowers. The berries turn from red to black as they mature – black pepper is the dried, fully grown, unripe fruit.

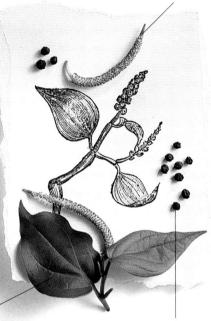

fruit

fresh cutting

dried peppercorn

AROMATHERAPY/ HOME USE

Not compatible with homeopathic treatment.
Skin Care: *Chilblains.*
Circulation, Muscles and Joints: *Anemia, arthritis, muscular aches and pains, neuralgia, poor circulation, poor muscle tone (muscular atonia), rheumatic pain, sprains, stiffness.*
Respiratory System: *Catarrh, chills.*
Digestive System: *Colic, constipation, diarrhea, flatulence, heartburn, loss of appetite, nausea.*
Immune System: *Colds, flu, infections and viruses.*

OTHER USES

Used in certain tonic and rubefacient preparations. Used for unusual effects in perfumery work; for example, with rose or carnation in oriental or floral fragrances. The oil and oleoresin are used extensively in the food industry, as well as in alcoholic drinks.

DISTRIBUTION

Native to south-west India; cultivated extensively in tropical countries. Major producers are India, Indonesia, Malaysia, China and Madagascar. It is also distilled in Europe and the USA from the imported dried fruits.

OTHER SPECIES

The so-called white pepper is the dried ripe fruit with the outer pericarp removed. Not to be confused with cayenne pepper or paprika from the capsicum species, which are used to make an oleoresin.

EXTRACTION

Essential oil by steam distillation from the black peppercorns, dried and crushed. ('Light' and 'heavy' oils are produced by the extraction of the low or high boiling fractions respectively.) An oleoresin is also produced by solvent extraction, mainly for flavour use.

CHARACTERISTICS

A water-white to pale olive mobile liquid with a fresh, dry-woody, warm, spicy scent. It blends well with frankincense, sandalwood, lavender, rosemary, marjoram, spices and florals (in minute quantities).

ACTIONS

Analgesic, antimicrobial, antiseptic, antispasmodic, antitoxic, aperitif, aphrodisiac, bactericidal, carminative, diaphoretic, digestive, diuretic, febrifuge, laxative, rubefacient, stimulant (nervous, circulatory, digestive), stomachic, tonic.

PRINCIPAL CONSTITUENTS

Mainly monoterpenes (70–80 per cent): thujene, pinene, camphene, sabinene, carene, myrcene, limonene, phellandrene; and sesquiterpenes (20–30 per cent) and oxygenated compounds.

Pistacia lentiscus

Mastic

FAMILY: ANACARDIACEAE **SYNONYMS:** MASTICK TREE, MASTICK, MASTIX, MASTICH, LENTISK

Herbal/Folk Tradition

In the East it is used for the manufacture of confectionery and cordials; it is still used medicinally for diarrhea in children and is chewed to sweeten the breath. The oil was used in the West in a similar way to turpentine – 'It has many of the properties of coniferous turpentines and was formerly greatly used in medicine.'[80]

A small bushy tree or shrub up to 3m (10ft) high, which produces a natural oleoresin from the trunk. Incisions are made in the bark in order to collect the liquid oleoresin, which then hardens into brittle pea-sized lumps.

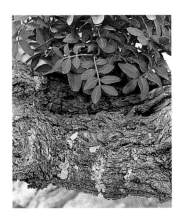

fresh mastic

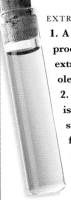

EXTRACTION

1. A resinoid is produced by solvent extraction from the oleoresin, and
2. an essential oil is produced by steam distillation from the oleoresin or occasionally directly from the leaves and branches.

CHARACTERISTICS

1. A pale amber or greenish viscous mass with a faint balsamic turpentine-like odour.
2. A pale yellow mobile liquid with a fresh balsamic turpentine-like odour. It blends well with lavender, mimosa, citrus and floral oils.

ACTIONS

Antimicrobial, antiseptic, antispasmodic, astringent, diuretic, expectorant, stimulant.

PRINCIPAL CONSTITUENTS

Mainly monoterpene hydrocarbons – mostly pinenes.

Pistacia lentiscus

AROMATHERAPY/ HOME USE

Use with care for:
Skin Care: *Boils, cuts, fleas, insect repellant, lice, ringworm, scabies, wounds.*
Circulation, Muscles and Joints: *Arthritis, gout, muscular aches and pains, rheumatism, sciatica.*
Respiratory System: *Bronchitis, catarrh, whooping cough.*
Genito-urinary System: *Cystitis, leucorrhea, urethritis.*
Immune System: *Colds.*
Nervous System: *Neuralgia.*

OTHER USES

Used in dentistry and in the production of varnish. The resinoid and oil are employed in high-class colognes and perfumes, and used as a flavouring agent, especially in liqueurs.

DISTRIBUTION

Native to the Mediterranean region (France, Spain, Portugal, Greece, Turkey) and also found in North Africa. Most mastic is produced on the Greek Island of Chios; some is also produced in Algeria, Morocco and the Canary Islands.

OTHER SPECIES

It belongs to the same family as Peruvian pepper or Peruvian mastic (Schinus molle). Mastic resembles the resin 'sanderach' but unlike the latter it can be chewed, rather than turning to powder.

Pogostemon cablin

Patchouli

FAMILY: LAMIACEAE (LABIATAE) **SYNONYMS:** *P. PATCHOULY*, PATCHOULY, PUCHAPUT

Herbal/Folk Tradition

The oil is used in the East generally to scent linen and clothes, and it is believed to help prevent the spread of disease (prophylactic). In China, Japan and Malaysia the herb is used to treat colds, headaches, nausea, vomiting, diarrhea, abdominal pain and halitosis. In Japan and Malaysia it is used as an antidote to poisonous snakebites.

A perennial bushy herb up to 1m (3ft) high with a sturdy, hairy stem, large, fragrant, furry leaves and white flowers tinged with purple.

fresh patchouli

AROMATHERAPY/ HOME USE

Skin Care: *Acne, athlete's foot, cracked and chapped skin, dandruff, dermatitis, eczema (weeping), fungal infections, hair care, impetigo, insect repellent, oily hair and skin, open pores, sores, wounds, wrinkles.*
Nervous System: *Frigidity, nervous exhaustion and stress-related complaints.*

OTHER USES

Extensively used in cosmetic preparations, and as a fixative in soaps and perfumes. Extensively used in the food industry, in alcoholic and soft drinks. It makes a good masking agent for unpleasant tastes and smells.

DISTRIBUTION

Native to tropical Asia, especially Indonesia and the Philippines. It is extensively cultivated for its oil in its native regions as well as in India, China, Malaysia and South America. The oil is also distilled in Europe and the USA from the dried leaves.

OTHER SPECIES

Closely related to the Java patchouli (P. heyneanus), also known as false patchouli, which is also occasionally used to produce an essential oil.

Pogostemon cablin

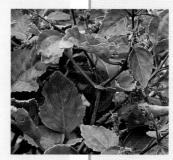

EXTRACTION

Essential oil by steam distillation of the dried leaves (usually subjected to fermentation previously). A resinoid is also produced, mainly as a fixative.

CHARACTERISTICS

An amber or dark orange viscous liquid with a sweet, rich, herbaceous-earthy odour – it improves with age. It blends well with labdanum, vetiver, sandalwood, cedarwood, oakmoss, geranium, clove, lavender, rose, orange blossom, bergamot, cassia, myrrh, opopanax, clary sage and oriental-type bases.

ACTIONS

Antidepressant, anti-inflammatory, anti-emetic, antimicrobial, antiphlogistic, antiseptic, antitoxic, antiviral, aphrodisiac, astringent, bactericidal, carminative, cicatrizant, deodorant, digestive, diuretic, febrifuge, fungicidal, nervine, prophylactic, stimulant (nervous), stomachic, tonic.

PRINCIPAL CONSTITUENTS

Patchouli alcohol (40 per cent approx.), pogostol, bulnesol, nor patchoulenol, bulnese, patchoulene, among others.

Polianthes tuberosa

Tuberose

FAMILY: AGAVACEAE SYNONYMS: TUBEROSA, TUBEREUSE

Herbal/Folk Tradition

The double-flowered variety is grown for ornamental purposes and for use by the cut flower trade. 'Pure absolute extraction of tuberose is perhaps the most expensive natural flower oil at the disposal of the modern perfumer.'[81]

EXTRACTION
A concrete and absolute by solvent extraction from the fresh flowers, picked before the petals open. (An essential oil is also obtained by distillation of the concrete.)

CHARACTERISTICS
The absolute is a dark orange or brown soft paste, with a heavy, sweet-floral, sometimes slightly spicy, tenacious

fragrance. It blends well with gardenia, violet, opopanax, rose, jasmine, carnation, orris, Peru balsam, orange blossom and ylang ylang.

ACTIONS
Narcotic.

PRINCIPAL CONSTITUENTS
Methyl benzoate, methyl anthranilate, benzyl alcohol, butyric acid, eugenol, nerol, farnesol, geraniol, among others.

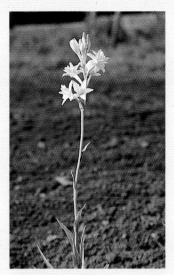

Polianthes tuberosa

AROMATHERAPY/ HOME USE
Perfume.

OTHER USES
Used in high-class perfumes, especially of an oriental, floral or fantasy type. Occasionally used for flavouring confectionery and some beverages.

DISTRIBUTION
Native of Central America, where it is found growing wild. Cultivated for its oil in southern France, Morocco, China, Taiwan and Egypt.

OTHER SPECIES
Related to the narcissus and jonquil. The Chinese species of tuberose is somewhat different from the French and Moroccan type, although both are single-flowered varieties.

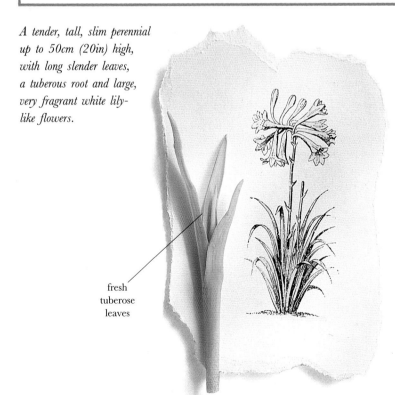

A tender, tall, slim perennial up to 50cm (20in) high, with long slender leaves, a tuberous root and large, very fragrant white lily-like flowers.

fresh tuberose leaves

Prunus dulcis var. amara

Bitter almond

FAMILY : ROSACEAE SYNONYMS: *P. AMYGDALUS VAR. AMARA, AMYGDALUS COMMUNIS VAR. AMARA, A. DULCIS, P. COMMUNIS*

Herbal/Folk Tradition

A 'fixed' oil commonly known as 'sweet almond oil' is make by pressing the kernels from both the sweet and bitter almond trees. Unlike the essential oil, this fixed oil does not contain any benzaldehyde or prussic acid, and has many medical and cosmetic uses. It is used as a laxative, for bronchitis, coughs, heartburn and for disorders of the kidneys, bladder and biliary ducts. It helps relieve muscular aches and pains, softens the skin and promotes a clear complexion.

The almond tree grows to a height of about 7m (23ft) and is popular as a garden tree because of its pinky-white blossom. It is botanically classified as a drupe.

bitter almond kernels

EXTRACTION
Essential oil by steam distillation from the kernels. The nuts are first pressed and macerated in warm water for 12 to 24 hours before the oil is extracted. It is during this process that the prussic acid is formed; it is not present in the raw seed. Most commercial bitter almond oil is rectified to remove all prussic acid, i.e. free from prussic acid (FFPA).

CHARACTERISTICS
Light colourless liquid with a characteristic 'marzipan' scent (FFPA).

ACTIONS
Anesthetic, antispasmodic, narcotic, vermifuge (FFPA).

PRINCIPAL CONSTITUENTS
Benzaldehyde (95 per cent), prussic acid (3 per cent).

AROMATHERAPY/ HOME USE
None. 'Should not be used in therapy either internally or externally.' [82]

OTHER USES
Bitter almond oil is no longer used for internal medication. Rectified bitter almond oil is used for flavouring foods, mainly confectionery; the most common uses are 'almond essence' and marzipan. The oil (FFPA) is increasingly being replaced by synthetic benzaldehyde in food flavourings.

DISTRIBUTION
Native to western Asia and North Africa, it is now extensively cultivated throughout the Mediterranean region, Israel and California.

OTHER SPECIES
There are two main types of almond trees — bitter and sweet. The sweet almond does not produce any essential oil.

Rosa x *centifolia*

Cabbage rose

FAMILY: ROSACEAE SYNONYMS: ROSE MAROC, FRENCH ROSE, PROVENCE ROSE, HUNDRED-LEAVED ROSE, MOROCCAN OTTO OF ROSE (OIL), FRENCH OTTO OF ROSE (OIL), ROSE DE MAI (ABSOLUTE OR CONCRETE)

Herbal/Folk Tradition

Up to the Middle Ages the rose played an essential part in the materia medica, being used for a wide range of disorders, including digestive and menstrual problems, headaches and nervous tension, liver congestion, poor circulation, fever (plague), eye infections and skin complaints.

'The symbolism connected with the rose is perhaps one of the richest and most complex associated with any plant . . . traditionally associated with Venus, the Goddess of love and beauty, and in our materialistic age the Goddess is certainly alive and well in the cosmetics industry for rose oil (mainly synthetic) is found as a component in 46% of men's perfumes and 98% of women's fragrances.'[83]

The French or Moroccan rose possesses narcotic properties and has the reputation for being aphrodisiac. For further distinctions between the different properties of rose types, see damask rose.

The rose that is generally used for oil production is strictly a hybrid involving R. x centifolia, R. gallica *and a few other roses. Known as rose de mai, it grows to 2.5m (8ft) high and has a mass of pink or rosy-purple flowers.*

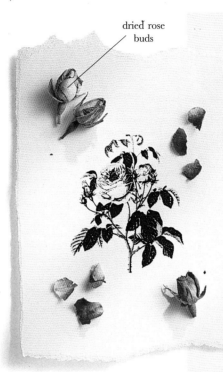

dried rose buds

AROMATHERAPY/ HOME USE

See damask rose.

OTHER USES

See damask rose.

DISTRIBUTION

The birthplace of the cultivated rose is believed to be ancient Persia; now cultivated mainly in Morocco, Tunisia, Italy, France, former Yugoslavia and China. The concrete, absolute and oil are produced mainly in Morocco; the absolute in France, Italy and China.

OTHER SPECIES

There are over 10,000 types of cultivated rose! There are several subspecies of R. centifolia, *depending on the country of origin. Other therapeutic species are the red rose or apothecary rose (*R. gallica*) of traditional Western medicine, the oriental or tea rose (*R. indica*), the Chinese or Japanese rose (*R. rugosa*) and the Turkish or Bulgarian rose (*R. damascena*), which is also extensively cultivated for its oil. Recently rosehip seed oil from* R. rubiginosa *has been found to be a very effective skin treatment; it promotes tissue regeneration and is good for scars, burns and wrinkles. See also entry on damask rose and the Botanical Classification section.*

EXTRACTION
See damask rose.

CHARACTERISTICS
**1. The oil is a pale yellow liquid with a deep, sweet, rosy-floral, tenacious odour.
2. The absolute is a reddish-orange viscous liquid with a deep, rich, sweet, rosy-spicy, honey-like fragrance. It blends well with jasmine, cassie, mimosa, orange blossom, geranium, bergamot, lavender, clary sage, sandalwood, guaiacwood, patchouli,**

benzoin, chamomile, Peru balsam, clove and palmarosa.

ACTIONS
See damask rose.

PRINCIPAL CONSTITUENTS
It has over 300 constituents, some in minute traces. Mainly citronellol (18–22 per cent), phenyl ethanol (63 per cent), geraniol and nerol (10–15 per cent), stearopten (8 per cent), farnesol (0.2–2 per cent), among others.

Rosa x *damascena*

Damask rose

SAFETY DATA *Non-toxic, non-irritant, non-sensitizing*

FAMILY: ROSACEAE SYNONYMS: SUMMER DAMASK ROSE, BULGARIAN ROSE, TURKISH ROSE (ANATOLIAN ROSE OIL), OTTO OF ROSE (OIL), ATTAR OF ROSE (OIL)

Herbal/Folk Tradition

'The damask rose, on account of its fragrance, belongs to the cephalics . . oil of roses is used by itself to cool hot inflammations or swellings, and to bind and stay fluxes of humours to sores.'[84] Rose hips are still current in the British Herbal Pharmacopoeia, mainly because of their high Vitamin C content. See also cabbage rose.

Small prickly shrub between 1–2m (3–6ft) high, with pink fragrant blooms and whitish hairy leaves.

damask rose petals

AROMATHERAPY/ HOME USE

Skin Care: *Broken capillaries, conjunctivitis (rose water), dry skin, eczema, herpes, mature and sensitive complexions, wrinkles.*
Circulation, Muscles and Joints: *Palpitations, poor circulation.*
Respiratory System: *Asthma, coughs, hay fever.*
Digestive System: *Cholecystitis, liver congestion, nausea.*
Genito-urinary System: *Irregular menstruation, leucorrhea, menorrhagia, uterine disorders.*
Nervous System: *Depression, impotence, insomnia, frigidity, headache, nervous tension and stress-related complaints − 'But the rose procures us one thing above all: a feeling of well being, even of happiness.'[85]*

OTHER USES

Rose water is used as a household cosmetic and culinary article. The concrete, absolute and oil are employed extensively in soaps, cosmetics, toiletries and perfumes of all types. Some flavouring uses.

DISTRIBUTION

Believed to be a native of the Orient, now cultivated mainly in Bulgaria, Turkey and France. Similar types are grown in China, India and Russia; however, India produces only rose water and aytar − a mixture of rose otto and sandalwood.

OTHER SPECIES

Many different subspecies: the Turkish variety is known simply as R. x damascena. 'Trigintipetala' is the principal cultivar in commercial cultivation, known as the 'Kazanlik rose'. Bulgaria also grows the white rose (R. x damascena var. alba) and a musk rose (R. x centifolia 'Muscosa'). See also cabbage rose and the Botanical Classification section.

EXTRACTION

1. Essential oil or otto by water or steam distillation from the fresh petals. (Rose water is produced as a byproduct of this process.)
2. Concrete and absolute by solvent extraction from the fresh petals. (A rose leaf absolute is also produced in small quantities in France.)

CHARACTERISTICS

1. A pale yellow or olive yellow liquid with a very rich, deep, sweet-floral, slightly spicy scent. 2. The absolute is a reddish-orange or olive viscous liquid with a rich, sweet, spicy-floral, tenacious odour. It blends well with most oils and is useful for 'rounding off' blends. The Bulgarian type is considered superior in perfumery work, but in therapeutic practice it is more a matter of differing properties between the types of rose.

ACTIONS

Antidepressant, antiphlogistic, antiseptic, antispasmodic, anti-tubercular agent, antiviral, aphrodisiac, astringent, bactericidal, choleretic, cicatrizant, depurative, emmenagogue, hemostatic, hepatic, laxative, regulator of appetite, sedative (nervous), stomachic, tonic (heart, liver, stomach, uterus).

PRINCIPAL CONSTITUENTS

Mainly citronellol (34–55 per cent), geraniol and nerol (30–40 per cent), stearopten (16–22 per cent), phenyl ethanol (1.5–3 per cent) and farnesol (0.2–2 per cent), with many other trace constituents.

Rosmarinus officinalis

Rosemary

SAFETY DATA *Non-toxic, non-irritant (in dilution only), non-sensitizing. Avoid during pregnancy. Not to be used by epileptics. Contra-indicated in cases of high blood pressure*

FAMILY: LAMIACEAE (LABIATAE) **SYNONYMS:** *R. CORONARIUM*, COMPASS PLANT, INCENSIER

Herbal/Folk Tradition

One of the earliest plants to be used for food, medicine and magic. Sprigs of rosemary were burned at shrines in ancient Greece, fumigations were used in the Middle Ages to drive away evil spirits, and to protect against plague.

It has been used for a wide range of complaints including respiratory and circulatory disorders, liver congestion, digestive and nervous complaints, muscular and rheumatic pain, skin and hair problems. It is current in the British Herbal Pharmacopoeia as a specific for 'depressive states with general debility and indications of cardiovascular weakness'.[86]

A shrubby evergreen bush up to 2m (6ft) high with silvery-green, needly-shaped leaves and pale blue flowers. The whole plant is strongly aromatic.

fresh rosemary

EXTRACTION
Essential oil by steam distillation of the fresh flowering tops or (in Spain) the whole plant (poorer quality).

CHARACTERISTICS
A colourless or pale yellow mobile liquid with a strong, fresh, minty-herbaceous scent and a woody-balsamic undertone. Poor-quality oils have a strong camphoraceous note. It blends well with olibanum, lavender, lavandin, citronella, oregano, thyme, pine, basil, peppermint, labdanum, elemi, cedarwood, petitgrain, cinnamon and other spice oils.

ACTIONS
Analgesic, antimicrobial, antioxidant, antirheumatic, antiseptic, antispasmodic, aphrodisiac, astringent, carminative, cephalic, cholagogue, choleretic, cicatrizant, cordial, cytophylactic, diaphoretic, digestive, diuretic, emmenagogue, fungicidal, hepatic, hypertensive, nervine, parasiticide, restorative, rubefacient, stimulant (circulatory, adrenal cortex, hepatobiliary), stomachic, sudorific, tonic (nervous, general), vulnerary.

PRINCIPAL CONSTITUENTS
Mainly pinenes, camphene, limonene, cineol, borneal with camphor, linalol, terpineol, octanone, bornyl acetate, among others.

AROMATHERAPY/ HOME USE

Skin Care: *Acne, dandruff, dermatitis, eczema, greasy hair, insect repellent, lice, promotes hair growth, regulates seborrhea, scabies, stimulates scalp, varicose veins.*

Circulation, Muscles and Joints: *Arteriosclerosis, fluid retention, gout, muscular pain, palpitations, poor circulation, rheumatism.*

Respiratory System: *Asthma, bronchitis, whooping cough.*

Digestive System: *Colitis, dyspepsia, flatulence, hepatic disorders, hypercholesterolemia, jaundice.*

Genito-urinary System: *Dysmenorrhea, leucorrhea.*

Immune System: *Colds, flu, infections.*

Nervous System: *Debility, headaches, hypotension, neuralgia, mental fatigue, nervous exhaustion and stress-related disorders.*

OTHER USES

Used extensively in soaps, detergents, cosmetics, household sprays and perfumes and as a masking agent. Employed in most major food categories, as well as drinks.

DISTRIBUTION

Native to the Mediterranean, now grown in California, Russia, the Middle East, Britain, France, Spain, Portugal, former Yugoslavia, Morocco, China, etc. The main oil-producing countries are France, Spain and Tunisia.

OTHER SPECIES

R. officinalis *is the type used for oil production, although there are many different cultivars. See also Botanical Classification section.*

Ruta graveolens

Rue

FAMILY: RUTACEAE   **SYNONYMS:** GARDEN RUE, HERB-OF-GRACE, HERBYGRASS

Herbal/Folk Tradition

A favoured remedy of the ancients, especially as an antidote to poison. It was seen as a magic herb by many cultures and as a protection against evil. It was also used for nervous afflictions. 'It helps disorders in the head, nerves and womb, convulsions and hysteric fits, the colic, weakness of the stomach and bowels; it resists poison and cures venomous bites.' [87]

An ornamental, shrubby herb with tough, woody branches, small, smooth, bluish-green leaves and greeny-yellow flowers. The whole plant has a strong, aromatic, bitter or acrid scent.

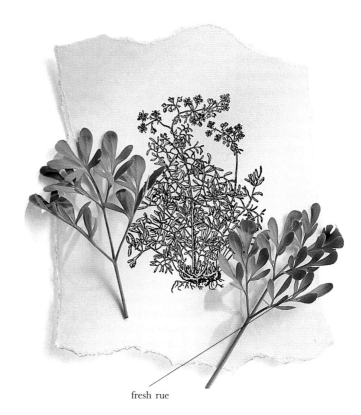

fresh rue

EXTRACTION
Essential oil by steam distillation from the fresh herb.

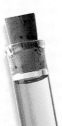

CHARACTERISTICS
A yellow or orange viscous mass that generally solidifies at room temperature, with a sharp, herbaceous-fruity acrid odour. The winter rue oil does not solidify at room temperature.

ACTIONS
Antitoxic, antitussive, antiseptic, antispasmodic, diuretic, emmenagogue, insecticidal, nervine, rubefacient, stimulant, tonic, vermifuge.

PRINCIPAL CONSTITUENTS
Mainly methyl nonyl ketone (90 per cent in summer rue oil).

AROMATHERAPY/
HOME USE
None. 'Should not be used at all in aromatherapy.' [89]

OTHER USES
Employed as a source of methyl nonyl ketone.

DISTRIBUTION
Native to the Mediterranean region; found growing wild extensively in Spain, Morocco, Corsica, Sardinia and Algeria. It is cultivated mainly in France and Spain for its oil; also in Italy and former Yugoslavia.

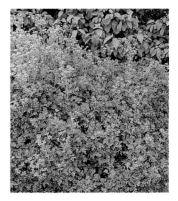

Ruta graveolens

OTHER SPECIES
There are several different types of rue, such as the summer rue (R. montan), winter rue (R. chalepansis) and Sardinian rue (R. angustifolia), which are also used to produce essential oils.

Salvia lavandulifolia

Spanish sage

FAMILY: LAMIACEAE (LABIATAE)   **SYNONYM:** LAVENDER-LEAVED SAGE

Herbal/Folk Tradition

In Spain it is regarded as something of a 'cure-all'. Believed to promote longevity and protect against all types of infection (such as plague). Used to treat rheumatism, digestive complaints, menstrual problems, infertility and nervous weakness.

EXTRACTION
Essential oil by steam distillation from the leaves.

CHARACTERISTICS
A pale yellow mobile liquid with a fresh-herbaceous, camphoraceous, slightly pine-like odour. It blends well with rosemary, lavandin, lavender, pine, citronella, eucalyptus, juniper, clary sage and cedarwood.

ACTIONS
Antidepressant, anti-inflammatory, antimicrobial, antiseptic, antispasmodic, astringent, carminative, deodorant, depurative, digestive, emmenagogue, expectorant, febrifuge, hypotensive, nervine, regulator (of seborrhea), stimulant (hepatobiliary, adrenocortical glands, circulation), stomachic, tonic (nerve and general).

PRINCIPAL CONSTITUENTS
Camphor (up to 34 per cent), cineol (up to 35 per cent), limonene (up to 41 per cent), camphene (up to 20 per cent), pinene (up to 20 per cent) and other minor constituents.

AROMATHERAPY/HOME USE

Skin Care: *Acne, cuts, dandruff, dermatitis, eczema, excessive sweating, hair loss, gingivitis, gum infections, sores.*

Circulation, Muscles and Joints: *Arthritis, debility, fluid retention, muscular aches and pains, poor circulation, rheumatism.*

Respiratory System: *Asthma, coughs, laryngitis.*

Digestive System: *Jaundice, liver congestion.*

Genito-urinary System: *Amenorrhea, dysmenorrhea, sterility.*

Immune System: *Colds, fever, flu.*

Nervous System: *Headaches, nervous exhaustion and stress-related conditions.*

OTHER USES

Used extensively as a fragrance component in soaps, cosmetics, toiletries and perfumes, especially 'industrial'-type fragrances. Employed extensively in foods (especially meat products), as well as alcoholic and soft drinks.

DISTRIBUTION

Native to the mountains in Spain, it also grows in south-west France and former Yugoslavia. The oil is produced mainly in Spain.

OTHER SPECIES

A very similar oil is distilled in Turkey from a Greek species, S. fruticosa, which is used for pharmaceutical purposes. See also entries on clary sage and common sage for other types of sage.

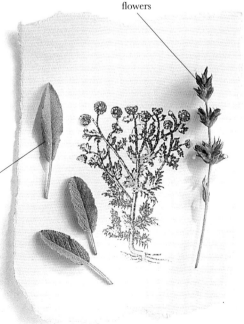

An evergreen shrub, similar to the garden sage but with narrower leaves and small purple flowers. The whole plant is aromatic with a scent reminiscent of spike lavender.

small purple flowers

fresh leaf

Salvia officinalis

Common sage

FAMILY: LAMIACEAE (LABIATAE) **SYNONYMS:** GARDEN SAGE, TRUE SAGE, DALMATIAN SAGE

Herbal/Folk Tradition

A herb of ancient repute, valued as a culinary and medicinal plant – called *herba sacra*, 'sacred herb', by the Romans. It has been used for a variety of disorders including respiratory infections, menstrual difficulties and digestive complaints. It was also believed to strengthen the senses and the memory.

It is still current in the British Herbal Pharmacopoeia as a specific for inflammations of the mouth, tongue and throat.

An evergreen, shrubby, perennial herb up to 80cm (32in) high with a woody base, soft, silver, oval leaves and a mass of deep blue or violet flowers.

fresh
common
sage

AROMATHERAPY/
HOME USE

None.
Use with care or avoid in therapeutic work altogether – Spanish sage or clary sage are good alternatives.

OTHER USES

Used in some pharmaceutical preparations such as mouthwashes, gargles, toothpastes, etc. Employed as a fragrance component in soaps, shampoos, detergents, anti-perspirants, colognes and perfumes, especially men's fragrances.
The oil and oleoresin are used extensively for flavouring foods (mainly meat products), soft drinks and alcoholic beverages, especially vermouth. It also serves as a source of natural anti-oxidants.

DISTRIBUTION

Native to the Mediterranean region; cultivated worldwide especially in Albania, former Yugoslavia, Greece, Italy, Turkey, France, China and the USA.

OTHER SPECIES

There are several different species and cultivars that have been developed, such as the Mexican sage (S. azurea grandiflora) and the red sage (S. colorata) both of which are used medicinally. Essential oils are also produced from other species including the Spanish sage (S. lavendulifolia) and clary sage (S. sclarea). See separate entries and Botanical Classification section.

EXTRACTION
Essential oil by steam distillation from the dried leaves. (A so-called oleoresin is also produced from the exhausted plant material.)

CHARACTERISTICS
A pale yellow mobile liquid with a fresh, warm-spicy, herbaceous, somewhat camphoraceous odour. It blends well with lavandin, rosemary, rosewood, lavender, hyssop, lemon and other citrus oils. The common sage oil is preferred in perfumery work to the Spanish sage oil, which, although safer, has a less refined fragrance.

ACTIONS
Anti-inflammatory, antimicrobial, anti-oxidant, antiseptic, antispasmodic, astringent, digestive, diuretic, emmenagogue, febrifuge, hypertensive, insecticidal, laxative, stomachic, tonic.

PRINCIPAL CONSTITUENTS
Thujone (about 42 per cent), cineol, borneol, caryophyllene and other terpenes.

Salvia sclarea

Clary sage

SAFETY DATA *Non-toxic, non-irritant, non-sensitizing. Avoid during pregnancy. Do not use clary sage oil while drinking alcohol; it can induce a narcotic effect and exaggerate drunkenness*

FAMILY: LAMIACEAE (LABIATAE) **SYNONYMS:** CLARY, CLARY WORT, MUSCATEL SAGE, CLEAR EYE, SEE BRIGHT, COMMON CLARY, CLARRY, EYE BRIGHT

Herbal/Folk Tradition

This herb, highly esteemed in the Middle Ages, has now largely fallen out of use. It was used for digestive disorders, kidney disease, uterine and menstrual complaints, for cleansing ulcers and as a general nerve tonic. The mucilage from the seeds was used for treating tumours and for removing dust particles from the eyes.

Like garden sage, it cools inflammation and is especially useful for throat and respiratory infections.

Stout biennial or perennial herb up to 1m (3ft) high with large, hairy leaves, green with a hint of purple, and small blue flowers.

fresh leaf

EXTRACTION

Essential oil by steam distillation from the flowering tops and leaves. (A concrete and absolute are also produced by solvent extraction in small quantities.)

CHARACTERISTICS

A colourless or pale yellowy-green liquid with a sweet, nutty-herbaceous scent. It blends well with juniper, lavender, coriander, cardomon, geranium, sandalwood, cedarwood, pine, labdanum, jasmine, frankincense, bergamot and other citrus oils.

ACTIONS

Anticonvulsive, antidepressant, antiphlogistic, antiseptic, antispasmodic, aphrodisiac, astringent, bactericidal, carminative, cicatrizant, deodorant, digestive, emmenagogue, euphoric, hypotensive, nervine, regulator (of seborrhea), sedative, stomachic, tonic, uterine.

PRINCIPAL CONSTITUENTS

Linalyl acetate (up to 75 per cent), linalol, pinene, myrcene and phellandrene, among others. Constituents vary according to geographical origin – there are several different chemotypes.

AROMATHERAPY/ HOME USE

Clary sage is generally used in preference to the garden sage in aromatherapy due to its lower toxicity level.
Skin Care: *Acne, boils, dandruff, hair loss, inflamed conditions, oily skin and hair, ophthalmia, ulcers, wrinkles.*
Circulation, Muscles and Joints: *High blood pressure, muscular aches and pains.*
Respiratory System: *Asthma, throat infections, whooping cough.*
Digestive System: *Cramp, dyspepsia, flatulence.*
Genito-urinary System: *Amenorrhea, labour pain, dysmenorrhea, leucorrhea.*
Nervous System: *Depression, frigidity, impotence, migraine, nervous tension and stress-related disorders.*

OTHER USES

The oil and absolute are used as fragrance components and fixatives in soaps, detergents, cosmetics and perfumes. The oil is used extensively by the food and drink industry, especially in the production of wines with a muscatel flavour.

DISTRIBUTION

Native to southern Europe; cultivated worldwide especially in the Mediterranean region, Russia, the USA, Britain, Morocco and central Europe. The French, Moroccan and English clary are considered of superior quality for perfumery work.

OTHER SPECIES

Closely related to the garden sage (S. officinalis) and the Spanish sage (S. lavendulifolia), which are both used to produce essential oils. Other types of sage include meadow clary (S. pratensis) and vervain sage (S. verbenaca). Clary sage should not be confused with the common wayside herb eyebright (Euphrasia).

Santalum album

Sandalwood

FAMILY: SANTALACEAE **SYNONYMS:** WHITE SANDALWOOD, YELLOW SANDALWOOD, EAST INDIAN SANDALWOOD, SANDALWOOD MYSORE, SANDERS-WOOD, SANTAL (OIL), WHITE SAUNDERS (OIL), YELLOW SAUNDERS (OIL)

Herbal/Folk Tradition

One of the oldest known perfume materials, with at least 4,000 years of uninterrupted use. It is used as a traditional incense, as a cosmetic, perfume and embalming material all over the East. It is also a popular building material, especially for temples.

In Chinese medicine it is used to treat stomach ache, vomiting, gonorrhea, choleraic difficulties and skin complaints. In the Ayurvedic tradition it is used mainly for urinary and respiratory infections, for acute and chronic diarrhea. In India it is often combined with rose in the famous scent *aytar*.

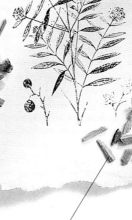

sandalwood
chippings

A small evergreen, parasitic tree up to 9m (30ft) high with brown-grey trunk and many smooth, slender branches. It has leathery leaves and small pinky-purple flowers. The tree must be over thirty years old before it is ready for the production of sandalwood oil.

EXTRACTION
Essential oil by water or stream distillation from the roots and heartwood, powdered and dried.

CHARACTERISTICS
A pale yellow, greenish or brownish viscous liquid with a deep, soft, sweet-woody balsamic scent of excellent tenacity. It blends well with rose, violet, tuberose, clove, lavender, black pepper, bergamot, rosewood, geranium, labdanum, oakmoss, benzion, vetiver, patchouli, mimosa, cassie, costus, myrrh and jasmine.

ACTIONS
Antidepressant, antiphlogistic, antiseptic (urinary and pulmonary), antispasmodic, aphrodisiac, astringent, bactericidal, carminative, cicatrizant, diuretic, expectorant, insecticidal, sedative, tonic.

PRINCIPAL CONSTITUENTS
About 90 per cent santalols, 6 per cent sesquiterpene hydrocarbons: santene, teresantol, borneol, santalone, tri-cyclo-ekasantalal, among others.

AROMATHERAPY/ HOME USE

Skin Care: *Acne, dry, cracked, and chapped skin, aftershave (barber's rash), greasy skin, moisturizer.*
Respiratory System: *Bronchitis, catarrh, coughs (dry, persistent), laryngitis, sore throat.*
Digestive System: *Diarrhea, nausea.*
Genito-urinary System: *Cystitis.*
Nervous System: *Depression, insomnia, nervous tension and stress-related complaints.*

OTHER USES

Formerly used as a pharmaceutical disinfectant, now largely abandoned. Extensively employed as a fragrance component and fixative in soaps, detergents, cosmetics and perfumes — especially oriental, woody, aftershaves, chyprès, etc. Extensively used in the production of incense. Employed as a flavour ingredient in most major food categories, including soft and alcoholic drinks.

DISTRIBUTION

Native to tropical Asia. India is the main essential oil producer; the region of Mysore exports the highest-quality oil, although some oil is distilled in Europe and the USA.

OTHER SPECIES

The Australian sandalwood (S. spicatum or Eucarya spicata) produces a very similar oil, but with a dry-bitter top note. The so-called West Indian sandalwood or amyris (Amyris balsamifera) is a poor substitute and bears no botanical relation to the East Indian sandalwood.

Santolina chamaecyparissus

Santolina

FAMILY: ASTERACEAE (COMPOSITAE) **SYNONYMS:** *LAVANDULA TAEMINA*, COTTON LAVENDER

Herbal/Folk Tradition

It was used as an antidote to all sorts of poison, and to expel worms; also 'good against obstruction of the liver, the jaundice and to promote menses'.[90] It was used to keep away moths from linen, to repel mosquitoes, and as a remedy for insect bits, warts, scabs and veruccae. The Arabs are said to have used the juice for bathing the eyes.

An evergreen, woody shrub with whitish-grey foliage and small, bright yellow, ball-shaped flowers borne on long single stalks. The whole plant has a strong rank odour, a bit like chamomile.

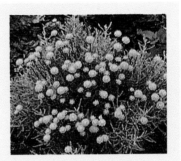

Santolina chamaecyparissus

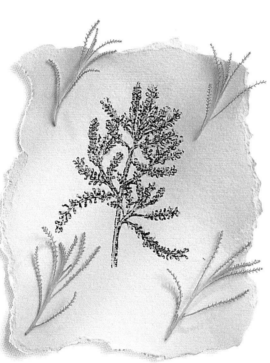

fresh santolina leaves

AROMATHERAPY/ HOME USE

None.
'There is no safety data available ... likely to be dangerously toxic.'[91]

OTHER USES

Little used in flavour or perfumery work due to toxicity.

DISTRIBUTION

Native to Italy, now common throughout the Mediterranean region. Much grown as a popular border herb.

OTHER SPECIES

There are several varieties such as S. fragrantissima. *It is not related to true lavender* (Lavandula angustifolia) *despite the common name.*

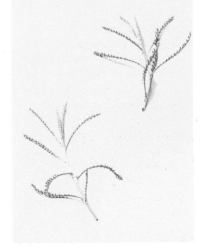

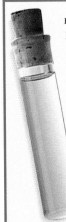

EXTRACTION
Essential oil by steam distillation from the seeds.

CHARACTERISTICS
A pale yellow liquid with a strong, acrid, herbaceous odour.

ACTIONS
Antispasmodic, antitoxic, anthelminthic, insecticidal, stimulant, vermifuge.

PRINCIPAL CONSTITUENTS
Only one principal constituent: santolinenone.

Sassafras albidum

Sassafras

SAFETY DATA *Highly toxic – ingestion of even small amounts has been known to cause death. Carcinogen. Irritant. Abortifacient*

FAMILY: LAURACEAE **SYNONYMS:** *S. OFFICINALE, LAURUS SASSAFRAS, S. VARIIFOLIUM,* COMMON SASSAFRAS, NORTH AMERICAN SASSAFRAS, SASSAFRAX

Herbal/Folk Tradition

It has been used for treating high blood pressure, rheumatism, arthritis, gout, menstrual and kidney problems, and for skin complaints. 'Sassafras pith – used as a demulcent, especially for inflammation of the eyes, and as a soothing drink in catarrhal affection.' [92] The wood and bark yield a bright yellow dye.

A deciduous tree up to 40m (131ft) high with many slender branches, a soft and spongy orange-brown bark and small yellowy-green flowers. The bark and wood are aromatic.

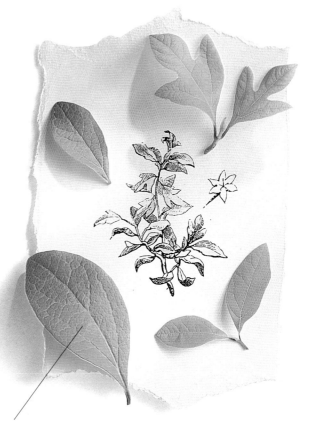

fresh
sassafras

EXTRACTION
Essential oil by steam distillation from the dried root bark chips.

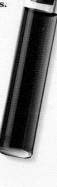

CHARACTERISTICS
A yellowy-brown, oily liquid with a fresh, sweet-spicy, woody-camphoraceous odour. (A safrol-free sassafras oil is produced by alcohol extraction.)

ACTIONS
Antiviral, diaphoretic, diuretic, carminative, pediculicide (destroys lice), stimulant.

PRINCIPAL CONSTITUENTS
Safrole (80–90 per cent), pinenes, phellandrenes, asarone, camphor, thujone, myristicin and menthone, among others.

AROMATHERAPY/ HOME USES

None. 'Should not be used in therapy, whether internally or externally.' [93]

OTHER USES

Sassafras oil and crude are banned from food use; safrol-free extract is used to a limited extent in flavouring work. Safrol is used as a starting material for the fragrance item 'heliotropin'.

DISTRIBUTION

Native to eastern parts of the USA; the oil is produced mainly from Florida to Canada and in Mexico.

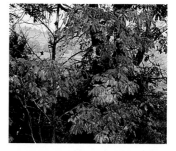

Sassafras albidum

OTHER SPECIES

There are several other species, notably the Brazilian sassafras (Ocotea pretiosa), which is also used to produce an essential oil (also highly toxic). See also Botanical Classification section.

Satureja hortensis

Summer savory

FAMILY: LAMIACEAE (LABIATAE) SYNONYMS: *SATUREIA HORTENSIS*, *CALAMINTHA HORTENSIS*, GARDEN SAVORY

Herbal/Folk Tradition

A popular culinary herb, with a peppery flavour. It has been used therapeutically mainly as a tea for various ailments including digestive complaints (cramp, nausea, indigestion; intestinal parasites), menstrual disorders and respiratory conditions (asthma, catarrh, sore throat). Applied externally, the fresh leaves bring instant relief from insect bites, bee and wasp stings.

'This kind is both hotter and drier than the winter kind . . . it expels tough phlegm from the chest and lungs, quickens the dull spirits in the lethargy'.[94]

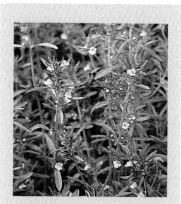

Satureja hortensis

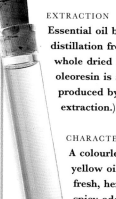

EXTRACTION

Essential oil by steam distillation from the whole dried herb. (An oleoresin is also produced by solvent extraction.)

CHARACTERISTICS

A colourless or pale yellow oil with a fresh, herbaceous, spicy odour. It blends well with lavender, lavandin, pine needle, oakmoss, rosemary and citrus oils.

ACTIONS

Anticatarrhal, antiputrescent, antispasmodic, aphrodisiac, astringent, bactericidal, carminative, cicatrizant, emmenagogue, expectorant, fungicidal, stimulant, vermifuge.

PRINCIPAL CONSTITUENTS

Carvacrol, pinene, cymene, camphene, limonene, phellandrene and borneol, among others.

AROMATHERAPY/ HOME USE

None. 'Should not be used on the skin at all.'[95]

OTHER USES

Occasionally used in perfumery work for its fresh herbaceous notes. The oil and oleoresin are used in most major food categories, especially meat products and canned food.

DISTRIBUTION

Native to Europe, naturalized in North America. Extensively cultivated, especially in Spain, France, former Yugoslavia and the USA for its essential oil.

OTHER SPECIES

Closely related to the thyme family, with which it shares many characteristics. There are several different types of 'savory', including S. thymbra, found in Spain, which contains mainly thymol, and the winter savory (S. montana) - see separate entry.

An annual herb up to 45cm (18in) high with slender, erect, slightly hairy stems, linear leaves and small, pale lilac flowers.

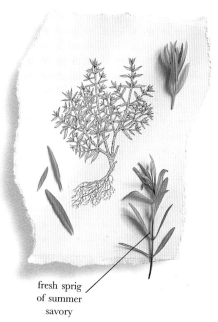

fresh sprig of summer savory

Satureja montana

Winter savory

FAMILY: LAMIACEAE (LABIATAE) SYNONYMS: *S. OBOVATA, CALAMINTHA MONTANA*

Herbal/Folk Tradition

It has been used as a culinary herb since antiquity, much in the same way as summer savory. It was used as a digestive remedy especially good for colic, and in Germany it is used particularly for diarrhea. When compared with many varieties of thyme, rosemary and lavender, recent research has shown 'the net superiority of the anti-microbial properties of essence of savory'.[96]

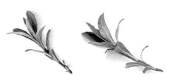

A bushy perennial sub-shrub up to 40cm (16in) high with woody stems at the base, linear leaves and pale purple flowers.

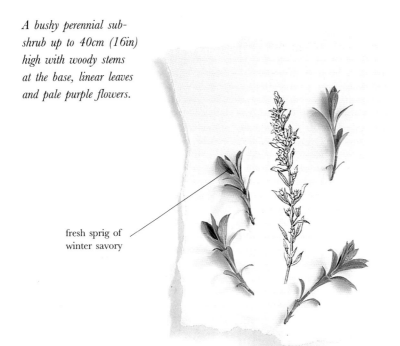

fresh sprig of winter savory

AROMATHERAPY/ HOME USE

None. 'Should not be used on the skin at all.' [97]

OTHER USES

Occasionally used in perfumery work. The oil and oleoresin are employed to some extent in flavouring, mainly meats and seasonings.

DISTRIBUTION

Native to the Mediterranean region, now found all over Europe, Russia and Turkey. The oil is produced mainly in Spain, Morrocco and former Yugoslavia.

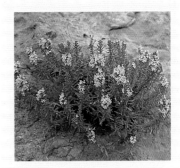

Satureja montana

OTHER SPECIES

The creeping variety of the winter savory (S. montana subspicata) *is also a well-known garden herb. See also summer savory* (S. hortensis) *and Botanical Classification section.*

EXTRACTION
Essential oil by steam distillation from the whole herb. (An oleoresin is also produced by solvent extraction.)

CHARACTERISTICS
A colourless or pale yellow liquid with a sharp, medicinal, herbaceous odour.

ACTIONS
Anticatarrhal, antiputrescent, antispasmodic, aphrodisiac, astringent, bactericidal, carminative, cicatrizant, emmenagogue, expectorant, fungicidal, stimulant, vermifuge.

PRINCIPAL CONSTITUENTS
Mainly carvacrol, cymene, thymol, with lesser amounts of pinenes, limonene, cineol, borneol and terpineol.

Saussurea costus

Costus

FAMILY: ASTERACEA (COMPOSITAE) **SYNONYMS:** *S. LAPPA, AUCKLANDIA COSTUS, APLOTAXIS LAPPA, A. AURICULATA*

Herbal/Folk Tradition

The root has been used for millennia in India and China for digestive complaints, respiratory conditions, as a stimulant and for infection including typhoid and cholera. It is also used as an incense.

A large, erect, perennial plant up to 2m (6ft) high with a thick tapering root and numerous almost black flowers.

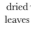
dried
leaves

EXTRACTION
The dried roots are macerated in warm water, then subjected to steam distillation followed by solvent extraction of the distilled water. (A concrete and absolute are also produced in small quantities.)

CHARACTERISTICS
A pale yellow or brownish viscous liquid of soft, woody-musty, extremely tenacious odour. It blends well with patchouli, opopanax, ylang ylang, oriental and floral fragrances.

ACTIONS
Antiseptic, antispasmodic, antiviral, bactericidal, carminative, digestive, expectorant, febrifuge, hypotensive, stimulant, stomachic, tonic.

PRINCIPAL CONSTITUENTS
Mainly sesquiterpene lactones, including dihydrocostus lactone and costunolide (together up to 50 per cent), other sesquiterpenes such as costols, caryophyllene and selinene, as well as costic and oleic acids, among others.

AROMATHERAPY/ HOME USE
Costus is not recommended for aromatherapy or home use because it is a common and severe dermal sensitizer. In a recent skin test, it produced sensitization reactions in all 25 volunteers.

OTHER USES
Fixative and fragrance component in cosmetics and perfumes. Used as a flavour ingredient by the food industry, especially in confectionery, alcoholic and soft drinks.

DISTRIBUTION
Native to northern India; cultivated in India and south-west China. The oil is produced mainly in India.

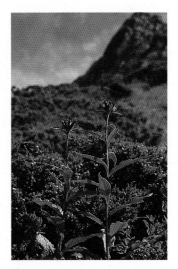
Saussurea costus

OTHER SPECIES
*Closely related to elecampane (*Inula helenium*), whose roots are also used to produce an essential oil.*

Schinus molle

Schinus molle

FAMILY: ANACARDIACEAE **SYNONYMS:** PERUVIAN PEPPER, PERUVIAN MASTIC, CALIFORNIAN PEPPER TREE

Herbal/Folk Tradition

In Greece and other Mediterranean countries an intoxicating beverage is made from the fruits of the tree. The fruit is also used as a substitute for black pepper in the growing areas. During World War II, the oil of black pepper was unavailable and was consequently replaced by schinus molle.

EXTRACTION
Essential oil by steam distillation from the fruit or berries. (An oil from the leaves is also produced in small quantities.)

CHARACTERISTICS
A pale green or olive, oily liquid with a warm, woody-peppery scent with a smoky undertone. It blends well with oakmoss, clove, nutmeg, cinnamon, black pepper and eucalyptus.

ACTIONS
Antiseptic, antiviral, bactericidal, carminative, stimulant, stomachic.

PRINCIPAL CONSTITUENTS
Mainly phellandrene, also caryophyllene, pinene and carvacrol.

A tropical evergreen tree up to 20m (65ft) high with graceful, drooping branches, feathery foliage and fragrant yellow flowers. The berries or fruit have an aromatic, peppery flavour.

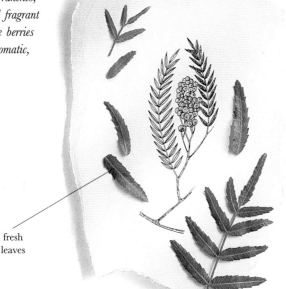

fresh leaves

AROMATHERAPY/ HOME USE
Not compatible with homeopathic treatment.
Skin Care: *Chilblains.*
Circulation, Muscles and Joints: *Anemia, arthritis, muscular aches and pains, neuralgia, poor circulation, poor muscle tone (muscular atonia), rheumatic pain, sprains, stiffness.*
Respiratory System: *Catarrh, chills.*
Digestive System: *Colic, constipation, diarrhea, flatulence, heartburn, loss of appetite, nausea.*
Immune System: *Colds, flu, infections and viruses.*

OTHER USES
Used as a substitute for black pepper in perfumery and flavouring work.

DISTRIBUTION
Native to South America; found growing wild in Mexico, Peru, Guatemala and other tropical regions, including California. It has been introduced into North Africa and the Mediterranean region. The fruits are collected for essential oil production in Spain, Guatemala and Mexico.

Schinus molle

OTHER SPECIES
Closely related to the mastic tree (Pistacia lentiscus) – see entry on mastic.

Spartium junceum

Spanish broom

FAMILY: FABACEAE (LEGUMINOSAE) SYNONYMS: *GENISTA JUNCAE*, GENISTA, WEAVERS BROOM, BROOM (ABSOLUTE), GÊNET (ABSOLUTE)

Herbal/Folk Tradition

The twigs and bark have been used since ancient times to produce a strong fibre that can be made into cord or a coarse cloth. The branches were also used for thatching, basketwork, fencing and, of course, for making brooms. Spanish broom has similar therapeutic properties to the common broom, which is still current in the British Herbal Pharmacopoeia for cardiac dropsy, myocardial weakness, tachycardia, and profuse menstruation. However, the Spanish broom is said to be five to six times more active than the common broom, and even that must be used with caution by professional herbalists due to the strength of the active ingredients: 'A number of cases of poisoning have occurred from the substitution of the dried flowers of Spartium for those of true Broom.'[98]

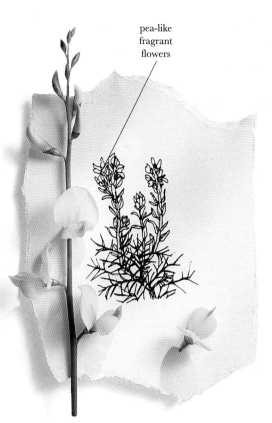

pea-like fragrant flowers

A decorative plant, often cultivated as an ornamental shrub, up to 3m (10ft) high with upright woody branches and tough flexible stems. It has bright green leaves and large, yellow, pea-like fragrant flowers, also bearing its seed pods or legumes.

AROMATHERAPY/ HOME USE

None.
In large doses, it causes vomiting, renal irritation, weakens the heart, depresses the nerve cells and lowers the blood pressure, and in extreme cases causes death.

OTHER USES

Used in soaps, cosmetics and high-class perfumery; also as a flavour ingredient in sweet rich 'preserves', alcoholic and soft drinks.

DISTRIBUTION

Native to southern Europe, especially southern Spain and southern France; cultivated mainly in Spain, France, Italy

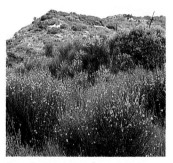

Spartium junceum

and the USA (as a garden shrub). The absolute is produced in southern France.

OTHER SPECIES

Closely related to dyer's greenweed (Genista tinctoria) and the common or green broom (Cytisus scoparius), which flowers in late spring and early summer. There are also several other related species of broom, which are rich in their folk tradition.

EXTRACTION

An absolute is obtained by solvent extraction from the dried flowers.

CHARACTERISTICS

A dark brown, viscous liquid with an intensely sweet, floral, hay-like scent with a herbaceous undertone. It blends well with rose, tuberose, cassie, mimosa, violet, vetiver, and herbaceous-type fragrances.

ACTIONS

Antihemorrhagic, cardioactive, diuretic, cathartic, emmenagogue, narcotic, vasoconstrictor.

PRINCIPAL CONSTITUENTS

The absolute contains capryllic acid, phenols, aliphatics, terpenes, esters, scoparin and sparteine, as well as wax, etc.

Styrax benzoin

Benzoin

FAMILY: STYRACACEAE   **SYNONYMS:** GUM BENZOIN, GUM BENJAMIN, STYRAX BENZOIN

Herbal/Folk Tradition

Used for thousands of years in the East as a medicine and incense. In the West, best known in the form of compound tincture of benzoin or Friars Balsam, used for respiratory complaints. Externally it is used for cuts and irritable skin conditions; internally it is used as a carminative for indigestion, etc.

A large tropical tree up to 20m (65ft) high with pale green citrus-like leaves, whitish underneath, bearing hard-shelled flattish fruit.

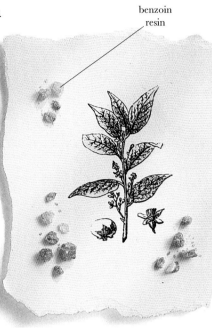

benzoin resin

EXTRACTION
The crude benzoin is collected from the trees directly. Benzoin resinoid, or 'resin absolute', is prepared from the crude using solvents, for example benzene and alcohol, which are then removed. Commercial benzoin is usually sold dissolved in ethyl glycol or a similar solvent. A 'true' absolute is also produced in small quantities.

CHARACTERISTICS
**1. Sumatra crude benzoin occurs as greyish-brown brittle lumps with reddish streaks, with a styrax-like odour. There are several different qualities available; the so-called almond grade is considered superior.
2. Siam benzoin comes in pebble or tear-shaped orange-brown pieces, with a sweet-balsamic vanilla-like scent, this type having a more refined odour than the Sumatra type. Benzoin resinoid is**

produced from either the Siam or Sumatra types, or a mix of the two. It is an orange-brown viscous mass with an intensely rich sweet-balsamic odour. It blends well with sandalwood, rose, jasmine, copaiba balsam, frankincense, myrrh, cypress, juniper, lemon, coriander and other spice oils.

ACTIONS
Anti-inflammatory, anti-oxidant, antiseptic, astringent, carminative, cordial, deodorant, diuretic, expectorant, sedative, styptic, vulnerary.

PRINCIPAL CONSTITUENTS
1. Sumatra Benzoin: mainly coniferyl cinnamate and sumaresinolic acid, with benzoic acid, cinnamic acid, and traces of styrene, vanillin and benzaldehyde. 2. Siam benzoin: mainly coniferyl benzoate (65–75 per cent), with benzoic acid, vanillin, siaresinolic acid and cinnamyl benzoate.

AROMATHERAPY/HOME USE

Skin Care: *Cuts, chapped skin, inflamed and irritated conditions.*
Circulation, Muscles and Joints: *Arthritis, gout, poor circulation, rheumatism.*
Respiratory System: *Asthma, bronchitis, chills, colic, coughs, laryngitis.*
Immune System: *Flu.*
Nervous System: *Nervous tension and stress-related complaints. It warms and tones the heart and circulation, both physically and metaphorically: 'This essence creates a kind of euphoria; it interposes a padded zone between us and events.'* [100]

OTHER USES
Compound benzoin tincture is used in pharmaceuticals and in dentistry to treat gum inflammation. The resinoid and absolute are used extensively as fixatives and fragrance components in soaps, cosmetics, toiletries and perfumes, especially Siam benzoin. Both types are used in most food categories, including alcoholic and soft drinks.

DISTRIBUTION
Native to tropical Asia; the two main regions of production are Sumatra, Java and Malaysia for 'Sumatra' benzoin, and Laos, Vietnam, Cambodia, China and Thailand for 'Siam' benzoin.

OTHER SPECIES
There are many different varieties within the Styrax family that produce benzoin, but these are generally classified under either Sumatra benzoin (S. paralleloneurus) or Siam benzoin (S. tonkinensis). See also Botanical Classification section.

Syzygium aromaticum

Clove

FAMILY: MYRTACEAE **SYNONYMS:** *EUGENIA AROMATICA, E. CARYOPHYLLATA, E. CARYOPHYLLUS*

Herbal/Folk Tradition

Extensively used as a domestic spice worldwide. Tincture of cloves has been used for skin infections (scabies, athlete's foot); for digestive upsets; to dress the umbilical cord; for intestinal parasites; to ease the pain of childbirth (steeped in wine); and notably for toothache. The tea is used to relieve nausea.

In Chinese medicine the oil is used for diarrhea, hernia, bad breath and bronchitis as well as for those conditions mentioned above.

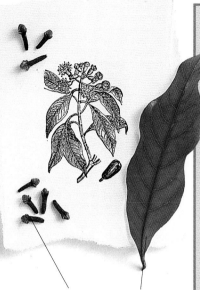

dried cloves   fresh leaf

A slender evergreen tree with a smooth grey trunk, up to 12m (39ft) high. It has large bright green leaves standing in pairs on short stalks. At the start of the rainy season long buds appear with a rosy-pink corolla at the tip; as the corolla fades the calyx slowly turns deep red. These are beaten from the tree and, when dried, provide the cloves of commerce.

AROMATHERAPY/ HOME USE

Only use clove bud oil, not the leaf or stem oil.
Skin Care: *Acne, athlete's foot, bruises, burns, cuts, insect repellent (mosquito), toothache, ulcers, wounds.*
Circulation, Muscles and Joints: *Arthritis, rheumatism, sprains.*
Respiratory System: *Asthma, bronchitis.*
Digestive System: *Colic, dyspepsia, nausea.*
Immune System: *Colds, flu, minor infections.*

OTHER USES

Used in dental preparations, and as a fragrance component in toothpastes, soaps, toiletries, cosmetics and perfumes.

Extensively employed as a flavour ingredient in major food categories, alcoholic and soft drinks. Used in the production of printing ink, glue and varnish; clove leaf oil is used as the starting material for the isolation of eugenol.

DISTRIBUTION

Believed to be native to Indonesia; now cultivated worldwide, especially in the Philippines, the Molucca Islands and Madagascar. The main oil-producing countries are Madagascar and Indonesia.

OTHER SPECIES

The clove tree has been cultivated in plantations for over 2,000 years. The original wild trees in the Moluccas produce an essential oil that contains no eugenol at all.

EXTRACTION

Essential oil by water distillation from 1. the buds and 2. the leaves, and by steam distillation from 3. the stalks or stems. A concrete, absolute and oleoresin are also produced from the buds in small quantities.

CHARACTERISTICS

1. Clove bud is a pale yellow liquid with a sweet-spicy odour and a fruity-fresh top note. The bud oil is favoured in perfumery work. It blends well with rose, lavender, vanillin, clary sage, bergamot, bay leaf, lavandin, allspice, ylang ylang and cananga. 2. Clove leaf is a dark brown oil with a crude, burnt-woody odour. 3. Clove stem oil is a pale yellow liquid with a strong spicy-woody odour.

ACTIONS

Anthelminthic, antibiotic, anti-emetic, antihistaminic, antirheumatic, antineuralgic, anti-oxidant, antiseptic, antiviral, aphrodisiac, carminative, counter-irritant, expectorant, larvicidal, spasmolytic, stimulant, stomachic, vermifuge.

PRINCIPAL CONSTITUENTS

1. Bud: 60–90 per cent eugenol, eugenol acetate, caryophyllene and other minor constituents. 2. Leaf: 82–88 per cent eugenol with little or no eugenol acetate, and other minor constituents. 3. Stem: 90–95 per cent eugenol, with other minor constituents.

Tagetes minuta

Tagetes

> **SAFETY DATA** *'It is quite possible that "tagetone" (the main constituent) is harmful to the human organism.'*[101] *Some reported cases of dermatitis with the tagetes species. Use with care, in moderation*

FAMILY: ASTERACEAE (COMPOSITAE) **SYNONYMS:** *T. GLANDULIFERA*, TAGETTE, TAGET, MARIGOLD, MEXICAN MARIGOLD, WRONGLY CALLED 'CALENDULA' (OIL)

Herbal/Folk Tradition

In India the locally grown flowering tops of the French marigold are distilled into a receiver that contains a solvent, often sandalwood oil, to produce 'attar genda' – a popular Indian perfume material. In China the flowers of the African marigold are used for whooping cough, colds, colic, mumps, sore eyes and mastitis – usually as a decoction.

A strongly scented annual herb about 30cm (12in) high with bright orange, daisy-like flowers and soft green oval leaves.

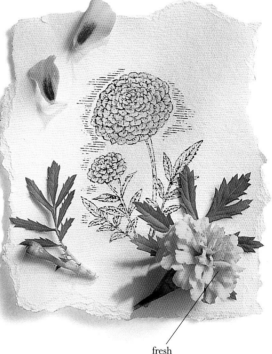

fresh tagetes flower

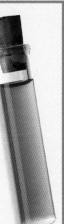

EXTRACTION
1. An essential oil by steam distillation from the fresh flowering herb. 2. An absolute (and concrete) by solvent extraction from the fresh flowering herb.

CHARACTERISTICS
1. A dark orange or yellow mobile liquid that slowly solidifies on exposure to air and light, with a bitter-green, herby odour. 2. An orange, olive or brown semi-liquid mass with an intense, sweet, green-fruity odour. It blends well with clary sage, lavender, jasmine, bergamot and other citrus oils in very small percentages.

ACTIONS
Anthelminthic, antispasmodic, bactericidal, carminative, diaphoretic, emmenagogue, fungicidal, stomachic.

PRINCIPAL CONSTITUENTS
Mainly tagetones, with ocimene, myrcene, linalol, limonene, pinenes, carvone, citral, camphene, valeric acid and salicylaldehyde, among others.

AROMATHERAPY/ HOME USE

Skin Care: *Bunions, calluses, corns, fungal infections.*

OTHER USES

Used in some pharmaceutical products. The absolute and oil are employed to a limited extent in herbaceous and floral perfumes. Used for flavouring tobacco and in most major food categories, including alcoholic and soft drinks.

DISTRIBUTION

Native in South America and Mexico. Now grows wild in Africa, Europe, Asia and North America. The oil is produced mainly in South Africa, France,

Argentina and Egypt, the absolute in Nigeria and France.

OTHER SPECIES

There are several other types of tagetes that share similar characteristics and are used to produce essential oils, notably the French marigold (T. patula) and the African or Aztec marigold (T. erecta) – see also Botanical Classification section. NB: Not to be confused with the 'pot' marigold (Calendula officinalis), which has very different properties and constituents and is used extensively in herbal medicine (and occasionally to make an absolute). See entry on marigold.

Tanacetum vulgare

Tansy

FAMILY: ASTERACEAE (COMPOSITAE) **SYNONYMS:** *CHRYSANTHEMUM VULGARE, C. TANACETUM,* BUTTONS, BITTER BUTTONS, BACHELOR'S BUTTONS, SCENTED FERN, CHEESE

Herbal/Folk Tradition

Traditionally used to flavour eggs and omelettes. It has a long history of medicinal use, especially among gypsies, and is regarded as something of a 'cure all'. It was used to expel worms, to treat colds and fever, prevent possible miscarriage and ease dyspepsia and cramping pains. Externally, the distilled water was used to keep the complexion pale, and the bruised leaves employed as a remedy for scabies, bruises, sprains and rheumatism. It was also used generally for nervous disorders and to keep flies and vermin away.

Tansy flowers are still current in the British Herbal Pharmacopoeia as a specific (used externally) for worms in children.

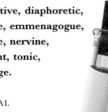

fresh
tansy

A hardy perennial wayside herb, up to 1m (3ft) high with a smooth stem, dark ferny leaves and small, round brilliant yellow flowers borne in clusters. The whole plant is strongly scented.

AROMATHERAPY/ HOME USE

None. 'Should not be used in aromatherapy whether internally or externally.' [102]

OTHER USES

Occasionally used in herbaceous-type perfumes. The oil was formerly used in alcoholic drinks – it is no longer used for flavouring.

DISTRIBUTION

Native to central Europe; naturalized in North America and now found in most temperate regions of the world. The essential oil is produced mainly in France, Germany, Hungary, Poland and the USA.

OTHER SPECIES

Closely related to the medicinal herb feverfew (Tanacetum parthenium), the marigolds and daisy family.

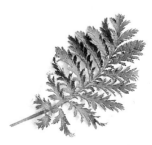

Tanacetum vulgare

EXTRACTION
Essential oil by steam distillation from the whole herb (aerial parts).

CHARACTERISTICS
A yellow, olive or orange liquid (darkening with age) with a warm, sharp-spicy herbaceous odour.

ACTIONS
Anthelminthic, anti-inflammatory, antispasmodic, **carminative, diaphoretic, digestive, emmenagogue, febrifuge, nervine, stimulant, tonic, vermifuge.**

PRINCIPAL CONSTITUENTS
Thujone (66–81 per cent), camphor, borneol, among others.

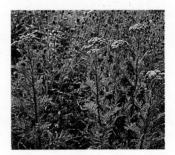

Thuja occidentalis

Thuja

SAFETY DATA *Oral toxin – poisonous due to high thujone content. Abortifacient*

FAMILY: CUPRESSACEAE SYNONYMS: SWAMP CEDAR, WHITE CEDAR, NORTHERN WHITE CEDAR, EASTERN WHITE CEDAR, TREE OF LIFE, AMERICAN ARBORVITAE, CEDARLEAF (OIL)

Herbal/Folk Tradition

Used as an incense by ancient civilizations for ritual purposes. A decoction of leaves has been used for coughs, fever, intestinal parasites, cystitis and venereal diseases. The ointment has been used for rheumatism, gout, warts, veruccae, psoriasis and other ailments.

The twigs are current in the British Herbal Pharmacopoeia, used specifically for bronchitis with cardiac weakness, and warts.

EXTRACTION
Essential oil by steam distillation from the leaves, twigs and bark.

CHARACTERISTICS
A colourless to pale yellowy-green liquid with a sharp, fresh, camphoraceous odour.

ACTIONS
Antirheumatic, astringent, diuretic, emmenagogue, expectorant, insect repellent, rubefacient, stimulant (nerves, uterus and heart muscles), tonic, vermifuge.

PRINCIPAL CONSTITUENTS
Thujone (approx. 60 per cent), fenchone, camphor, sabinene and pinene, among others.

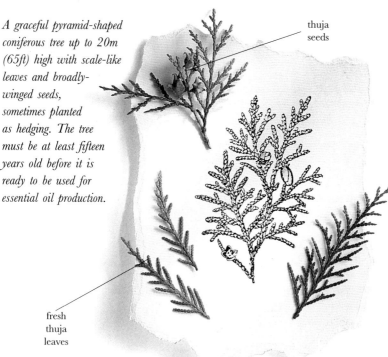

A graceful pyramid-shaped coniferous tree up to 20m (65ft) high with scale-like leaves and broadly-winged seeds, sometimes planted as hedging. The tree must be at least fifteen years old before it is ready to be used for essential oil production.

thuja seeds

fresh thuja leaves

AROMATHERAPY/HOME USE

None. 'Should not be used in aromatherapy either internally or externally.' [103]

OTHER USES

Used in pharmaceutical products such as disinfectants and sprays; also as a counter-irritant in analgesic ointments and liniments. A fragrance component in some toiletries and perfumes. Employed as a flavour ingredient in most major food categories (provided that the finished food is recognized thujone-free).

DISTRIBUTION

Native to north-eastern North America; cultivated in France. The oil is produced mainly in Canada and the USA, similar oils are also produced in the East – see below.

OTHER SPECIES

There are many forms and cultivated varieties of this tree: the western red cedar or Washington cedar (T. plicata); the Chinese or Japanese cedar (T. orientalis or Biota orientalis); the North African variety (T. articulata), which yields a resin known as 'sanderac'.
The hiba tree (Thujopsis dolobrata) is used to produce hiba wood oil and hiba leaf oil in Japan. Hiba wood oil, according to available data, is non-toxic, non-irritant and non-sensitizing (unlike the other thuja oils), and has excellent resistance to fungi and bacteria due to the ketonic substances found in the oil. It is used extensively in Japan as an industrial perfume.

Thymus capitatus

Spanish oregano

SAFETY DATA *Dermal toxin, skin irritant, mucous membrane irritant*

FAMILY: LAMIACEAE (LABIATAE) **SYNONYMS:** *T. CAPITANS, CORIDOTHYMUS CAPITATUS, SATUREJA CAPITATA, THYMBRA CAPITATA,* OREGANUM (OIL), ISRAELI OREGANUM (OIL), CRETAN THYME, CORIDO THYME, CONEHEAD THYME, HEADED SAVORY, THYME OF THE ANCIENTS

Herbal/Folk Tradition

According to Mrs Grieve the properties and oil of Spanish oregano (*Thymus capitatus*) are similar to the common thyme (*T. vulgaris*); it also shares many qualities with the common oregano or wild marjoram (*Origanum vulgare*).

A perennial creeping herb with a woody stem, small dark green leaves and pink or white flowers borne in clusters.

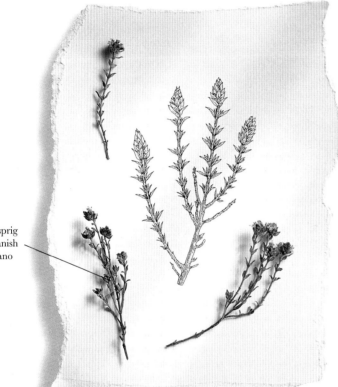

fresh sprig of Spanish oregano

AROMATHERAPY/ HOME USE

None. 'Should not be used on the skin at all.' [104]

OTHER USES

Used as a fragrance component in soaps, colognes and perfumes, especially men's fragrances. Employed to some extent as a flavouring agent, mainly in meat products and pizzas.

DISTRIBUTION

Native to the Middle East and Asia Minor; grows wild in Spain. The oil is produced mainly in Spain, Israel, Lebanon, Syria and Turkey.

OTHER SPECIES

Although this herb is strictly a thyme, it serves as the source for most so-called oregano oil. For other related species see entries on common thyme, common oregano and sweet marjoram; see also Botanical Classification section.

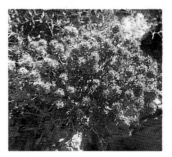

Thymus capitatus

EXTRACTION
Essential oil by steam distillation from the dried flowering tops.

CHARACTERISTICS
A dark brownish-red or purple oil with a strong tar-like, herbaceous, refreshing odour.

ACTIONS
See common oregano.

PRINCIPAL CONSTITUENTS
Carvacrol, thymol, cymene, caryophyllene, pinene, limonene, linalol, borneol, myrcene, thujone, terpinene.

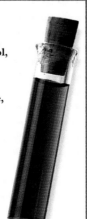

Thymus vulgaris

Common thyme

FAMILY: LAMIACEAE (LABIATAE) **SYNONYMS:** *T. AESTIVUS,*
T. ILERDENSIS, T. WEBBIANUS, T. VALENTIANUS, FRENCH THYME,
GARDEN THYME, RED THYME (OIL), WHITE THYME (OIL)

Herbal/Folk Tradition

One of the earliest
medicinal plants in
Western herbal medicine,
its main areas of
application are respiratory
problems, digestive
complaints and the
prevention and treatment
of infection. In the British
Herbal Pharmacopoeia it
is indicated for dyspepsia,
chronic gastritis,
bronchitis, pertussis,
asthma, children's
diarrhea, laryngitis,
tonsillitis and enuresis in children.

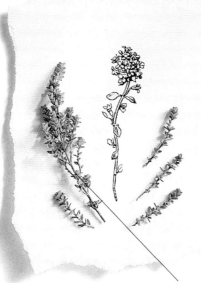

fresh thyme

*A perennial evergreen subshrub up to 45cm(18in) high with a woody root and much-
branched stem. It has grey-green, aromatic leaves and pale purple or white flowers.*

SAFETY DATA *Contra-indicated in cases
of high blood pressure. Red thyme oil, serpolet
(from wild thyme), 'thymol' and 'carvacrol' type
oils all contain quite large amounts of toxic
phenols (carvacrol and thymol). See below. White
thyme is not a 'complete' oil and is often
adulterated. Lemon thyme and 'linalol' types
are in general less toxic, non-irritant, with
less possibility of sensitization – safe for use
on the skin and with children.*

EXTRACTION
**Essential oil by water or steam
distillation from the fresh or
partially dried leaves and
flowering tops. 1. 'Red thyme
oil' is the crude distillate.
2. 'White thyme oil' is
produced by further
redistillation or rectification.
(An absolute is also produced
in France by solvent extraction
for perfumery use.)**

CHARACTERISTICS
**1. A red, brown or orange
liquid with a warm, spicy-
herbaceous, powerful odour.
2. A clear, pale yellow liquid
with a sweet, green-fresh,
milder scent. It blends well
with bergamot, lemon,
rosemary, melissa, lavender,
lavandin, marjoram, Peru
balsam, pine, etc.**

ACTIONS
**Anthelminthic, antimicrobial,
anti-oxidant, antiputrescent,
antirheumatic, antiseptic**
**(intestinal, pulmonary,
genito-urinary), antispasmodic,
antitussive, antitoxic, aperitif,
astringent, aphrodisiac,
bactericidal, balsamic,
carminative, cicatrizant,
diuretic, emmenagogue,
nervine, revulsive, rubefacient,
parasiticide, stimulant
(immune system, circulation),
sudorific, tonic, vermifuge.**

PRINCIPAL
CONSTITUENTS
**Thymol and carvacrol
(up to 60 per cent),
cymene, terpinene,
camphene, borneol, linalol;
depending on the source it
can also contain geraniol,
citral and thuyanol, etc.
There are many chemotypes
of thyme oil: notably the
'thymol' and 'carvacrol' types
(warming and active); the
'thuyanol' type (penetrating
and antiviral); and the milder
'linalol' or 'citral' types (sweet-
scented, non-irritant).**

AROMATHERAPY/ HOME USE

*Can irritate mucous membranes,
cause dermal irritation and may
cause sensitization in some
individuals. Use in moderation,
in low dilution only. Best
avoided during pregnancy.*
Skin Care: *Abscess, acne,
bruises, burns, cuts, dermatitis,
eczema, insect bites, lice, gum
infections, oily skin, scabies.*
**Circulation, Muscles and
Joints:** *Arthritis, cellulitis, gout,
muscular aches and pains, obesity,
edema, poor circulation, rheumatism,
sprains, sports injuries.*
Respiratory System:
*Asthma, bronchitis, catarrh,
coughs, laryngitis, sinusitis,
sore throat, tonsillitis.*
Digestive System:
Diarrhea, dyspepsia, flatuence.
Genito-urinary System:
Cystitis, urethritis.
Immune System: *Chills,
colds, flu, infectious diseases.*
Nervous System: *Headaches,
insomnia, nervous debility and
stress-related complaints.*

OTHER USES

*The oil is used in mouthwashes,
gargles, toothpastes and cough
lozenges. 'Thymol' is used in
surgical dressings, disinfectants, etc.
Used as a fragrance component in
soaps, toiletries, aftershaves, etc.
Extensively employed by the food
and drink industry.*

DISTRIBUTION

*Native to Spain and the
Mediterranean region; now
found throughout Asia Minor,
Algeria, Turkey, Tunisia,
Israel, the USA, Russia, China
and central Europe.*

Tilia x *vulgaris*
Linden

FAMILY: TILIACEAE **SYNONYMS:** *T.* x *EUROPAEA*, LIME TREE, COMMON LIME, LYNE, TILLET, TILEA

Herbal/Folk Tradition

Linden tea, known as 'tilleul', is drunk a great deal in continental Europe, especially in France, as a general relaxant. The flowers are also used for indigestion, palpitations, nausea, hysteria and catarrhal symptoms following a cold. The honey from the flowers is highly regarded, and used in medicines and liqueurs. According to Culpeper the flowers are a 'good cephalic and nervine, excellent for apoplexy, epilepsy, vertigo and palpitation of the heart'. [105] Lime flowers are current in the British Herbal Pharmacopoeia, indicated for migraine, hysteria, arteriosclerotic hypertension and feverish colds.

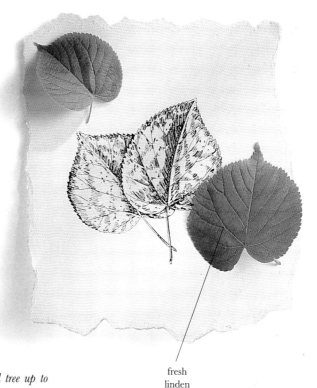

fresh
linden

A tall graceful tree up to 30m (98ft) high with a smooth bark, spreading branches and bright green, heart-shaped leaves. It has yellowy-white flowers borne in clusters, which have a very powerful scent.

EXTRACTION
A concrete and absolute by solvent extraction from the dried flowers.

CHARACTERISTICS
The concrete is a hard, brittle, dark green mass with a herbaceous, dry, hay-like odour. The absolute is a yellow semi-solid mass with a green-herbaceous, dry, characteristic odour.

ACTIONS
Astringent (mild), antispasmodic, bechic, carminative, cephalic, diaphoretic, diuretic, emollient, nervine, sedative, tonic.

PRINCIPAL CONSTITUENTS
Mainly farnesol – the concrete is very rich in waxes.

AROMATHERAPY/ HOME USE

Digestive System: *Cramps, indigestion, liver pains.*
Nervous System: *Headaches, insomnia, migraine, nervous tension and stress-related conditions.*

OTHER USES
Occasionally used in high-class perfumery.

DISTRIBUTION
Native to Europe and the northern hemisphere. Common in Britain, France, the Netherlands, etc.

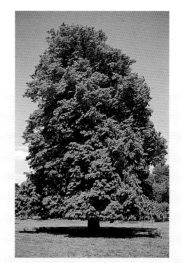

Tilia x *vulgaris*

OTHER SPECIES
Several related types such as the broad-leaved lime (T. platyphyllos) and the small-leaved lime (T. cordata).

Trachyspermum copticum

Ajowan

FAMILY: APIACEAE (UMBELLIFERAE) **SYNONYMS:** *T. AMMI, AMMI COPTICUM, CARUM AJOWAN, C. COPTICUM, PTYCHOTIS AJOWAN,* AJUAN, OMUM, AJVAN, TRUE BISHOP'S WEED.

Herbal/Folk Tradition

The seeds are used extensively in curry powders and as a general household remedy for intestinal problems. The tincture, essential oil and 'thymol' are used in Indian medicine, particular for cholera. The oil, which is sometimes know as 'Oman water', is also used as an antiseptic and to aid digestion. The crushed seeds are dried for use in scented powders and pot pourri. Almost the whole of the export of ajowan seed from India, Egypt, Persia and Afghanistan went to Germany for the distillation of the oil and extraction of thymol, the annual export of the seed from India being about 1,200 ton(ne)s. On the outbreak of war the export of ajowan seed dropped to 2 ton(ne)s per month and there was a shortage of thymol, an excellent antiseptic, just when it was needed.

An annual herb with a greyish-brown seed, which resembles parsley in appearance. It has bright green leaves and an erect habit of growth usually not exceeding 50cm (20in) in height. It is an umbelliferous plant, a kind of Indian caraway, being widely cultivated in India for medicinal properties.

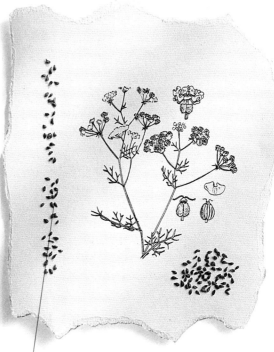

ajowan
seeds

AROMATHERAPY/ HOME USE

Not recommended.

OTHER USES

It has been used extensively for the isolation of thymol, but this has largely been replaced by synthetic thymol. Thymol finds no place in perfumery but the residual oil, after extracting the crystalline thymol from ajowan oil, which amounts to about 50 per cent of the original oil, is generally sold as a cheap perfume for soap-making and similar purposes under the name 'Thymene'. The oil is occasionally used in the production of soap.

DISTRIBUTION

Chiefly India, also Afghanistan, Egypt, the West Indies and the Seychelle Islands.

OTHER SPECIES

See Botanical Classification section.

EXTRACTION
Essential oil by steam distillation from the seed.

CHARACTERISTICS
A yellow-orange or reddish liquid with a herbaceous-spicy medicinal odour, much like thyme.

ACTIONS
Powerful antiseptic and germicide, carminative.

PRINCIPAL CONSTITUENTS
Thymol, pinene, cymene, dipentene, terpinene and carvacrol, among others. Ajowan contains 40–55 per cent of thymol. The extraction of thymol is produced by treating the oil with a warm solution of sodium hydroxide; this alkali dissolves the thymol and on dilution with hot water the undissolved oil (terpenes, etc.) rises to the surface.

Tsuga canadensis

Hemlock spruce

SAFETY DATA *Non-toxic, non-irritant, non-sensitizing*

FAMILY: PINACEAE **SYNONYMS:** *PINUS CANADENSIS*, *ABIES CANADENSIS*, SPRUCE, EASTERN HEMLOCK, COMMON HEMLOCK, HEMLOCK (OIL), SPRUCE (OIL), FIR NEEDLE (OIL)

Herbal/Folk Tradition

The bark of the hemlock spruce (which contains tannins and resin as well as volatile oil) is current in the British Herbal Pharmacopoeia indicated for diarrhea, cystitis, mucous colitis, leucorrhea, uterine prolapse, pharyngitis, stomatitis and gingivitis. An extract of the bark is also used in the tanning industry.

A large evergreen tree up to 50m (164ft) tall, with slender horizontal branches, finely toothed leaves and smallish brown cones, which yields a natural exudation from its bark.

newly formed cones

fresh hemlock spruce

fresh leaves

EXTRACTION
Essential oil by steam distillation from the needles and twigs.

CHARACTERISTICS
A colourless or pale yellow liquid with a pleasing, fresh-balsamic, sweet-fruity odour. It blends well with pine, oakmoss, cedarwood, galbanum, benzoin, lavender, lavandin and rosemary.

ACTIONS
Antimicrobial, antiseptic, antitussive, astringent, diaphoretic, diuretic, expectorant, nervine, rubefacients, tonic.

PRINCIPAL CONSTITUENTS
Mainly pinenes, limonene, bornyl acetate, tricyclene, phellandrene, myrcrene, thujone, dipentene and cadinene, among others. Constituents vary according to source and exact botanical species (sometimes mixed).

AROMATHERAPY/ HOME USE

Circulation, Muscles and Joints: *Muscular aches and pains, poor circulation, rheumatism.*
Respiratory System: *Asthma, bronchitis, coughs, respiratory weakness.*
Immune System: *Colds, flu, infections.*
Nervous System: *Anxiety, stress-related conditions – 'opening and elevating though grounding . . . excellent for yoga and meditation'.[106]*

OTHER USES

Used in veterinary liniments. Extensively used for room spray perfumes, household detergents, soaps, bath preparations and toiletries, especially in the USA.

DISTRIBUTION

Native to the west coast of the USA. The oil is produced in Vermont, New York, New Hampshire, Virginia and Wisconsin.

OTHER SPECIES

Numerous cultivars of this species exist; often the oil is produced from a mixture of different types. Similar oils, also called simply 'spruce oil', are produced from the black spruce (Picea nigra or P. mariana), the Norway spruce (P. abies) and the white or Canadian spruce (P. glauca). The essential oil from the western hemlock (Tsuga heterophylla) contains quite different constituents. Hemlock spruce is also closely related to the Douglas fir (Pseudotsuga taxifolia), which is also used to produce an essential oil and a balsam.

Valeriana fauriei

Valerian

FAMILY: VALERIANACEAE **SYNONYMS:** *V. OFFICINALIS, V. OFFICINALIS VAR. ANGUSTIFOLIUM, V. OFFICINALIS VAR. LATIFOLIA,* EUROPEAN VALERIAN, COMMON VALERIAN, BELGIAN VALERIAN, FRAGRANT VALERIAN, GARDEN VALERIAN

Herbal/Folk Tradition

This herb has been highly esteemed since medieval times, and used to be called 'all heal'. It has been used in the West for a variety of complaints, especially where there is nervous tension or restlessness, such as insomnia, migraine, dysmenorrhea, intestinal colic, rheumatism, and as a pain reliever.

In Europe the oil has been used for cholera, epilepsy and for skin complaints. In China it is used for backache, colds, menstrual problems, bruises and sores.

The root is current in the British Herbal Pharmacopoeia as a specific for 'conditions presenting nervous excitability'.[107]

A perennial herb up to 1.5m (5ft) high with a hollow, erect stem, deeply dissected dark leaves and many purplish-white flowers. It has short, thick, greyish roots, largely showing above ground, which have a strong odour.

root of
valerian

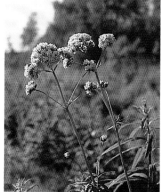

Valeriana fauriei

AROMATHERAPY/ HOME USE

Nervous System: *Insomia, nervous indigestion, migraine, restlessness and tension states.*

OTHER USES

Used in pharmaceutical preparations as a relaxant and in herbal teas. The oil and absolute are used as fragrance components in soaps and in 'moss' and 'forest' fragrances. Used to flavour tobacco, root beer, liqueurs and apple flavourings.

DISTRIBUTION

Native to Europe and parts of Asia; naturalized in North America. It is cultivated mainly in Belgium for its oil, also in France, the Netherlands, Britain, Scandinavia, former Yugoslavia, Hungary, China and Russia.

OTHER SPECIES

*There are over 150 species of valerian found in different parts of the world. The Eastern varieties are slightly different from the Western types: the oil from the Japanese plant called 'kesso root' (*V. officinalis*) is more woody; the oil from the Indian valerian (*V. wallichii*) is more musky. Also closely related to spikenard (*Nardostachus jatamansi*) – see entry.*

EXTRACTION

1. Essential oil by steam distillation from the rhizomes. 2. An absolute (and concrete) by solvent extraction of the rhizomes.

CHARACTERISTICS

1. An olive to brown liquid (darkening with age) with a warm-woody, balsamic, musky odour; a green top note in fresh oils. 2. An olive-brown viscous liquid with a balsamic-green, woody bitter-sweet strong odour. It blends well with patchouli, costus, oakmoss, pine, lavender, cedarwood, mandarin, petitgrain and rosemary.

ACTIONS

Anodyne (mild), antidandruff, diuretic, antispasmodic, bactericidal, carminative, depressant of the central nervous system, hypnotic, hypotensive, regulator, sedative, stomachic.

PRINCIPAL CONSTITUENTS

Mainly bornyl acetate and isovalerate, with caryophyllene, pinenes, valeranone, ionone, eugenyl isovalerate, borneol, patchouli alcohol and valerianal, among others.

Vanilla planifolia

Vanilla

FAMILY: ORCHIDACEAE **SYNONYMS:** *V. FRAGRANS*, COMMON VANILLA, MEXICAN VANILLA, BOURBON VANILLA, REUNION VANILLA

Herbal/Folk Tradition

When vanilla is grown in cultivation the deep trumpet-shaped flowers have to be hand-pollinated – except in Mexico where the native humming birds do most of the work!

EXTRACTION

A resinoid (often called an oleoresin) by solvent extraction from the 'cured' vanilla beans. (An absolute is occasionally produced by further extraction from the resinoid.)

CHARACTERISTICS

A viscous dark brown liquid with a rich, sweet, balsamic, vanilla-like odour. It blends well with sandalwood, vetiver, opopanax, benzoin, balsams and spice oils.

ACTIONS

Balsamic.

PRINCIPAL CONSTITUENTS

Vanillin (1.3–2.9 per cent) with over 150 other constituents, many of them traces: hydroxybenzaldehyde, acetic acid, isobutyric acid, caproic acid, eugenol and furfural, among others.

AROMATHERAPY/ HOME USE

None.

OTHER USES

Used in pharmaceutical products as a flavouring agent. Used as a fragrance ingredient in perfumes, especially oriental types. Widely used to flavour tobacco and as a food flavouring, mainly ice-cream, yoghurt and chocolate.

DISTRIBUTION

Native to Central America and Mexico; cultivated mainly in Madagascar and Mexico; also Tahiti, the Comoro Islands, East Africa and Indonesia, although the pods are often processed in Europe or the USA.

OTHER SPECIES

There are several different species of vanilla, such as the Tahiti vanilla (V. tahitensis), which is a smaller bean, and the 'vanillons' type (V. pompona), which produces an oil of inferior quality.

A perennial herbaceous climbing vine up to 25m (82ft) high, with green stems and large white flowers that have a deep narrow trumpet. The green capsules or fruits are ready to pick after eight or nine months on the plant, and then have to be 'cured'. The immature vanilla 'pod' or 'bean', which is from 14–22cm (5.5–9in) long, has to be fermented and dried to turn it into the fragrant brown vanilla pods of commerce – a process that can take up to six months to complete. During the drying process vanillin can accumulate as white crystals on the surface of the bean.

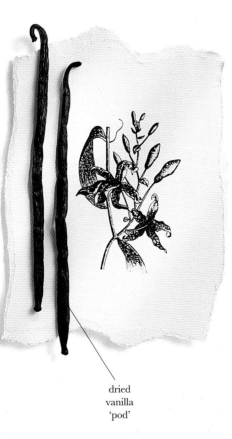

dried
vanilla
'pod'

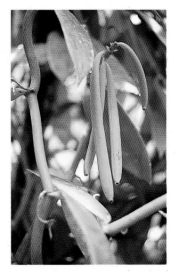

Vanilla planifolia

Vetiveria zizanioides

Vetiver

FAMILY: POACEAE (GRAMINEAE)   **SYNONYMS:** *ANDROPOGON MURICATUS*, VETIVERT, KHUS KHUS

Herbal/Folk Tradition

The rootlets have been used in the East for their fine fragrance since antiquity. They are used by the locals to protect domestic animals from vermin, and the fibres of the grass are woven into aromatic matting. It is grown in India to protect against soil erosion during the tropical rainy season.

In India and Sri Lanka the essence is known as 'the oil of tranquillity'.

A tall, tufted, perennial, scented grass, with a straight stem, long narrow leaves and an abundant complex lacework of underground white rootlets.

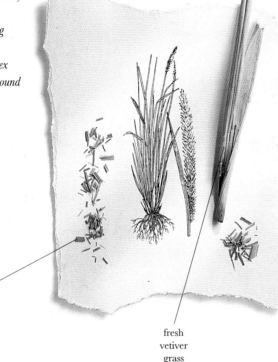

dried
vetiver
grass

fresh
vetiver
grass

EXTRACTION
Essential oil by steam distillation from the roots and rootlets – washed, chopped, dried and soaked. (A resinoid is also produced by solvent extraction for perfumery work.)

CHARACTERISTICS
A dark brown, olive or amber viscous oil with a deep smoky, earthy-woody odour with a sweet persistent undertone. The colour and scent can vary according to the source – Angola produces a very pale oil with a dry-woody odour. It blends well with sandalwood, rose, violet, jasmine, opopanax, patchouli, oakmoss, lavander, clary sage, mimosa, cassie and ylang ylang.

ACTIONS
Antiseptic, antispasmodic, depurative, ruberfacient, sedative (nervous system), stimulant (circulatory, production of red corpuscles), tonic, vermifuge.

PRINCIPAL CONSTITUENTS
Vetiverol, vitivone, terpenes, e.g. vetivenes, among others.

AROMATHERAPY/ HOME USE

Skin Care: *Acne, cuts, oily skin, wounds.*

Circulation, Muscles and Joints: *Arthritis, muscular aches and pains, rheumatism, sprains, stiffness.*

Nervous System: *Debility, depression, insomnia, nervous tension – 'Vetiver is deeply relaxing, so valuable in massage and baths for anybody experiencing stress.'[108]*

OTHER USES

Employed as a fixative and fragrance ingredient in soaps, cosmetics and perfumes, especially oriental types. The oil is used in food preservatives, especially for asparagus.

DISTRIBUTION

Native to south India, Indonesia and Sri Lanka. Also cultivated in Reunion, the Philippines, the Comoro Islands, Japan, West Africa and South America. The oil is produced mainly in Java, Haiti and Reunion; some is distilled in Europe and the USA.

OTHER SPECIES

Botanically related to lemongrass, citronella, litsea cubeba and flouve oil (also from the roots of a tropical grass).

Viola odorata

Violet

SAFETY DATA *Non-toxic, non-irritant, possible sensitization in some individuals*

FAMILY: VIOLACEAE   **SYNONYMS:** ENGLISH VIOLET, GARDEN VIOLET, BLUE VIOLET, SWEET-SCENTED VIOLET

Herbal/Folk Tradition

Both the leaf and flowers have a long tradition of use in herbal medicine, mainly for congestive pulmonary conditions and sensitive skin conditions, including capillary fragility. The leaf has also been used to treat cystitis and as a mouthwash for infections of the mouth and throat. It is reported to have mild pain-killing properties, probably due to the presence of salicylic acid (as in 'aspirin').

The flowers are still used to make a 'syrup of violet', which is used as a laxative and colouring agent. The dried leaf and flowers are current in the British Herbal Pharmacopoeia as a specific for 'eczema and skin eruptions with serious exudate, particularly when associated with rheumatic symptoms'.[109]

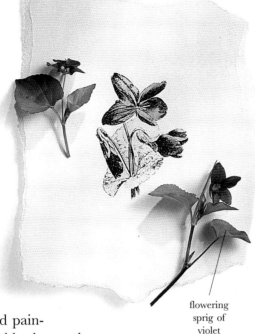

flowering sprig of violet

A small, tender, perennial plant with dark green, heart-shaped leaves, fragrant violet-blue flowers and an oblique underground rhizome.

EXTRACTION
A concrete and absolute from 1. fresh leaves, and 2. flowers.

CHARACTERISTICS
1. The leaf absolute is an intense dark green viscous liquid with a strong green-leaf odour and a delicate floral undertone.
2. The flower absolute is a yellowish-green viscous liquid with a sweet, rich, floral fragrance, characteristic of the fresh flowers. It blends well with tuberose, clary sage, boronia, tarragon, cumin, hop, basil, hyacinth and other florals.

ACTIONS
Analgestic (mild), anti-inflammatory, antirheumatic, antiseptic, decongestant (liver), diuretic, expectorant, laxative, soporific, stimulant (circulation).

PRINCIPAL CONSTITUENTS
Both leaves and petals contain nonadienal, parmone, hexyl alcohol, bezyl alcohol, ionone and viola quercitin, among others.

AROMATHERAPY/ HOME USE

Skin Care: *Acne, eczema, refines the pores, thread veins, wounds.*
Circulation, Muscles and Joints: *Fibrosis, poor circulation, rheumatism.*
Respiratory System: *Bronchitis, catarrh, mouth and throat infections.*
Nervous System: *Dizziness, headaches, insomnia, nervous exhaustion – the scent was believed to 'comfort and strengthen the heart'.[110]*

OTHER USES

Used in high-class perfumery work; occasionally used in flavouring, mainly confectionery.

DISTRIBUTION

Native to Europe and parts of Asia; cultivated in gardens worldwide. It is grown mainly in southern France (Grasse) and to a lesser extent in Italy and China for perfumery use.

OTHER SPECIES

There are over 200 species of violet; the main types cultivated for aromatic extraction are the 'Parma' and the 'Victoria' violets.

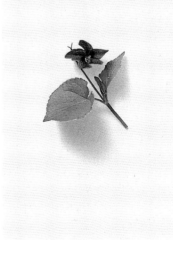

Zingiber officinale

Ginger

FAMILY: ZINGIBERACEAE **SYNONYMS:** COMMON GINGER, JAMAICA GINGER

Herbal/Folk Tradition

Ginger has been used as a domestic spice and as a remedy for thousands of years, especially in the East. Fresh ginger is used in China for many complaints including rheumatism, bacterial dysentery, toothache, malaria, and for cold and moist conditions such as excess mucus and diarrhea.

It is best known as a digestive aid, especially in the West: in the British Herbal Pharmacopoeia it is specifically indicated for flatulent intestinal colic. Preserved and crystallized ginger is a popular confectionery, in the East and West.

An erect perennial herb up to 1m (3ft) high with a thick, spreading, tuberous rhizome root, which is very pungent. Each year it sends up a green reed-like stalk with narrow spear-shaped leaves and white or yellow flowers on a spike direct from the root.

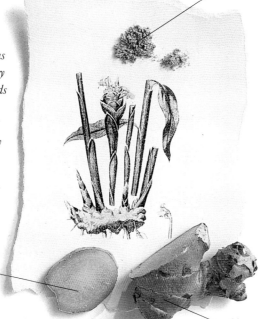

ground ginger

section of root

rhizome root

AROMATHERAPY/ HOME USE

Circulation, Muscles and Joints: *Arthritis, fatigue, muscular aches and pains, poor circulation, rheumatism, sprains, strains, etc.*
Respiratory System: *Catarrh, congestion, coughs, sinusitis, sore throat.*
Digestive System: *Diarrhea, colic, cramp, flatulence, indigestion, loss of appetite, nausea, travel sickness.*

Nervous System: *Debility, nervous exhaustion.*

OTHER USES

The oleoresin is used in digestive, carminative and laxative preparations; used as a fragrance component in cosmetics and perfumes, especially oriental and men's fragrances; extensively employed in all major food categories, alcoholic and soft drinks.

DISTRIBUTION

Native to southern Asia, extensively cultivated all over the tropics, particularly in Nigeria, the West Indies, China, Jamaica and Japan. Most oil is distilled in Britain, China and India.

OTHER SPECIES

Several varieties according to location which are all used to produce oils with slight variation in their constituents; for example the Africa oil is generally darker. Another member of the same family, galangal (Alpinia officinarum), is also known as ginger root or Chinese ginger.

EXTRACTION
Essential oil by steam distillation from the unpeeled, dried, ground root. (An absolute and oleoresin are also produced for use in perfumery.)

CHARACTERISTICS
A pale yellow, amber or greenish liquid with a warm, slightly green, fresh, woody-spicy scent. It blends well with sandalwood, vetiver, patchouli, frankincense, rosewood, cedarwood, coriander, rose, lime, orange blossom, orange and other citrus oils.

ACTIONS
Analgesic, anti-oxidant, antiseptic, anti-spasmodic, antitussive, aperitif, aphrodisiac, bactericidal, carminative, cephalic, diaphoretic, expectorant, febrifuge, laxative, rubefacient, stimulant, stomachic, tonic.

PRINCIPAL CONSTITUENTS
Gingerin, gingenol, gingerone, zingiberine, linalol, camphene, phellandrene, citral, cineol, borneol, among others.

General Glossary

Abortifacient: capable of inducing abortion.

Absolute: a highly concentrated viscous, semi-solid or solid perfume material, usually obtained by alcohol extraction from the concrete.

Acrid: leaving a burning sensation in the mouth.

Aerophagy: swallowing of air.

Allergy: hypersensitivity caused by a foreign substance, small doses of which produce a violent bodily reaction.

Alliaceous: garlic or onion-like.

Alopecia: baldness, loss of hair.

Alterative: corrects disordered bodily function.

Amebicidal: a substance with the power of destroying amebae.

Amenorrhea: absence of menstruation.

Analgesic: remedy or agent that deadens pain.

Anaphrodisiac: reduces sexual desire.

Anemia: deficiency in either quality or quantity of red corpuscles in the blood.

Anemic: relating to anemia, caused by or suffering from anemia.

Anesthetic: loss of feeling or sensation; substance that causes such a loss.

Annual: refers to a plant that completes its life cycle in one year.

Anodyne: stills pain and quiets disturbed feelings.

Anorexia: condition of being without, or having lost the appetite for, food.

Anthelmintic: a vermifuge, destroying or expelling intestinal worms.

Anti-anemic: an agent that combats anemia.

Anti-arthritic: an agent that combats arthritis.

Antibilious: an agent that helps remove excess bile from the body.

Antibiotic: prevents the growth of, or destroys, bacteria.

Anticatarrhal: an agent which helps remove excess catarrh from the body.

Anticonvulsant: helps arrest or prevent convulsions.

Antidepressant: helps alleviate depression.

Antidiarrheal: efficacious against diarrhea.

Anti-emetic: an agent which reduces the incidence and severity of nausea or vomiting.

Antihemorrhagic: an agent that prevents or combats hemorrhage or bleeding.

Antihistamine: treats allergic conditions; counteracts effects of histamine (which produces capillary dilation and, in larger doses, hemoconcentration).

Anti-inflammatory: alleviates inflammation.

Antilithic: prevents the formation of a calculus or stone.

Antimicrobial: an agent that resists or destroys pathogenic micro-organisms.

Antineuralgic: relieves or reduces nerve pain.

Anti-oxidant: a substance used to prevent or delay oxidation or deterioration, especially with exposure to air.

Antiphlogistic: checks or counteracts inflammation.

Antipruritic: relieves sensation of itching or prevents its occurrence.

Antiputrescent: an agent that prevents and combats decay or putrefaction.

Antipyretic: reduces fever; *see also* febrifuge.

Antirheumatic: helps prevent and relieve rheumatism.

Antisclerotic: helps prevent the hardening of tissue.

Antiscorbutic: a remedy for scurvy.

Antiscrofula: combats the development of tuberculosis of lymph nodes (scrofula).

Antiseborrheic: helps control the products of sebum, the oily secretion from sweat glands.

Antiseptic: destroys and prevents the development of microbes.

Antispasmodic: prevents and eases spasms or convulsions.

Antitoxic: an antidote or treatment that counteracts the effects of poison.

Antitussive: relieves coughs.

Antiviral: substance that inhibits the growth of a virus.

Aperient: a mild laxative.

Aperitif: a stimulant of the appetite.

Aphonia: loss of voice

Aphrodisiac: increases or stimulates sexual desire.

Apoplexy: sudden loss of consciousness, a stroke or sudden severe hemorrhage.

Aril: the husk or membrane covering the seed of a plant.

Aromatherapy: the therapeutic use of essential oils.

Aromatic: a substance with a strong aroma or smell.

Arteriosclerosis: loss of elasticity in the walls of the arteries due to thickening and calcification.

Arthritis: inflammation of a joint or joints.

Asthenia: *see* debility.

Astringent: causes contraction of organic tissues.

Atony: lessening or lack of muscular tone or tension.

Axil: upper angle between a stem and leaf or bract.

Bactericidal: an agent that destroys bacteria (a type of microbe or organism).

Balsam: a resinous semi-solid mass or viscous liquid exuded from a plant, which can be either a pathological or physiological product. A 'true' balsam is characterized by its high content of benzoic acid, benzoates, cinnamic acid or cinnamates.

Balsamic: a soothing medicine or application having the qualities of a balsam.

Bechic: anything that relieves or cures coughs; or referring to cough.

Biennial: a plant which completes its life cycle in two years, without flowering in the first year.

Bilious: a condition caused by an excessive secretion of bile.

Bitter: a tonic component which stimulates the appetite and promotes the secretion of saliva and gastric juices by exciting the taste buds.

General Glossary

Blenorrhea: abnormally free secretion and discharge of mucus, sometimes from the genitals (as in gonorrhea).

Blepharitis: inflammation of the eyelids.

Calculus: a soild pathological concentration (or 'stone'), usually of inorganic matter in a matrix of protein and pigment, formed in any part of the body.

Calmative: a sedative.

Calyx: the sepals or outer layer of floral leaves.

Capsule: a dry fruit, opening when ripe, composed of more than one carpel.

Cardiac: pertaining to the heart.

Cardiotonic: having a stimulating effect on the heart.

Carminative: settles the digestive system, relieves flatulence.

Catarrh: inflammation of mucous membranes, usually associated with an increase in secretion of mucus.

Cathartic: purgative, capable of causing a violent purging or catharsis of the body.

Cellulite: accumulation of toxic matter in the form of fat in the tissue.

Cephalic: remedy for disorders of the head; referring or directed towards the head.

Cerebral: pertaining to the largest part of the brain, the cerebrum.

Chemotype: the same botanical species occurring in other forms due to different conditions of growth, such as climate, soil, altitude, etc.

Chlorosis: a form of anemia rarely encountered nowadays.

Cholagogue: stimulates the secretion and flow of bile into the duodenum.

Cholecystokinetic: agent that stimulates the contraction of the gall bladder.

Choleretic: aids excretion of bile by the liver, so there is a greater flow of bile.

Cholesterol: a steroid alcohol found in nervous tissue, red blood cells, animal fat and bile. Excess can lead to gallstones.

Cicatrizant: an agent that promotes healing by the formation of scar tissue.

Cirrhosis: degenerative change in any organ (especially liver), caused by various poisons, bacteria or other agents, resulting in fibrous tissue overgrowth.

Colic: pain due to contraction of the involuntary muscle of the abdominal organs.

Colitis: inflammation of the colon.

Compress: a lint or substance applied hot or cold to an area of the body, for relief of swelling and pain, or to produce localized pressure.

Concrete: a concentrate, waxy, solid or semi-solid perfume material prepared from previously live plant matter, usually using a hydrocarbon type of solvent.

Constipation: congestion of the bowels; incomplete or infrequent action of the bowels.

Contagious disease: a disease spreading from person to person by direct contact.

Cordial: a stimulant and tonic.

Corolla: the petals of a flower considered as a whole.

Counter-irritant: applications to the skin that relieve deep-seated pain, usually applied in the form of heat; *see also* rubefacient.

Cutaneous: pertaining to the skin.

Cystitis: bladder inflammation, usually characterized by pain on urinating.

Cytophylactic: referring to cytophylaxis – the process of increasing the activity of leucocytes in defence of the body against infection.

Cytotoxic: toxic to all cells.

Debility: weakness, lack of tone.

Decoction: a herbal preparation, where the plant material (usually hard or woody) is boiled in water and reduced to make a concentration extract.

Decongestive: an agent for the relief or reduction of congestion, e.g. mucus.

Demulcent: a substance that protects mucous membranes and allays irritation.

Depurative: helps combat impurity in the blood and organs; detoxifying.

Deodorant: an agent that corrects, masks or removes unpleasant odours.

Dermal: pertaining to the skin.

Dermatitis: inflammation of the skin; many causes.

Diaphoretic: *see* sudorific.

Diarrhea: frequent passage of unformed liquid stools.

Digestive: substance that promotes or aids the digestion of food.

Disinfectant: prevents and also combats the spread of germs.

Diuretic: aids production of urine, promotes urination, increases flow.

Dropsy: excess of fluid in the tissues; *see also* edema.

Drupe: a fleshy fruit, with one or more seeds, each surrounded by a stony layer.

Dysmenorrhea: painful and difficult menstruation.

Dyspepsia: difficulty with digestion associated with pain, flatulence, heartburn and nausea.

Edema: a painless swelling caused by fluid retention beneath the skin's surface.

Elliptical: shaped like an ellipse, or regular curve.

Emetic: induces vomiting.

Emmenagogue: induces or assists menstruation.

Emollient: softens and soothes the skin.

Emphysema: condition in which the alveoli of the lungs are dilated, or an abnormal amount of air is present in tissues of body cavities.

Engorgement: congestion of a part of the tissues, or fullness (as in the breasts).

Enteritis: inflammation of the mucous membrane of the intestine.

Enzyme: complex proteins that are produced by the living cells, and catalyse specific biochemical reactions.

Erythema: a superficial redness of the skin due to excess of blood.

Essential oil: a volatile and aromatic liquid (sometimes semi-solid), which generally constitutes the odorous principles of a plant. It is obtained by a process of expression or distillation from a single botanical form or species.

Estrogen: a hormone produced by the ovary, necessary for the development of female secondary sexual characteristics.

Expectorant: helps promote the removal of mucus from the respiratory system.

Febrifuge: combats fever.

Fixative: a material that slows down the rate of evaporation of the more volatile components in a perfume composition.

Fixed oil: a name given to a vegetable oil obtained from plants that, in contradistinction to essential oils, are fatty, dense and non-volatile, such as olive or sweet almond oil.

Florets: the small individual flowers in the flowerheads of the Compositae family.

Follicle: a dry, one-celled, many seeded fruit.

Fungicidal: prevents and combats fungal infection.

Galactagogue: increases secretion of milk.

Gastritis: inflammation of stomach lining.

Genito-urinary: referring to both genital and reproductive systems.

Germicidal: destroys germs or micro-organisms such as bacteria, etc.

Gingivitis: inflammation of the gum, manifested by swelling and bleeding.

Gout: a disease that involves excess uric acid in the blood.

Gums: 'true' gums are little used in perfumery, being virtually odourless. However, the term 'gum' is often applied to 'resins', especially with relation to turpentines, as in the Australian 'gum tree'. Strictly speaking, gums are natural or synthetic water-soluble materials, such as gum arabic.

Halitosis: offensive breath.

Hallucinogenic: causes visions or delusions.

Heartwood: the central portion of a tree trunk.

Hematuria: blood in the urine.

Hemorrhoids: piles, dilated rectal veins.

Hemostatic: arrests bleeding.

Hepatic: relating to the liver (tones and aids its function).

Herpes: inflammation of the skin or mucous membrane with clusters of deep-seated vesicles.

Hormone: a product of living cells that produces a specific effect on the activity cells remote from its point of origin.

Hybrid: a plant orginating by fertilization of one species or subspecies by another.

Hypertension: raised blood pressure.

Hypertensive: agent which raises blood pressure.

Hypnotic: causing sleep.

Hypocholesterolemia: lowering the cholesterol content of the blood.

Hypoglycemia: lowered blood sugar levels or concentration.

Hypotension: low blood pressure, or a fall in blood pressure below the normal range.

Hypotensive: agent that lowers blood pressure.

Hysteria: a psychoneurosis manifesting itself in various disorders of the mind and body.

Inflorescence: flowering structure above the last stem leaves (including bracts and flowers).

Infusion: a herbal remedy prepared by steeping the plant material in water.

Insecticide: repels insects.

Insomnia: inability to sleep.

Lanceolate: lance-shaped, oval and pointed at both ends (usually a leaf shape).

Larvicidal: an agent that prevents and kill larvae.

Laxative: promotes evacuation of the bowels.

Legume: a fruit consisting of one carpel, opening on one side, such as a pea.

Leucocyte: white blood cells responsible for fighting disease.

Leucocytosis: an increase in the number of white blood cells above the normal limit.

Leucorrhea: white discharge from the vagina.

Ligulet: a narrow protection from the top of a leaf sheath in grasses.

Linear: of leaves, narrow and more or less parallel-sided.

Lipolytic: causing lipolysis, the chemical disintegration or splitting of fats.

Lithuria: a morbid condition marked by the presence of excessive amounts of uric acid in the urine.

Lumbago: a painful rheumatic affliction of the muscles and fibrous tissue of the lumbar region of the back.

Lymphatic: pertaining to the lymph system.

Macerate: soak until soft.

Menopause: the normal cessation of menstruation, a life change for women.

Menorrhagia: excessive menstruation.

Metrorrhagia: uterine bleeding outside the menstrual cycle.

Microbe: a minute living organism, especially pathogenic bacteria, viruses, etc.

Mucilage: a substance containing gelatinous constituents that are demulcent.

Mucolytic: dissolving or breaking down mucus.

Narcotic: a substance that induces sleep; intoxicating or poisonous in large doses.

General Glossary

Nervine: strengthening and toning to the nerves and nervous system.

Nephritis: inflammation of the kidneys.

Neuralgia: a stabbing pain along a nerve pathway.

Neurasthenia: nervous exhaustion.

Oleo gum resin: a natural exudation from trees and plants that consists mainly of essential oil, gum and resin.

Oleoresin: a natural resinous exudation from plants, or an aromatic liquid preparation, extracted from botanical matter using solvents. They consist almost entirely of a mixture of essential oil and resin.

Olfaction: the sense of smell.

Ophthalmia: inflammation of the eye, a term usually applied to conjunctivitis.

Otitis: inflammation of the ear.

Ovate: egg-shaped.

Palpitation: undue awareness of the heartbeat, occasioned by anxiety. Rapid heartbeats or abnormal rhythm.

Panacea: a cure-all.

Pappus: the calyx in a composite flower having feathery hairs, scales or bristles.

Parasiticide: prevents and destroys parasites such as fleas, lice, etc.

Parturient: aiding childbirth.

Pathogenic: causing or producing disease.

Pathological: unnatural or destructive process on living tissue.

Pediculicide: an agent that destroys lice.

Peptic: applied to gastric secretions and areas affected by them.

Perennial: a plant that lives for more than two years, normally flowering every year.

Petiole: the stalk of a leaf.

Pharmacology: medical science of drugs that deals with their actions, properties and characteristics.

Pharmacopeia: an official publication of drugs in common use, in a given country.

Physiological: describes the natural biological processes of a living organism.

Phytohormones: plant substances that mimic the action of human hormones.

Phytotherapy: the treatment of disease by plants; herbal medicine.

Pinnate: a leaf composed of more than three leaflets arranged in two rows along a common stalk.

Pomade: a prepared perfume material obtained by the enfleurage process.

Poultice: the therapeutic application of a soft moist mass (such as fresh herbs) to the skin, to encourage local circulation and to relieve pain.

Prophylactic: preventative of disease or infection.

Prostatitis: any inflammatory condition of the prostate gland.

Prurigo: chronic skin disease with irritation, itching and papular eruption.

Pruritis: itching.

Psoriasis: a skin disease characterized by red patches and silver scaling.

Psychosomatic: the manifestation of physical symptoms resulting from a mental state.

Pulmonary: pertaining to the lungs.

Purgative: a substance stimulating an evacuation of the bowels.

Pyelitis: inflammation of the kidney.

Pyorrhea: bleeding or a discharge of pus.

Raceme: an inflorescence, usually conical in outline in which the lowest flowers open first.

Receptacle: the upper part of the stem from which the floral parts arise.

Rectification: the process of redistillation applied to essential oils to rid them of certain constituents.

Refrigerant: cooling – reduces fever.

Regulator: an agent that helps balance and regulate the functions of the body.

Relaxant: soothing, causing relaxation, relieving strain or tension.

Renal: pertaining to the kidney.

Resins: a natural or prepared product, either solid or semi-solid in nature. Natural resins are exudations from trees, such as mastic; prepared resins are oleoresins from which essential oil has been removed.

Resinoids: a perfumery material prepared from natural resinous matter, such as balsams, gum resins, etc., by extraction with a hydrocarbon type of solvent.

Resolvent: an agent that disperses swelling, or effects absorption of a new growth.

Restorative: an agent that helps strengthen and revive the body systems.

Revulsive: relieves pain by means of the diversion of blood or disease from one part of the body to another; *see also* counter-irritant.

Rhinitis: inflammation of the mucous membrane of the nose.

Rhizome: an underground stem lasting more than one season.

Rosette: leaves that are closely arranged in a spiral.

Rubefacient: a substance that causes redness of the skin, possibly irritation.

Sciatica: pain down the back of the legs, in the area supplied by the sciatic nerve, due to various causes including pressure on the nerve roots.

Sclerosis: hardening of tissue due to inflammation.

Scrofula: an outdated name for tuberculosis.

Seborrhea: increased secretion of sebum, usually associated with excessive oil secretion from the sweat glands.

Sedative: an agent that reduces functional activity; calming.

Sessile: without a stalk.

Sialogogue: an agent that stimulates the secretion of saliva.

Soporific: a substance that induces sleep.

Spasmolytic: *see* antispasmodic.

Spike: an inflorescence in which the sessile flowers are arranged in a raceme.

Splenic: relating to the spleen, the largest endocrine gland.

Splenitis: inflammation of the spleen.

Stimulant: an agent that quickens the physiological functions of the body.

Stomachic: digestive aid and tonic; improving appetite.

Styptic: an astringent agent that stops or reduces external bleeding.

Sudorific: an agent that causes sweating.

Synergy: agents working together harmoniously; co-ordination in the action of muscles, organs or substances such as drugs.

Tachycardia: abnormally increased heartbeat and pulse rate.

Tannin: a substance that has an astringent action, and helps seal the tissue.

Thrombosis: formation of a thrombus or blood clot.

Thrush: an infection of the mouth or vaginal region caused by a fungus (candida).

Tincture: a herbal remedy, or perfumery material prepared in an alcohol base.

Tonic: strengthens and enlivens the whole or specific parts of the body.

Tracheitis: inflammation of the windpipe.

Trifoliate: a plant having three distinct leaflets.

Tuber: a swollen part of an underground stem of one year's duration, capable of new growth.

Umbel: umbrella-like; a flower where the petioles all arise from the top of the stem.

Uterine: pertaining to the uterus.

Urticaria: hives, nettle rash, acute or chronic affection of the skin characterized by the formation of weals, attended by itching, stinging or burning.

Vasoconstrictor: an agent that causes narrowing of the blood vessels.

Vasodilator: an agent that dilates the blood vessels.

Vermifuge: expels intestinal worms.

Vesicant: causing blistering to the skin; a counter-irritant.

Vesicle: a small blister or sac containing fluid.

Volatile: unstable, evaporates easily, as in 'volatile oil'; *see* essential oil.

Vulnerary: an agent that helps heal wounds and sores by external application.

Whorl: a circle of leaves around a node.

Botanical Classification

The following list is based on the work of Arthur O. Tucker and Brian M. Lawerence published in *Herbs, Spices and Medicinal Plants, Vol II*, Oryx Press, 1987, as the 'Botanical Nomenclature of Commercial Sources of Essential Oils, Concretes and Absolutes'. It represents a survey of aromatic materials currently produced commercially, in which the botanical names are in accordance with the recent guidelines set out by the International Organization for Standardization.

Agavaceae
Polianthes tuberosa (Polyanthes tuberosa): Tuberose.

Amaryllidaceae
Narcissus jonquilla: Jonquil.
Narcissus poeticus: Poet's narcissus, pheasant's eye; two subspecies exist: *var. poeticus; var. radiiflorus.*

Anacardiaceae
Pistacia lenticus: Mastic, mastick tree, mastix, mastich, lentisk.
Schinus molle: Peruvian pepper tree, Peruvian mastic, California pepper tree.

Annonaceae
Cananga odorata (Canangium odoratum): two forms exist:
var. odorata (var. genuina, Unona odorantissimum): Ylang Ylang;
var. macrophylla: Cananga.

Apiaceae (Umbelliferae)
Ammi visnaga: Khella seed, visnaga.
Anethum graveolens (Peucedanum graveolens, Fructus anethi): Dill, European dill, American dill.
Anethum sowa: Indian dill.
Angelica archangelica (A. officinalis): Angelica, European angelica, garden angelica; two subspecies exist.
Angelica atropurpurea: Purple angelica, American angelica.
Angelica keiskei: Japanese angelica.
Angelica ursina: Japanese angelica.
Anthricus cerefolium (A. longirostris): Chervil, garden chervil, salad chervil.
Apium graveolens: Celery; there are at least four varieties, including: *var. dulce:* Sweet celery; *var. rapaceum:* Celeriac.
Carum carvi (Apium carvi): Caraway, carum.
Carum roxburghianum: Ajmud (Indian).
Coriandrum maritimum: Samphire, rock samphire.
Coriandrum sativum: Coriander, Chinese parsley.
Cuminum cyminum (C. odorum): Cumin, cummin, Roman caraway.
Daucus carota: Carrot, wild carrot, Queen Anne's lace, bird's nest, carrot seed (oil); there are at least twelve subspecies.
Dorema ammoniacum: Ammoniac, Bombay sumbul, boi.
Ferula asa-foetida: Asafetida, asafoetida, gum asafetida, devil's dung, food of the gods, giant fennel.
Ferula diversittata (F. suavolens): Sumbul, muskroot.
Ferula foetida: Asafetida.
Ferula galbaniflua (F. gummosa): Galbanum, 'bubonion'.
Ferula jaeschkeana: four varieties exist.
Ferula moschata (F. sumbul): Sumbul, muskroot.
Foeniculum vulgare (F. officinale, cappilaceum, Anethum foeniculum): Fennel, fenkel; its subspecies include: *var. azoricum:* Florence fennel; *var. dulce:* Sweet fennel; *var. amara:* Bitter fennel.
Levisticum mutellina: Alpine lovage.
Levisticum officinale (Angelica levisticum, Ligusticum levisticum): Lovage, garden lovage, common lovage, old English lovage, Italian lovage, maggi herb, smellage, Cornish lovage.
Ligusticum scoticum: Sea lovage.
Pastinaca sativa: Parsnip; these are four subspecies.
Petroselinum sativum (P. hortense, Apium petroselinum, Carum petroselinum): Parsley; there are four varieties including: *Petroselinum crispum:* Curly-leaved parsley.

Pimpinella anisum (Anisum officinalis, A. vulgare): Aniseed, anise, sweet cumin.
Pimpinella major: Great burnet, saxifrage.
Pimpinella saxifraga: Burnet saxifraga, black caraway.
Trachyspermum copticum (T. ammi, Carum copticum, Carum ajowan, Ptychotis ajowan, Ammi copticum): Ajowan, ajuan, omum.

Aquifoliaceae
Ilex paraguayensis: Paraguay tea.

Araceae
Acorus calamus var. angustatus (Calamus aromaticus): Sweet flag, calamus, sweet sedge, sweet root, sweet rush, sweet cane, sweet myrtle, myrtle grass, myrtle sedge, cinnamon sedge; several varieties exist.

Araucariaceae
Agathis australis: Kauri, kauri pine, New Zealand kauri.

Aristolochiaceae
Aristolochia serpentaria: Virginian snakeroot, serpentaria (oil).
Asarum canadense: Canadian snakeroot, wild ginger, Indian ginger.

Asteraceae (Compositae)
Achillea erba-rotta (A. moschata): Iva, musk yarrow.
Achillea ligustica: Ligurian yarrow.
Achillea millefolium: Common yarrow, milfoil, nosebleed, thousand leaf; at least two subspecies exist.
Arnica montana (A. fulgens, A. sororia): Arnica, leopard's bane, wolf's bane,; two subspecies exist.
Artemisia abrotanum: Southern wood, old man, lad's love.
Artemisia absinthium: Wormwood, common wormwood, green ginger, armoise, absinthium (oil).
Artemisia afra: African wormwood, lanyana, wildeals.
Artemisia annua: Annual wormwood, sweet Annie.
Artemisia dracunculus: French taraggon, Russian tarragon, estragon (oil).
Artemisia genipi (A. spicata, A. laxa, A. mutellina, A. glacialis): Genipi.
Artemisia herba-alba (A. sieversiana): Armoise.
Artemisia judaica: Semen contra.
Artemisia maritima (A. cina): Levant wormseed.
Artemisia pallens: Davana.
Artemisia pontica: Roman wormwood, small absinthe.
Artemisia princeps: Japanese mugwort.
Artemisia vestita.
Artemisia vulgaris: Mugwort, Indian wormwood.
Atractylodes lancea: Atractylis; two varieties exist.
Baccharis dracunculifolia: Vassoura.
Baccharis gennistelloides: Carqueja.
Balsamita major (Chrysanthemum balsamita, Pyrethrum majus): Costmary, mint geranium, sweet Mary, Bible leaf, balsamite.
Blumea balsamifera: Ngai camphor.
Blumea chinensis: Tombak-tombak.
Blumea lacera.
Blumea myriocephala (B. lanceolaria).
Brachylaena hutchinsii: Muhuhu.
Calendula officinalis: Poet's marigold, pot marigold, calendula, marygold, gold-bloom, hollygold, common marigold, marybud.
Carphephorus odoratissimus, Trilisa odoratissima, Liatris odoratissima, Frasera speciosa: Deertongue, hound's tongue, deer's tongue, Carolina vanilla, vanilla leaf, wild vanilla, vanilla trilisa, whart's tongue, liatris (oil).
Chamaemelum nobile (Anthemis nobilis): Roman chamomile, camomile, English chamomile, garden chamomile, sweet chamomile, true chamomile.
Chameamelum suaveolens (Matricaria matricarioides): Pineapple weed.
Conyza canadensis (Erigeron canadensis): Fleabane, horseweed.
Eriocephalus punctulatus: Eriocephalee.
Helichrysum angustifolium: Immortelle, everlasting, helichrysum.

Helichrysum italicum: Curry plant, white-leaved everlasting.

Helichrysum stoechas: Everlasting, immortelle; at least two subspecies exist.

Helichrysum orientale: Everlasting, immortelle.

Inula helenium (Helenium grandiflorum, Aster officinalis, A. helenium): Elecampane, scabwort, alant, horseheal, yellow starwort, elf dock, wild sunflower, velvet dock.

Matricaria recutita (M. chamomilla): German chamomile, Hungarian chamomile, sweet false chamomile, camomile, blue chamomile, single chamomile, wild chamomile.

Ormentis mixta (Anthemis mixta): Moroccan chamomile.

Ormentis multicaulis: Moroccan chamomile.

Pteronia incana: Pteronia, blue dog.

Santolina chameacyparissus (Lavendula taemina): Santolina, cotton lavender.

Saussaurea costus (S. lappa, Aucklandia costus, Aplotaxis lappa, A. auriculata): Costus.

Solidago odora: Sweet goldenrod, fragrant goldenrod.

Tagetes erecta: African marigold, Aztec marigold.

Tagetes lucida: Sweet marigold, sweet mace, Mexican tarragon.

Tagetes minuta (T. glandulifera): Taget (oil), tagetes, tagette.

Tagetes patula: French marigold, taget (oil).

Tanacetum vulgare (Chrysanthemum vulgare, C. tanacetum): Tansy, bitter buttons, bachelor's buttons, cheese, scented fern.

Betulaceae

Betula alba (B. odorata, B. alba var. pubescens, B. pendula): White birch, silver birch, European white birch.

Betula alleghaniensis: Yellow birch.

Betula lenta (B. capinefolia): Sweet birch, southern birch, cherry birch, mountain mahogany, mahogany birch.

Betula nigra: Black birch.

Betula papyrifera: Paper birch, birch bud (oil); several subspecies exist.

Betula verrucosa: Birch bud (oil), birch tar (oil); many cultivars exist.

Boraginaceae

Heliotropium arborescens (H. peruvianum): Heliotrope.

Brassicaceae (Cruciferae)

Armoracia rusticana (A. lapathifolia, Cochlearia armoracia): Horseradish, red cole, raifort.

Brassica juncea: Indian mustard, brown mustard.

Brassica nigra: Black mustard.

Cheiranthus cheiri: Wallflower.

Burseraceae

Boswellia bhau-dajiana: Frankincense.

Boswellia carteri: Frankincense, olibanum, gum thus.

Boswellia frereana: African elemi, elemi frankincense.

Boswellia papyrifera: Sudanese frankincense.

Boswellia sacra (B. thurifera sensu): Saudi frankincense.

Boswellia serrata: Indian frankincense, Indian olibanum.

Bursera aloexylon: Linaloe.

Bursera fagaroides: Linaloe.

Bursera glabrifolia (B. delpechiana): Linaloe, Mexican linaloe, 'copal lemon'.

Bursera penicillata: Linaloe.

Bursera simaruba (Elaphrium simaruba): West Indian birch, West Indian elemi, gumbo limbo, incense tree.

Canarium luzonicum (C. commune): Elemi, Manila elemi, elemi gum, elemi resin.

Commiphora erythraea: Opopanax, bisabol myrrh.

Commiphora madagascariensis (C. abyssinica, Balsamodendron habessinica): Abyssinian myrrh.

Commiphora molmol: Somalian myrrh.

Commiphora myrrha: Common myrrh, hirabol myrrh.

Byttneriaceae

Theobroma cacoa: Cocoa, chocolate; several cultivars exist.

Caprifoliaceae

Lonocera etrusca (L. gigantea): Honeysuckle.

Lonicera periclymenum: Common honeysuckle.

Sambucus nigra: Elderberry, elderflower.

Caryophyllaceae

Dianthus caryophllus: Carnation, clove pink.

Dianthus plumarius: Pink.

Chenopodiaceae

Chenopodium album: Lamb's quarters.

Chenopodium ambrosioides (var. anthelminticum): Wormseed, American wormseed, chenopodium, Californian spearmint, Jesuit's tea, Mexican tea, herb sancti mariae, Baltimore (oil).

Chenopodium bonus-henricus: Allgood, Good King Henry.

Cistaceae

Cistus incanus (C. villosus, C. polymorphus): Labdanum; three subspecies exist: *C. polymorphus, C. corsicus* and *C. creticus.*

Cistus ladaniferus: Labdanum, cistus, ciste, cyste, ambreine, European rock rose.

Cupressaceae

Chamaecyparis funebris (Cupressus funebris): Mourning cypress, Chinese weeping cypress, Chinese cedarwood (oil).

Chamaecyparis lawsoniana: Port Orford cedar, Oregon cedar, Lawson false cypress; numerous cultivars exist.

Chamaecyparis nootkatensis: Alaska cedar, Alaska yellow cedar, yellow cedar.

Chamaecyparis obtusa exists in two varieties: *var. obtusa:* Hinoki false cypress; *var. formosana (C. taiwanensis):* Formosan hinoki.

Cupressus lusitanica: Kenya cypress.

Cupressus sempervirens: Mediterranean cypress; many cultivars exist, the most common being 'Stricta', the Italian cypress.

Cupressus torulosa: Himalayan cypress.

Juniperus ashei (J. mexicana): Mountain cedar, rock cedar, Mexican cedar, Mexican juniper.

Juniperus communis: Juniper, common juniper; many cultivars exist such as *var. depressa:* Canadian juniper; *var. communis (var. erecta).*

Juniperus oxycedrus: Prickly juniper, cade juniper, juniper tar, cade (oil), prickly cedar, medlar tree.

Juniperus phoenicea: Phoenician juniper, Phoenician savin (oil).

Juniperus sabina (Sabina cacumina): Savin juniper, savin (oil); many cultivars exist.

Juniperus smerka: Yugoslavian juniper.

Juniperus squamata (J. recurva var. squamata): Single-seed juniper, scaly-leaved Nepal juniper; several cultivars exist.

Juniperus virginiana: Eastern red cedar, red cedar, southern red cedar, Bedford cedarwood (oil), Virginian cedarwood (oil); many cultivars exist.

Neocallitropsis pancheri (N. araucarioides, Callitropsis araucarioides): Pancher neocallitropsis, araucaria (oil).

Thuja occidentalis: Northern white cedar, white cedar, eastern white cedar, American arborvitae, thuja, swamp cedar, cedarleaf (oil); many cultivars exist.

Thuja orientalis (Biota orientalis): Chinese or Japanese cedar.

Thuja plicata: Western red cedar, western arborvitae, Washington cedar.

Thujopsis dolobrata: Hiba; two varieties exist: *var. dolobrata:* Azunaro; *var. hondae:* Hinoki-asunaro.

Widdringtonia cupressoides (W. dracomontana, W. whytei): Mountain widdringtonia, mlange cedar.

Cyperaceae

Cyperus mitis (C. scariosus sensu): Nagar motha.

Cyperus rotundus: Nut-grass, coco-grass.

Dipterocarpaceae

Dipterocarpus alatus: Gurjun.

Dipterocarpus jourdainii: Gurjun.

Dipterocarpus tuberculatus: Gurjun.

Dipterocarpus turbinatus: Gurjun, East Indian copaiba balsam.

Dryobalanops aromatica (D. camphora): Borneo camphor, East Indian camphor, Baros camphor, Sumatra camphor, Malayan camphor, Borneol (oil).

Ericaceae

Gaultheria procumbens: Wintergreen, tea berry, checkerberry, aromatic wintergreen, gaultheria (oil).

Euphorbiaceae

Croton eluteria: Cascarilla, sweetwood bark, sweet bark, Bahama cascarilla, aromatic quinquina, false quinquina, cascarilla bark (oil).

Fabaceae (Leguminosae)

Copaifera coricea: Copaiba

Copaifera guyanensis: Copaiba.

Copaifera lansdorffinii: Copaiba.

Copaifera martii: Copaiba.

Copaifera multijuga: Copaiba.

Copaifera officinalis: Copaiba, copahu balsam, copaiva,

Botanical Classification

Jesuit's balsam, para balsam, Maracaibo balsam, balsam copaiba (oil).

Copaifera reticulata: Copaiba.

Daniellia thurifera: Ogea gum, illorin gum, balsam Sierra Leone, 'frankincense'.

Dipteryx odorata (Coumarouna odorata): Tonka, Dutch tonka bean, tonquin bean.

Glycyrrhiza glabra: Liquorice, licorice.

Melilotus officinalis: Yellow melilot, common melilot, white melilot, corn melilot, melilot trefoil, sweet clover, plaster clover, sweet lucerne, wild laburnum, king's clover, melilotin (oleoresin).

Myrocarpus fastigiatus: Cabreuva, cabureicica.

Mycrocarpus frondosus: Cabreuva.

Myroxylon balsamum: this group is divided into three main sub-species: *var. balsamum (var. geninum, Myrospermum toluiferum, Toluiferum balsamum, Balsamum americanum, Balsamum tolutanum)*: Opobalsam, Tolu balsam, Thomas balsam, resin tolu; *var. pereirae (Myrosperum pereirae, Toluifera pereirae, Myroxylon pereirae):* Peru Balsam, Peruvian balsam, Indian balsam, black balsam; *var. punctatum (Myroxylon punctatum).*

Robinia pseudo-acacia: Black locust, false acacia.

Spartium junceum (Genista juncea): Spanish broom, weaver's broom, genista, genet.

Trifolium pratense: Red clover; several varieties exist.

Trigonella foenum-graecum: Fenugreek.

Geraniaceae

Geranium macrorrhizum: Bulgarian geranium.

Pelargonium graveolens: Rose geranium, geranium; numerous other varieties and cultivars exist such as: *P. odoratissimum, P. radens, P. capitatum* and *P. x asperum.*

Grossulariaceae

Ribes nigrum: Blackcurrant, niribine (oil); several cultivars exist.

Hamamelidaceae

Liquidambar orientalis: Oriental sweetgum, Levant styrax, Asiatic styrax, storax, Turkish sweetgum, liquid storax.

Liquidambar styraciflua: Sweetgum, American styrax, storac, red gum.

Illiciaceae

Illicium verum: Star anise, Chinese anise, illicium, Chinese star anise.

Iridaceae

Iris florentina: Florentine orris, orris root.

Iris germanica: German iris, flag iris, orris root.

Iris pallida: Pale iris, orris root.

Lamiaceae (Labiatae)

Aeollanthus gamwelliae (A. graveolens): Ninde.

Calamintha officinalis (C. clinopodium, Melissa calminta): Calamintha, calamint, common calamint, mill mountain, mountain balm, mountain mint, basil thyme.

Hedeoma floribundum: Oregano.

Hedeoma patens: Oregano.

Hedeoma pulegioides: North American pennyroyal, squaw mint, stinking balm, tickweed, mosquito plant.

Hyssopus officinalis: Hyssop, 'azob'; four subspecies exist, including *var. decumbens.*

Lavandula angustifolia (L. officinalis, L. vera): Common lavender, true lavender, garden lavender; this variety is divided into two subspecies: *L. delphinensis* and *L. fragrans.* In addition many cultivars exist.

Lavendula x intermedia (L. hybrida, L. hortensis): Lavandin; several cultivars exist.

Lavendula latifolia (L. spica): Spike lavender, spike, aspic, broad-leaved lavender, lesser lavender.

Lavendula stoechas: French lavender, stoechas lavender; six subspecies exist.

Melissa officinalis: Lemon balm, balm, melissa, common balm, bee balm, sweet balm, heart's delight, honeyplant; two subspecies exist.

Mentha acquatica: Water mint, bergamot mint.

Mentha canadensis (M. arvensis var. villosa, M. arvensis var. glabrata, M. arvensis var. piperascens): Corn mint, Japanese peppermint, North American field mint.

Mentha x gracilis (M. gentilis): Scotch spearmint, red mint.

Mentha x piperita: Peppermint.

Mentha pulegium: Pennyroyal, European pennyroyal, pudding plant, pulegium.

Mentha spicata (M. viridis, M. longifolia): Spearmint.

Mentha suaveolens (M. rotundifolia): Pineapple mint.

Mentha x villosa var. alopecuroides: Woolly mint, apple mint, Bowles' mint, Egyptian mint.

Monarda citriodora: Lemon bee balm, lemon bergamot; two varieties exist.

Monarda clinopodia: Bee balm, wild bergamot.

Monarda didyma: Oswego tea, oswego bee balm, bergamot.

Monarda fistulosa: Wild bergamot, horsemint, bee balm; four varieties exist including *var. menthifolia.*

Monarda x media: several cultivars exist.

Monarda pectinata: Pony bee balm.

Nepeta cataria: Catnip, catmint.

Ocimum basilicum: Basil, sweet basil; numerous cultivars and chemotypes exist, including 'Comoran' basil (exotic or Reunion Basil) and the 'true' sweet basil (French, European or common basil).

Ocimum canum (O. americanum): Hoary basil, hairy basil.

Ocimum gratissimum (O. viride): East Indian basil, tree basil, shrubby basil.

Ocimum kilimanjaricum: Camphor basil.

Ocimum sanctum: Holy basil, sacred basil.

Origanum x applii: Oregano.

Origanum marjorana (Marjorana hortensis): Sweet marjoram, knotted marjoram.

Origanum x marjorana: Oregano, marjoram.

Origanum onites: Pot marjoram, French marjoram.

Origanum syriacum (O. maru): Syrian oregano.

Origanum vulgare: Common oregano; this is divided into six subspecies: *subsp. vulgare:* Wild marjoram, oreganum (oil), several cultivars exist; *subsp. glandulosum:* Oregano; *subsp. gracile (O. tytthanthum, O. kopetdaghense):* Russian oregano; *subsp. hirtum (O. hirtum, O. heracleoticum):* Winter, Greek or Italian oregano; *subsp. virent (O. virens):* Wild marjoram; *subsp. viride (O. heracleoticum):* Wild marjoram.

Perilla frutescens (P. ocymoides): Perilla, beefsteak plant; numerous varieties exist.

Pogostemon cablin (P. patchouly): Patchouli, patchouly, puchaput.

Pogostemon heyneanus (P. patchouli): False patchouly.

Rosmarinus officinalis: Rosemary; other varieties exist including: *var. officinalis:* Common rosemary; numerous cultivars and forms exist; *var. angustifolia (R. tenuifolius):* Pine-scented rosemary, pine-needled rosemary; *var. lavendulaceus (R. officinalis f. humulis, f. procumbens):* Prostrate rosemary, numerous cultivars exist.

Salvia clevelandii: Blue sage.

Salvia dorisiana: Peach-scented sage, British Honduran sage.

Salvia elegans (S. rutilans): Pineapple-scented sage.

Salvia fruticosa (S. triloba): Greek sage.

Salvia lavendulidefolia: Spanish sage, lavender-leaved sage.

Salvia leucophylla: Grey sage, purple sage.

Salvia officinalis: Common sage, dalmation sage, garden sage; many cultivars exist.

Salvia pomifera (S. calycina): Apple sage.

Salvia sclarea: Clary, clary sage, muscatel sage, clary wort, clear eye, see bright, common clary, clarry, eye bright.

Salvia verbenacea (S. clandestina, S. horminoides): Vervain sage, wild clary.

Salvia viridis (S. horminum): Bluebeard sage, Joseph sage, red-topped sage.

Satureja douglasii (Micromeria chamissonis, M. douglasii): Yerba buena (Spanish).

Satureja hortensis (Satureia hortensis, Calamintha hortensis): Summer savory, garden savory.

Satureja montana (S. obovata, Calamintha montana): Winter savour; at least five subspecies.

Satureja thymbra: Za'atar rumi (Arabic).

Thymis caespititius (T. micans, T. serpyllum): Tiny thyme, tufted thyme.

Thymus capitatus (Satureja capitata, Thymbra capitata, Coridothymus capitatus): Conehead thyme, corido thyme, Cretan thyme, thyme of the ancients, headed savory, Spanish oreganum (oil), Israeli oreganum (oil).

Thymus cephalatos.

Thymus x citriodorus (T. lanuginosus var. citriodorum, T. serpyllum var. citriodorus, T. 'Limoneum'): Lemon thyme.

Thymus herba-barona: Caraway thyme.

Thymus hirtus.

Thymus hyemalis: often wrongly cited as the source of Spanish verbena oil.

Thymus loscosii: two subspecies exist.

Thymus mastichina: Mastic thyme, Spanish marjoram.

Thymus praecox: Creeping thyme; five subspecies exist and several cultivars.

Thymus pulegoides: Wild thyme, Dutch tea thyme; several subspecies and cultivars exist.

Thymus quinquecostatus: Japanese thyme; two forms are known.

Thymus serpyllum: Wild thyme, mother-of-thyme; two subspecies exist.

Thymus vulgaris (T. aestivus, T. ilerdensis, T. webbianus, T. valentianus): garden thyme, common thyme, French thyme, red thyme (oil), white thyme (oil).

Thymus zygis (T. sabulicola, T. sylvestris): Spanish sauce thyme, red thyme (oil).

Other lesser known species and cultivars also exist in the *Thymus* group.

Lauraceae

Aniba duckei: Brazilian rosewood, bois de rose.

Aniba parviflora: Brazilian rosewood, bois de rose.

Aniba rosaeodora var. amazonica: Brazilian rosewood, bois de rose.

Cinnamomum burmanii (C. pedunculata): Indonesian cassia, padang cassia, padang cinnamon, Batavia cassia, Java cassia, Korintje cassia.

Cinnamonmum camphora (Laurus camphora): Camphor tree, true camphor, laurel camphor, gum camphor, Japanese camphor, Formosa camphor; several subvarieties exist.

Cinnamomum cassia (C. aromaticum, Laurus cassia): Cassia, Chinese cinnamon, false cinnamon, cassia cinnamon, cassia lignea.

Cinnamomum cecidodaphne: Nepalese tejpat.

Cinnamomum culiliban (C. culiliwan): Lawang.

Cinnamomum loueirii: Saigon cinnamon.

Cinnamomum micranthum: Chinese sassafras.

Cinnamomum tamala: Indian cassia.

Cinnamomum zeylanicum (C. verum, Laurus cinnamomum): Cinnamon, Ceylon cinnamon, Seychelles cinnamon, Madagascar cinnamon, true cinnamon.

Cryptocarya massoy (Massoia aromatica): Massoi.

Laurus nobilis: Grecian laurel, sweet bay, laurel, true bay, Mediterranean bay, Roman laurel, noble laurel, laurel leaf (oil); three subspecies exist.

Lindera umbellata var. umbellata: Kuru-moji; several other subspecies exist.

Litsea cubeba (L. citrata): May-chang, exotic verbena, tropical verbena.

Nectandra elaiophora: Louro nhamuy.

Ocotea caudata (Licaria guianensis): Cayenne rosewood.

Ocotea cymbarum (Mespilodaphne sassafras): Amazonian sassafras.

Ocotea pretiosa: Brazilian sassafras.

Phoebe nanmu.

Sassafras albidum (S. officinale, Laurus sassafras, S. variifolium): Common sassafras, North American sassafras, sassafrax.

Liliaceae

Allium cepa: Onion; numerous cultivars exist.

Allium fistulosum: Welsh onion, cibol, stone leek.

Allium kurrat (A. porrum var. aegyptiacum): kurrat.

Allium sativum: Garlic, allium, poor man's treacle; three

varieties exsist: *var. sativum:* Cultivated garlic; *var. ophioscorodon:* Serpent garlic, giant garlic, rocambole; *var. pekinense:* Peking garlic.

Allium schoenoprasum: Chives, cive; two varieties exist: *var. schoenoprasum:* Cultivated chives; *var alpinum (A. sibiricum):* Large chives.

Allium scorodoprasum: Sand leek; several subspecies exist.

Allium tricoccum: Ramps, wild leek.

Allium tuberosum (A. odorum): Chinese chives, garlic chives, oriental garlic.

Hyacinthus orientalis (Scilla nutans): Hyacinth, bluebell.

Magnoliaceae

Michelia champaca: Champaca.

Michelia figo.

Malvaceae

Abelmoschus moschatus (Hibiscus abelmoschus): Ambrette seed, musk seed, Egyptian alcee, target-leaved hibiscus, muskmallow.

Meliaceae

Aglaia odorata.

Cabralea cangerana: Cangerana.

Cedrela odorata: West Indian cedar, Spanish cedar, cigar-box cedar, Barbados cedar.

Mimosaceae

Acacia caven (A. cavenia): Roman cassie.

Acacia dealbata (A. decurrens var. dealbata): Mimosa, Sydney black wattle.

Acacia farnesiana (Cassia ancienne): Sweet acacia, cassie, huisache, popinac, opopanax.

Monimiaceae

Peumus boldus (Boldu boldus, Boldoa fragrans): Boldo, boldus, boldu.

Moraceae

Ficus carica: Fig.

Humulus lupulus: Hops, common hop, European hop, lupulus.

Myristicaceae

Myristica fragrans (M. officinalis, M. moschana, M. aromatica, M. amboinensis): Nutmeg and mace.

Myrtaceae

Eucalyptus citriodora: Lemon-scented gum, citron-scented gum, spotted gum.

Eucalyptus cneorifolia: Kangaroo Island narrow-leaved mallee.

Eucalyptus dives: Broad-leaved peppermint, blue peppermint, peppermint.

Eucalyptus dumosa: Mallee, Congo mallee.

Eucalyptus elata (E. andreana, E. lindleyana, E. longifolia, E. numerosa): River peppermint, river white gum.

Eucalyptus globulus (var. globulus): Blue gum, Tasmanian blue gum, southern blue gum, fever tree, gum tree, eucalyptus, stringy bark.

Eucalyptus goniocalyx (E. elaeophora): Long-leaved box, bundy, apple jack, olive-barked box.

Eucalyptus leucoxylon: Yellow gum, white ironbark, white gum; three subspecies exist.

Eucalyptus macarthurii: Camden woolybut, Paddy's river box.

Eucalyptus oleosa: Red mallee, glossy-leaved red mallee.

Eucalyptus piperita: Peppermint eucalyptus.

Eucalyptus polybractea: Blue-leaved mallee.

Eucalyptus radiate (E. australiana, E. phellandra): Narrow-leaved peppermint, grey peppermint; two subspecies exist.

Eucalyptus sideroxylon: Red ironbark, ironbark, mugga; two subspecies exist.

Eucalyptus smithii: Gully gum, gully peppermint, blackbutt peppermint.

Eucalyptus staigerana.

Eucalyptus viminalis: two subspecies exist.

Eucalyptus viridis: Green mallee.

Melaleuca alternifolia (M. linariifolia var. alternifolia): Tea tree, narrow-leaved paperbark tea tree, ti-tree, ti-trol, melasol.

Melaleuca bracteata: Tea tree.

Melaleuca cajeputi: Cajuput, cajeput, white tea tree, white wood, swamp tea tree, punk tree, paperbark tree.

Melaleuca leucadendra (Myrtus leucodendra): Cajeput, cajuput, river tea tree, weeping tea tree.

Melaleuca linariifolia: Tea tree.

Melaleuca minor: Cajuput, cajeput.

Botanical Classification

Melaleuca quinquenervia: Cajeput, cajuput.
Melaleuca viridiflora: Niaouli.
Mytrus communis: Myrtle; at least two subspecies exist.
Pimenta dioica (P. officinalis): Allspice, pimento, pimenta, Jamaica pepper.
Pimenta racemosa (P. acris, Myrcia acris): Bay, West Indian bay, bay rum tree, wild cinnamon, bayberry, myrcia.
Syzygium aromaticum (Eugenia aromatica, E. caryophyllata, E. caryophyllus): Clove.

Oleaceae
Jasminum auriculatum: Indian jasmine.
Jasminum grandiflorum (J. officinale var. grandiflorum): Catalonian jasmine, Royal jasmine, jasmin, Spanish jasmine, Italian jasmine.
Jasminum officinale: Jasmine, common jasmine, poet's jessamine, jessamine.
Jasminum sambac: Arabian jasmine, sambac; there are two cultivars: 'Grand Duke' and 'Maid of Orleans'.
Osmanthus fragrans: Sweet olive, fragrant olive, tea olive.
Syringa vulgaris: Common lilac, numerous cultivars exist.

Orchidaceae
Vanilla planifolia (V. fragrans): Vanilla, Bourbon vanilla, Mexican vanilla, common vanilla, Reunion vanilla
Vanilla pompona: West Indian vanilla, vanillon, Pompona vanilla, Guadeloupe vanilla.
Vanilla tahitensis: Tahiti vanilla.

Pandanceae
Pandanus fascicularis (P. odoratissimus): Padang, attar of kewda (oil), attar of keora (oil).

Parmeliaceae
Parmelia cirrhata (P. nepalensis): Indian moss.

Pinaceae
Abies alba (A. pectinata): Silver fir, white fir, silver spruce, European silver fir, white spruce.
Abies balsamea (A. balsamifera, Pinus balsamea): Balsam fir, Canadian balsam, balsam tree, American silver fir, balm of gilead fir, Canada turpentine (oil).
Abies mayriana: Mayr Sakhalin fir, Japanese fir needle (oil).
Abies sachalinensis: Sachalin fir, Japanese fir needle (oil).
Abies sibirica: Siberian fir, Siberian 'pine' (oil).
Cedrus atlantica: Atlantic cedar, Atlas cedar, African cedar, Moroccan cedarwood (oil), libanol (oil).
Cedrus deodara (C. deodorata): Deodar cedar, Himalayan cedar.
Cedrus libani: Cedar of Lebanon.
Picea abies (P. excelsa): Norway spruce, common spruce, burgundy pitch (oil), Jura turpentine (oil).
Picea glauca (P. alba, P. canadensis): White spruce, Canadian spruce.
Picea jezoensis: Yeddo spruce, Yezo spruce.
Picea mariana (P. nigra): Black spruce, Canadian black 'pine'.
Pinus ayacahuite: Mexican white pine, turpentine (oil).
Pinus contorta var. latifolia: Lodgepole pine, turpentine (oil); other subspecies exist.
Pinus elliottii (P. caribaea): Slash pine, turpentine (oil); other subspecies exist.
Pinus halepensis: Aleppo pine, Jerusalem pine.
Pinus insularis (P. khasya, P. kesiya, P. khasyana, P. langbianensis): Khasi pine, Benguet pine, Indian turpentine (oil).
Pinus koraiensis: Korean pine.
Pinus massoniana: Masson pine, southern red pine, turpentine (oil).
Pinus merkusii (P. latteri): Merkus pine.
Pinus mugo (P. montana): Mountain pine, Swiss mountain pine; other subspecies exist including *var. mughus (P. mughus):* mugho pine; *var. pumilio (P. pumilio):* Dwarf pine, pine needle (oil).
Pinus nigra: Austrian pine, black pine; other subspecies exist.
Pinus palustris: Longleaf pine, longleaf yellow pine, southern yellow pine, pitch pine, gum turpentine (oil).

Pinus pinaster: Sea pine, turpentine (oil).
Pinus ponderosa: Ponderosa pine, western yellow pine; other subspecies exist.
Pinus radiata: Monterey pine, New Zealand turpentine (oil).
Pinus roxburghii: Chir pine, Indian turpentine (oil).
Pinus strobus: White pine, Canadian white pine; many subspecies exist.
Pinus sylvestris: Scotch pine, turpentine (oil); many subspecies and cultivars exist.
Pinus tabulaeformis: Chinese pine.
Pinus yunnanensis: Yunnan pine, Chinese pine.
Pseudotsuga menziesii (P. taxifolia): Douglas fir, Oregon balsam (oil); two main subspecies exist *var. menziesii:* Coast Douglas fir; *var. glauca:* Rocky Mountain Douglas fir.
Tsuga canadensis (Pinus canadensis, Abies canadensis): Hemlock, eastern hemlock, common hemlock, spruce (oil); many cultivars exist.

Piperaceae
Piper cubeba (Cubeba officinalis): Cubebs, cubeba, tailed pepper, cubeb pepper.
Piper nigrum: Pepper, black pepper, white pepper, piper.

Poaceae (Gramineae)
Anthoxanthum odoratum: Sweet vernalgrass, flouve (oil).
Cymbopogon citratus (Andropogon citratus, A. schoenathus): West Indian lemongrass, Madagascar lemongrass, Guatemala lemongrass.
Cymbopogon flexuosus (Andropogon flexuosus): East Indian lemongrass.
Cymbopogon martinii (Andropogon martinii): Rosha; this species occurs in two eco-chemotypes: *var. martinii (var. motia):* Palmarosa, motia, East Indian geranium, Turkish geranium, Indian; *rosha var. sofia:* Gingergrass, sofia.
Cymbopogon nardus (Andropogon nardus): Citronella; this exists in two varieties: *var. nardus:* Ceylon citronella, Lenabatu citronella; *var. confertiflorus.*
Cymbopogon pendulus (Andropogon pendulus): Jammu lemongrass.
Cymbopogon winterianus: Java citronella.
Vetiveria zizanoides (Andropogon muricatus): Vetiver, khus khus, vetivert (oil).

Podocarpaceae
Dacrydium franklinii: Huon pine, huon dacrydium.

Resedaceae
Reseda ordorata: Reseda, common mignonette.

Rosaceae
Prunus dulcis (P. communis, P. amygdalus, Amygdalus communis, A. dulcis): Almond: there are two varieties: *var. dulcis:* Sweet almond; *var. amara:* Bitter almond.
Rosa alba (R. damascena var. alba): White rose: the main cultivar is called 'Semiplena', similar to the Bulgarian 'Suaveolens'.
Rosa canina: Dogrose, doghip.
Rosa centifolia: Cabbage rose, Provence rose, French rose, rose de mai, hundred-leaved rose.
Rosa damascena: Summer damask rose, Turkish rose, Bulgarian rose; the main cultivar is 'Trigintipetala' or 'Kazanlik rose'. There are also several other subspecies including: *var. semperflorens:* Autumn damask rose.
Rosa gallica: French rose, Provins rose; the two main cultivars were once 'Conditorum' or the Hungarian rose, and 'Officinalis', 'Apothecary' rose or the red damask rose.
Rosa indica: Tea rose, oriental rose.
Rosa muscatta: Musk rose.
Rosa rubiginosa (R. elglanteria): Eglantine, sweet briar.
Rosa rugosa: Rugosa rose, ramanas rose, Japanese rose, Chinese rose.

Rubiaceae
Anthocephalus indicus (A. cadamba): Cadamba, kadamba.
Coffea arabica: Coffee, common coffee, Arabian coffee: many

cultivars exist.

Coffea canephora (C. robusta): Robusta coffee; many cultivars exist.

Gardenia jasminoides (G. florida, G. grandiflora, G. radicans): Common gardenia, Cape jasmine, gardinia.

Leptactina senegambica: Karo-karounde.

Rutaceae

Agathosma betulina (Barosma betulina): Buchu, mountain buchu, short buchu, bookoo, buku, bucco.

Agathosma crenulata (Barosma crenulata): Oval buchu, crenate buchu.

Amyris balsamifera (Schimmelia oleifera): Amyris, West Indian sandalwood, West Indian rosewood.

Boronia megastigma: Boronia, brown boronia.

Citrus aurantifolia (C. latifolia, C. medica var. acida): Lime, Mexican lime, West Indian lime, sour lime.

Citrus aurantium var. amara (C. vulgaris, C. bigaradia): Bitter orange, sour orange, Seville orange, bigarade (oil), neroli bigarade (oil), orange flower (oil), petitgrain orange (oil).

Citrus bergamia (C. aurantium subsp. bergamia): Bergamot; the two main cultivars are 'Castagnaro' and 'Femmenillo'.

Citrus hystrix: Leech-lime, Mauritius papeda, combava (oil).

Citrus jambhiri: Rough lemon (Java lemon); the two main cultivars are 'Estes' and 'Milam'.

Citrus limetta: Italian lime, limette (oil).

Citrus limon (C. limonum): Lemon, cedro (oil); there are many cultivars notably 'Berna', 'Eureka', 'Lisbon', 'Femminello Ovale' and 'Femminello Sfusato'.

Citrus medica: Citron, cedrat; the main cultivar is 'Diamante'.

Citrus x paradisi (C. maxima var. racemosa, C. racemosa): Grapefruit; there are many cultivars.

Citrus reticulata (C. deliciosa, C. nobilis, C. unshiu): Mandarin, tangerine, satsuma; there are many cultivars, the most common being 'Crava'.

Citrus sinensis (C. aurantium var. sinensis, C. aurantium var. dulcis): Sweet orange, Portugal orange, China orange; there are many cultivars notably 'Valencia'; also produces neroli Portugal or neroli petalae (oil).

Citrus jambhiri x C. aurantifolia: Lemon 'n' lime.

Citrus limon x C. sinensis: Lemonange.

Citrus reticulata x C. paradisi: Tangelo.

Dictamus albus: Dittany, fraxinella, burning bush, gas plant.

Galipea trifoliate (G. officinalis, G. cusparia, Cusparia trifoliata): Angustora.

Luvunga scandens: Sugandh kokila.

Pilocarpus jaborandi (Pernambuco jaborandi, P. pennatifolius): Jaborandi, Iaborandi, jamborandi.

Ruta angustifolia: Sardinian rue, North African rue.

Ruta chalepensis (R. bracteosa): Winter rue, Sicilian rue, North African rue.

Ruta graveolens: Rue, garden rue, herb-of-grace, herbygrass.

Ruta montana: Summer rue, Spanish rue, North African rue.

Skimmia laureola.

Zanthoxylum alatum: Tomarseed.

Zanthoxylum piperitum: Prickly ash, 'san-sho'.

Zanthoxylum rhetsa (Z. bodrunga): Mulilam.

Zanthoxylum schinifolium (Z. mantchuricum): Pepperbush.

Zanthoxylum simulans (z. bungei): Chinese pepper, Szechuan pepper.

Salicaceae

Populus balsamifera (P. tacamahacca): Poplar, tacamahac, hackmatack; two subspecies exist.

Santalacea

Santalum album: East Indian sandalwood, white sandalwood, white saunders, yellow sandalwood, yellow saunders, sanderswood, Mysore sandalwood, yellow sandalwood.

Santalum spicatum (Eucarya spicata): Australian sandalwood.

Smilaceae

Smilax medica (S. aristolochiaefolia): Mexican sarsaparilla; several subspecies exist.

Solanaceae

Nicotiana tabacum: Tobacco.

Stryacaceae

Styrax benzoin: Gum benzoin, styrax benzoin, gum benjamin, Sumatra benzoin.

Styrax macrothyrsus: Vietnam styrax.

Styrax paralleloneurus: Haminjon toba (Indonesian), Sumatra benzoin.

Styrax tonkinensis: Siam styrax, Siam benzoin.

Taxodiaceae

Cryptomeria japonica: Cryptomeria, Japanese cedar, sugi; many cultivars exist.

Theaceae

Camellia sinensis: Tea; there are two varieties: *var. sinensis:* China tea; *var. assamica:* Assam tea.

Thymelaeaceae

Aquilaria agallocha: Agarwood, aloes wood, agar.

Aquilaria malaccensis: Indonesian agarwood.

Tiliaceae

Tilia vulgaris (T. europaea): Lime tree, linden, common lime, lyne, tillet, tilea.

Turneraceae

Turnera diffusa (T. aphrodisiaca): Damiana.

Usneaceae

Evernia furfuraceae: Tree moss.

Evernia prunastri: Oakmoss.

Ramalina fastigiata: Chinese moss.

Ramalina subcomplanata: Indian moss.

Usnea barbata is harvested with *Evernia furfurcea* as Tree moss.

Usnea lucea is harvested with *Ramalina subcomplanata* as Haraphool.

Valerianaaceae

Nardostachys chinensis: Chinese spikenard.

Nardostachys jatamansi: Nard, spikenard, 'false' Indian valerian root.

Valeriana fauriei (V. officinalis, V. officinalis var. angustifolia, V. officinalis var. latifolia): Common valerian, European valerian, Belgian valerian, fragrant valerian, garden valerian; other chemotypes exist such as: Japanese valerian, 'kesso root'.

Valeriana wallichii: Indian valerian.

Verbenaceae

Aloysia triphylla (A. citriodora, Lippia citriodora, L. triphylla, Verbena triphylla): Lemon verbena, verbena, herb Louisa.

Lippia abyssinica (L. adoensis): Gambian tea bush.

Lippia affinis: Oregano.

Lippia cardiostegia: Oregano.

Lippia formosa: Oregano.

Lippia fragrans: Oregano.

Lippia graveolens (L. berlandieri): Mexican oregano.

Lippia micromeria: False thyme.

Lippia origanoides: Oregano.

Lippia palmeri: Mexican oregano.

Lippia pseudo-thea: Brazilian tea.

Lippia umbellata: Oregano.

Violaceae

Viola alba: Parma violet; there are three subspecies.

Viola odorata: Sweet violet, English violet, garden violet, blue violet.

Viola suavis: Russian violet.

Zingiberaceae

Alpinia officinarum (Languas officinarum, Radix galanga monoris): Galanga, lesser galangal, Chinese ginger, small ginger, East Indian ginger, colic root, ginger root.

Curcuma longa (C. domestica, Amomoum curcuma): Turmeric, curcuma, Indian saffron, Indian yellow root.

Elettaria cardamomum: Cardomom, cardomum, cardomon, there are two main varieties: *var. cardamomum (var. minus, var. minuscula):* Mysore cardamom; *var. major:* Wild cardamom.

Hedychium flavescens (H. flavum): Longoze.

Hedychium spicatum: Sanna, ekangi.

Zingiber officinale: Ginger, common ginger, Jamaica ginger.

Zygophyllaceae

Bulnesia sarmienti: Guauacwood, champaca wood (oil).

Botanical Index

The main entry for each oil is given in bold type.

References

PART I

1. Naves, Y.R. *Natural Perfume Materials*, p.3.
2. Davies, P. *Aromatherapy An A-Z*, p.7.
3. Tisserand, R. *The Art of Aromatherapy*, p. 21.
4. Naves, as above, p.5.
5. Chetwynd, T. *Dictionary of Symbols* p.9.
6. *Yearbook of Pharmacy and Transactions of the British Pharmaceutical Conference, 1907*, p.217.
7. Maury, M. *Guide to Aromatherapy*, p.7.
8. Valnet, J. *The Practice of Aromatherapy*, p.44.
9. *Agbiotech News and Information*, 1990, Vol. II, *No.2*, p.211.
10. Baerheim & Scheffer, *Essential Oils and Aromatic Plants*.
11. Davis, as above, p.173.
12. Baerheim & Scheffer, as above.
13. Tisserand, R. 'Psychology of Perfumery, '91 Conference Report'. *International Journal of Aromatherapy*, Vol.III, No.3., p.10.
14. Maury, as above, p.94.
15. Whitmont, E. *Psyche and Substance*, p.24.
16. Hoffman, D. *The New Holistic Herbal*, p.14.
17. Lavabre, M. *Aromatherapy Workbook*, p.98.
18. Steele, J. *International Journal of Aromatherapy*, Vol.II, No.2, p.8.

PART III

1. Lavabre, M. *Aromatherapy*, p.123.
2. Grieve, M. *A Modern Herbal*, p.79.
3. *British Herbal Pharmocopoeia 1983*, p.14.
4. Tisserand, R. *The Essential Oil Safety Data Manual*, p.79.
5. Grieve, as above, p.831.
6. Lavabre, as above, p.86.
7. de bairacli Levy, J. *The Illustrated Herbal Handbook*, p.54.
8. Tisserand, as above, p.85.
9. Tisserand, as above, p.98.
10. Culpeper, N. *Complete Herbal*, p.363.
11. Tisserand, as above, p.86.
12. Le Strange, R. *A History of Herbal Plants*, p.44.
13. Mills, S.Y. *The A-Z of Modern Herbalism*, p.36.
14. Leung, A.Y. *Encyclopedia of Common Natural Ingredients*, p.64.
15. Cribb, J.W. & A.B. *Useful Wild Plants in Australia*, p.36.
16. Davis, P. *Aromatherapy, An A-Z*, p.135.

17. Tisserand, as above, p.86.
18. Davis, as above, p.214.
19. Moncrieff, R.W. *Odours*, 1970.
20. Maury, M. *Guide to Aromatherapy*, p.104.
21. Leung, as above, p.155.
22. Le Strange, as above, p.72.
23. Tisserand, as above, p.96.
24. Tisserand, as above, p.81.
25. Tisserand, as above, p.81.
26. Tisserand, as above, p.82.
27. Younger, D. *Household Gods*, p.43.
28. Davis, as above, p.236.
29. Tisserand, as above, p.189.
30. Culpeper. as above, p.110.
31. Lautie, R. & Passebecq, A. *Aromatherapy, The Use of Plant Essences in Healing*, p.86.
32. Guenther, E. *The Essential Oils*, Vol. IV, p.5.
33. Maury, as above, p.89.
34. Arctander, S. *Perfume and Flavor Materials of Natural Origin*, p.170.
35. Grieve, as above, p.819.
36. Grieve, as above p.127.
37. Lassak, E.V. & McCarthy, T. *Australian Medicine Plants*, p.201.
38. Leung, as above, p.166.
39. Grieve, as above.
40. Maury, as above, p.104.
41. Tisserand, as above, p.112.
42. School of Herbal Medicine, *Materia Medica, Part II*, p.27.
43. Culpeper, as above, p.198.
44. Worwood, V.A. *The Fragrant Pharmacy*, p.107.
45. Tisserand, as above, p.84.
46. Franchomme, P. *Phytoguide I*, p.35.
47. Culpeper, as above, p.202.
48. Tisserand, R. *The Art of Aromatherapy*, p.238.
49. Arctander, as above, p.581.
50. Tisserand, R. *The Essential Oil Safety Data Manual*, p.92.
51. Culpeper, as above, p.211.
52. Mills, as above, p.59.
53. Davis, as above, p.328.
54. Davis, as above, p.221.
55. School of Herbal Medicine, as above, p.25.
56. Grieve, as above, p.626.
57. Tisserand, as above, p.89.
58. Culpeper, as above, p.234.
59. Grieve, as above, p.536.
60. *British Herbal Pharmacopoeia 1983*, p.148.
61. Hoffmann, D. *The New Holistic Herbal*, p.168.
62. Culpeper, as above, p.247.
63. Davis, as above, p.233.

64. Grieve, as above, p.573.
65. *The Holy Bible*, St John 12:3.
66. Tisserand, as above, p.102.
67. Tisserand, R. *The Art of Aromatherapy*, p.183.
68. Culpeper, as above, p.227.
69. Tisserand, R. *The Essential Oil Safety Data Manual*, p.88.
70. Arctander, as above, p.157.
71. Lavabre, M. *Aromatherapy Workbook*, p.117.
72. Tisserand, as above, p.78.
73. Grieve, as above, p.445.
74. Davis, P. *London School of Aromatherapy Notes*, 1983.
75. Ceres, *Herbs for Healthy Hair*, p.19.
76. Younger, as above, p.67.
77. Valnet, as above, p.188.
78. Leung, as above, p.149.
79. Maury, as above, p.90.
80. Grieve, as above, p.522.
81. Guenther, E. *The Essential Oil*, Vol. V, p.348.
82. Tisserand, as above, p.76.
83. Warren-Davis, D. 'The symbolism of the rose', *The Herbal Review*, Autumn 1989, p.2.
84. Culpeper, as above, p.298.
85. Maury, as above, p.87.
86. *British Herbal Pharmacopoeia 1983*, p.181.
87. Culpeper, as above, p.305.
88. Arctander, as above, p.563.
89. Tisserand, as above, p.107.
90. Culpeper, as above, p.211.
91. Culpeper, as above, p.211.
92. Grieve, as above, p.715.
93. Tisserand, as above, p.90.
94. Culpeper, as above, p.319.
95. Tisserand, as above, p.69.
96. Valnet, as above, p.186.
97. Tisserand, as above, p.69.
98. Grieve, as above, p.155.
99. Leung, as above, p.62.
100. Maury, as above, p.96.
101. Arctander, as above, p.607.
102. Tisserand, as above, p.94.
103. Tisserand, as above, p.96.
104. Tisserand, as above, p. 88.
105. Culpeper, as above, p.216.
106. Lavabre, as above, p.64.
107. *British Herbal Pharmacopoeia, 1983*, p.226.
108. Davis, P. *Aromatherapy, An A-Z*, p.342.
109. *British Herbal Pharmacopoeia, 1983*, p.233.
110. Grieve, as above, p.835.

Bibliography

Arber, A. *Herbals, Their Origin and Evolution*, Cambridge University Press, 1912.

Arctander, S. *Perfume and Flavor Materials of Natural Origin*, published by the author, Elizabeth, New Jersey, 1960.

de Bairacli, Levy, J. *The Illustrated Herbal Handbook*, Faber & Faber, 1982.

Baerheim, S.A. & Scheffer J.J.C. *Essential Oils and Aromatic Plants*, Dr. W. Junk Publications, 1989.

Beckett, S. *Herbs to Soothe Your Nerves*, Thorsons, 1977.

Beresford-Cooke, C. *Massage for Healing and Relaxation*, Arlington, 1986.

Bianchini, F. & Corbetta. F. *Health Plants of the World – Atlas of Medicinal Plants*, Newsweek Books, New York, 1977.

Blunt. W. *The Art of Botanical Illustration*, Collins, 1950.

Boulos, C. & Danin A. *Medicinal Plants of North Africa*, Reference Publications, 1983.

British Herbal Pharmacopoeia, British Herbal Medicine Association, 1983.

Buchman, D.D. *Feed Your Face*, Duckworth, 1980.

Buchman, D.D. *Herbal Medicine*, Rider, 1984.

Ceres, *Herbs for Healthy Hair*, Thorsons, 1977.

Chetwynd, T. *A Dictionary of Symbols*, Paladin, 1982.

Chiej, R. *The Macdonald Encyclopedia of Medicinal Plants*, Arnoldo Mondadori Editore, Milan, 1984.

Conway, D. *The Magic of Herbs*, Mayflower, 1973.

Coon, N. *The Dictionary of Useful Plants*, Rodale, Emmaus, Pa.,1974.

Cribb, A.B. & J.W. *Useful Wild Plants in Australia*, Fontana/Collins, 1982.

Culpeper, N. *Culpeper's Complete Herbal*, W. Foulsham & Co. Ltd, 1952.

Dastur, J.F. *Useful Plants of India and Pakistan*, D.B. Taraporevala Sons & Co. Ltd, India, 1985.

Davies W.C., *New Zealand Native Plant Studies*, A.H. & A.W. Reed, Wellington, 1961.

Davis P. *Aromatherapy An A–Z*, C.W. Daniel, 1988.

Fay, I. *Perfumery with Herbs*, Darton, Longman and Todd, 1979.

Douglas, J.S. *Making Your Own Cosmetics*, Pelham Books, 1979.

Downing, G. *The Massage Book*, Penguin, 1974.

Franchomme, P. *Phytoguide I*, International Phytomedical Foundation, La Courtête, France, 1985.

Furia, T.E. & Bellanca. N. *Fenaroli's Handbook of Flavour Ingredients. Vol.I*, 2nd ed, CRC Press, Cleveland, Ohio, 1975.

Gardner, J. *Healing Yourself During Pregnancy*, The Crossing Press, California, 1987.

Grieve, M. *A Modern Herbal*, Penguin, 1982.

Griggs, B. *The Home Herbal*, Pan, 1983.

Guenther, E. *The Essential Oils*, Van Nostrand, New York, 1948.

Hall, R., Klemme D. & Nienhaus J. *The H & R Book: Guide to Fragrance Ingredients*, Johnson Publishing, 1985.

Hepper, C. *Herbal Cosmetics*, Thorsons, 1987.

Heriteatu, J. *Potpourris and other Fragrant Delights*, Penguin, 1975.

Hoffman, D. *The New Holistic Herbal*, Element Books, 1990.

Huxley, A. *Natural Beauty With Herbs*, Darton, Longman and Todd, 1977.

Jessee, J.E. *Perfume Album*, Robert E. Krieger, 1974.

Khan. I. *The Development of Spiritual Healing*, Sufi Publishing Co., 1974.

Krochmal A.& C. *A Guide to the Medicinal Plants of the United States*, Quadrangle, The New York Times Book Co, 1974.

Lassak, E.V. & McCarthy, T. *Australian Medicinal Plants*, Methuen, Australia, 1983.

Launert, E. *Edible and Medicinal Plants of Britain and Northern Europe*, Hamlyn, 1981.

Lautie, R. & Passebecq, A. *Aromatherapy; the Use of Plant Essences in Healing*, Thorsons, 1982.

Lavabre, M. *Aromatherapy Workbook*, Healing Arts Press, Vermont, 1990.

Lawerence, B.M. *Essential Oils*, Allured Publishing Co., Wheaton, USA, 1978.

Leung, A.Y. *Encyclopedia of Common Natural Ingredients*, John Wiley, New York, 1980.

Little, K. *Kitty Little's Book of Herbal Beauty*, Penguin, 1980.

Maury, M. *Marguerite Maury's Guide to Aromatherapy*, C.W. Daniel, 1989.

Mabey, R. *The Complete New Herbal*, Elm Tree Books, 1988.

McIntyre, A. *Herbs for Pregnancy and Childbirth*, Sheldon Press, 1988.

Metcalfe, J. *Herbs and Aromatherapy*, Webb & Bower, 1989.

Meunier, C. *Lavandes et Lavandins*, Charle-Yves Chaudoreille, Edisud, Aix-en-Provence, France, 1985.

Mills, S.Y. *The A–Z of Modern Herbalism*, Thorsons, 1989.

Naves, Y.R. & Mazuyer, G. *Natural Perfume Materials*, Reinhold Publishing, New York, 1947.

Page, M. *The Observers Book of Herbs*, Frederick Warne, 1980.

Parvati, J. Hygieia, *A Woman's Herbal*, Wildwood House, 1979.

Phillips, R. *Wild Flowers of Britain*, Pan, 1977.

Poucher, W.A. *Perfumes, Cosmetics and Soaps Vol. II*, Chapman and Hall, 1932.

Price, S. *Practical Aromatherapy*, Thorsons, 1983.

Rapgay, L. *Tibetan Therapeutic Massage*, published by the author, India, 1985.

Ranson, F. *British Herbs*, Penguin, 1949.

Rose, F. *The Wild Flower Key*, Frederick Warne, 1981.

Ryman, D. *The Aromatherapy Handbook*, Century, 1984.

Stead, C. *The Power of Holistic Aromatherapy*, Javelin Books, 1986.

Stobart, T. *Herbs, Spices and Flavourings*, Penguin, 1979.

Le Strange, R. *A History of Herbal Plants*, Angus and Robertson, 1977.

Temple, A.A. *Flowers and Trees of Palestine*, SPCK, Macmillan, 1978.

Thomson, W.A.R. *Healing Plants – A Modern Herbal*, Macmillan, 1978.

Tisserand, R. *Aromatherapy for Women*, Thorsons, 1985.

Tisserand, R. *The Essential Oil Safety Data Manual*, The Association of Tisserand Aromatherapists, 1985.

Tisserand, R. *The Art of Aromatherapy*, C.W. Daniel, 1985.

Valnet, J. *The Practice of Aromatherapy*, C.W. Daniel (English Translation), 1982.

Weiss, R.F. *Herbal Medicine*, Arcanum, 1988.

Whitmont, E.C. *Psyche and Substance*, North Atlantic Books, 1980.

Williams, D. *Lecture Notes on Essential Oils*, Eve Taylor Ltd, 1989.

Worwood, V.A. *The Fragrant Pharmacy*, Macmillan, 1990.

Wren, R.C. *Potters New Cyclopaedia of Botanical Drugs and Preparations*, C.W. Daniel, 1988.

Yearbook of Pharmacy and Transactions of the British Pharmaceutical Conference, The Pharmaceutical Press, Bloomsbury, London, 1907.

Younger, D. *Household Gods*, E.W.Allen, 1898.

Where to Get Essential Oils:

USEFUL ADDRESSES

A wide selection of top quality essential oils, base oils aromatherapy books and other aromatic products is available from Aqua Oleum UK. International Mail Order (including Australia), professional and export lists are also offered on request. Safety information, quality control and up to date product data are outlined in 'The Essential Oil Catalogue' supplied free with price list.

AQUA OLEUM
Unit 3, Lower Wharf, Wallbridge,
Stroud, Glos GL5 3JA, UK
Tel (01453) 753555
Fax (01453) 752179

Aqua Oleum products are also available from:

CANADA & USA
NATURE TRADING LIMITED
Box 263, 1857 West 4th Avenue,
Vancouver, B.C. Canada V63 1M4

DENMARK & SWEDEN
URTEKRAM A/S
Klostermarken 20, DK-9550 Mariager,
Denmark

FINLAND
**LUONNONRUOKKATUKKU
ADUKI KY**
Kirvesmelhankatu 10, 00810 Helsinki,
Finland

IRELAND
WHOLEFOODS WHOLESALE
Unit 2D, Kylemore Industrial Estate,
Dublin 10, Republic of Ireland

SOAP OPERA LTD
Unit 3, Enterprise Centre, Stafford
Street, Nenagh, Co. Tipperary,
Republic of Ireland

JAPAN
MARUNAKE K.K.
1-12-4 Ginza Chuo-ku, Tokyo, Japan

HONG KONG
7 Old Bailey Street, Central,
Hong Kong

Information regarding qualified aromatherapists and training programmes can be obtained from:

UK
THE INTERNATIONAL FEDERATION OF AROMATHERAPISTS
Stamford House, 2/4 Chiswick High
Road, London W4 1TH, UK
Tel (0181) 742 2605

USA
THE AMERICAN ALLIANCE OF AROMATHERAPY
PO Box 750428, Petaluma, CA 94975,
USA Tel: (707) 778 6762

AUSTRALIA
THE INTERNATIONAL FEDERATION OF AROMATHERAPISTS
1/390 Burwood Road, Hawthorne,
Melbourne, Victoria 3122, Australia
Tel: (613) 819 2502
Fax: (613) 819 2399

Information regarding qualified medical herbalists and training programmes can be obtained from:

UK
THE SCHOOL OF HERBAL MEDICINE/PHYTOTHERAPY
Bucksteep Manor, Bodle Street Green,
Hailsham, Sussex BN27 4RJ, UK
Tel: (01323) 833 812/4

THE NATIONAL INSTITUTE OF MEDICAL HERBALISTS
56 Longbrook Street, Exeter, Devon
EX4 6AH, UK Tel: (01392) 426022

USA
AMERICAN BOTANICAL COUNCIL AND HERB RESEARCH FOUNDATION
PO Box 201660, Austin,
Texas 78720, USA

CALIFORNIA SCHOOL OF HERBAL STUDIES
9309 HWY 116, Forestville,
CA 95436, USA

AUSTRALIA
NATIONAL HERBALISTS ASSOCIATION OF AUSTRALIA
Suite 305, 3 Smail Street, Broadway,
New South Wales 2007, Australia
Tel: (02) 211 6437 Fax: (02) 211 6452

General information on holistic forms of treatment can be obtained from:

UK
BRITISH HOLISTIC MEDICAL ASSOCIATION
Trust House, Royal Shrewsbury
Hospital South, Shrewsbury, Shropshire
SY3 8XF, UK
Tel: (01743) 261155
Fax: (01743) 353637

USA
AMERICAN HOLISTIC MEDICAL ASSOCIATION
Suite 201, 4101 Lake Boone Trail,
Raleigh, North Carolina 27607, USA
Tel: (919) 787 5146 Fax: (919) 787 4916

CANADA
CANADIAN HOLISTIC MEDICAL ASSOCIATION
700 Bay Street, PO Box 101, Suite 604,
Toronto, Ontario M5G 1Z6, Canada

AUSTRALIA
AUSTRALIAN NATURAL THERAPISTS ASSOCIATION
PO Box 308, Melrose Park,
South Australia 5039
Tel: 8297 9533 Fax: 8297 0003

PICTURE CREDITS

A–Z BOTANICAL COLLECTION: 96, 123, 147, 196, 217. G. Archer: 120, 159; Ron Bass: 216; Andrea Bologh: 103; Anthony Cooper: 102; Michael Jones: 90, 98; Geoff Kidd: 210; Iris Lane: 229, G.A.Matthews: 168; Elsa M. Megson: 205; Mrs W. Monks: 95, 215; Moira Newman: 172; Maurice Nimmo: 80BR; Sylvia O'Toole: 139; Dan Sams: 86BR, 138, 174, 176; Bjorn Svenson: 84TR, 203; Sam Ke Tran: 131TR; Irene Windridge: 118; Nick Wiseman: 97.
THE BRIDGEMAN ART LIBRARY: British Library: 18C; Galleria dell'Accademia, Florence: 23; Phillips Auctioneers: 38; Musée d'Orsay, Paris: 40.
BRUCE COLEMAN LTD/CLIVE HICKS: 18B.
C.W.DANIAL PUBLISHERS: 22L + C.

DERBY MUSEUM AND ART GALLERY: 19R.
EDITIONS MALONE, PARIS: 22B.
E. T. ARCHIVE/Aleppo Museum, Syria: 14; British Museum: 15; Uffizi Gallery, Florence: 16TL; Biblioteca Etense Moderna: 20; Bibliotheque Nationale, Paris: 2.
FINE ART PHOTO LIBRARY: 42, 47.
GUERLAIN: 46BL.
HARRY SMITH HORTICULTURAL PHOTOS: 70BR, 71BR, 73BR, 89, 91, 92, 94, 107, 110, 114, 116, 127, 135, 146, 149, 158, 161, 165, 167, 180, 182, 192, 197, 206, 218, 219, 220, 225, 227, 232, 233; Eric Crichton: 221; Smith/Polunin: 74BR, 78BR, 88, 90, 124, 143, 150.
IMAGES COLOUR LIBRARY: 19B.
S. & O. MATTHEWS: 48L, 83.
OXFORD SCIENTIFIC FILMS/Jack Dermio: 198;

Deni Brown: 105, 170, 204; Patti Murray: 134.
PHOTOS HORTICULTURAL: 36C.
SCIENCE PHOTO LIBRARY/Jean Loup Charmet: 21BL; Damien Lovegrove: 34.

SPECIAL THANKS TO:
Darren Webster and the Royal Botanic Gardens, Kew, London, UK; Clayhill Nurseries, Sussex, UK; Martin Cooper at Country Gardens, Sussex, UK; Countryside Companions, Lincolnshire, UK; Culpeper Ltd, Sussex, UK; Neals Yard Remedies, Sussex, UK; Dave Masters at Nymans Gardens, Sussex, UK; Mazin Al-Khafaji at The Skin Clinic, Sussex, UK; Suffolk Herbs, Essex, UK; also to Sarah Mellish and David Squire.